Endovascular Intervention

Current Controversies

Edited by

Michael G Wyatt & Anthony F Watkinson

Publisher

tfm Publishing Limited
Castle Hill Barns
Harley
Shrewsbury
SY5 6LX
UK

Tel: +44 (0)1952 510061
Fax: +44 (0)1952 510192
E-mail: nikki@tfmpublishing.com
Web site: www.tfmpublishing.com

Design and layout:	Nikki Bramhill
Cover image:	Courtesy of Dr Jos C van den Berg MD PhD
First Edition	June 2004

ISBN 1 903378 31 1

Printed by Gutenberg Press Ltd., Gudja Road, Tarxien, PLA 19, Malta.

Tel: +356 21897037; Fax: +356 21800069.

Contents

PART III. Carotid disease

PART IV. Lower limb disease

PART V. Renal and mesenteric disease

PART VI. Imaging

PART VII. Venous disease

Contributors

Donald J Adam, MD FRCSEd Senior Lecturer in Vascular Surgery and Consultant Vascular Surgeon, Research Institute (Lincoln House), Birmingham Heartlands Hospital, Birmingham, UK

Lambertus W Bartels, PhD Physicist, Image Sciences Institute, University Medical Center, Utrecht, The Netherlands

Jonathan Beard, ChM FRCS Consultant Vascular Surgeon, The Sheffield Vascular Institute, The Northern General Hospital, UK

Jocelyn Bell, BSc MSc PhD BASIL Trial Co-ordinator, Research Institute (Lincoln House), Birmingham Heartlands Hospital, Birmingham, UK

Anna-Maria Belli, FRCR Consultant Radiologist, St George's Hospital, London, UK

Viktor Berczi, MD PhD Endovascular Fellow, The Sheffield Vascular Institute, The Northern General Hospital, Sheffield, UK

Jan D Blankensteijn, MD Professor and Chief Division of Vascular Surgery, University Medical Center Nijmegen, Nijmegen, The Netherlands

Philipp Bonhoeffer, MD Consultant Paediatric Cardiologist, Great Ormond Street Hospital for Sick Children, London, UK

Robert S Bonser, FRCP FRCS FESC Consultant Cardiothoracic Surgeon, Queen Elizabeth Hospital, University Hospital Birmingham NHS Trust, Birmingham, UK

Gerard E Boyle, PhD Principal Physicist, St. James's Hospital, Dublin, Ireland

Andrew W Bradbury, BSc MD FRCSEd Professor of Vascular Surgery and Consultant Vascular Surgeon, Research Institute (Lincoln House), Birmingham Heartlands Hospital, Birmingham, UK

John Brennan, MD FRCS(Gen) Consultant Vascular Surgeon, Royal Liverpool & Broadgreen University Hospital, Liverpool, UK

Louise C Brown, MSc EVAR Trials Manager, Imperial College of Science, Technology & Medicine, Charing Cross Hospital, London, UK

Bruce Campbell, MS FRCP FRCS Professor and Consultant Surgeon, Royal Devon and Exeter Hospital and Peninsula Medical School, Exeter, UK

Nick J Cheshire, MD MRCS Consultant Vascular Surgeon, Regional Vascular Unit, St Mary's Hospital, London, UK

Trevor Cleveland, FRCS FRCR Consultant Vascular Radiologist, The Sheffield Vascular Institute, The Northern General Hospital, Sheffield, UK

Jeremy S Crane, MRCS Research Fellow, Vascular Surgery, Regional Vascular Unit, St Mary's Hospital, London, UK

Philip Davey, MRCS Research Fellow, Vascular Surgery, Northern Vascular Centre, Freeman Hospital, Newcastle-upon-Tyne, UK

Michiel H de Haan, MD PhD Consultant Radiologist, University Hospital Maastricht, Maastricht, the Netherlands

Stephen D'Souza, MRCP FRCR Consultant Vascular Radiologist, Royal Preston Hospital, Lancashire Teaching Hospitals NHS Trust, Preston, UK

Jonothan J Earnshaw, DM FRCS Consultant Vascular Surgeon, Gloucestershire Royal Hospital, Gloucester, UK

Dominic Fay, FRCR Specialist Registrar, Interventional Radiology, Northern Vascular Centre, Freeman Hospital, Newcastle-upon-Tyne, UK

Christine M Flis, MRCP FRCR Specialist Registrar, Kings College Hospital, London, UK

Peter A Gaines, FRCP FRCR Consultant Vascular Radiologist, The Sheffield Vascular Institute, The Northern General Hospital, Sheffield, UK

Derek A Gould, FRCP FRCR Consultant Radiologist, Royal Liverpool and Broadgreen University Hospitals Trust, Liverpool, UK

Roger M Greenhalgh, MA MD FRCS MChir Professor of Surgery, Imperial College of Science, Technology & Medicine, Charing Cross Hospital, London, UK

Alison Halliday, MS FRCS Consultant Vascular Surgeon, St George's Hospital Medical School, London, UK

Ralph W Jackson, MRCP FRCR Consultant Vascular and Interventional Radiologist, Northern Vascular Centre, Freeman Hospital, Newcastle-upon-Tyne, UK

Michael J Jacobs, MD PhD Consultant Vascular Surgeon & Professor of Surgery, University Hospital Maastricht, Maastricht, the Netherlands

H Rolf Jäger, MD FRCR Reader in Neuroradiology, National Hospital for Neurology and Neurosurgery, London, UK

David Kessel MA, MRCP, FRCR Consultant Vascular Radiologist, St James's University Hospital, Leeds, UK

Andreas M Lazaris, MD Research Fellow in Vascular Surgery, Regional Vascular Unit, St Mary's Hospital, London, UK

Tim A Lees, MD FRCS Consultant Vascular Surgeon, Northern Vascular Centre, Freeman Hospital, Newcastle-upon-Tyne, UK

Thomas M Loosemore, MS FRCS Consultant Vascular Surgeon, St George's Hospital, London, UK

Sumaira Macdonald, MRCP FRCR Consultant Vascular Radiologist & Honorary Clinical Senior Lecturer, Northern Vascular Centre, Freeman Hospital, Newcastle-upon-Tyne, UK

Joanna Marro, BSc ACST Trial Co-ordinator, St George's Hospital Medical School, London, UK

Richard McWilliams, FRCS FRCR Consultant Radiologist, Royal Liverpool & Broadgreen University Hospital, Liverpool, UK

James FM Meaney, FRCR FFR(RCSI) Consultant Radiologist, St. James's Hospital, Dublin, Ireland

Robert Morgan, MRCP FRCR Consultant Radiologist, St. George's Hospital, London, UK

Jon G Moss, FRCS FRCR Consultant Interventional Radiologist, Interventional Radiology Unit, North Glasgow Hospitals University NHS Trust, Gartnavel Hospital, Glasgow, UK

Graham J Munneke, MRCP FRCR Clinical Fellow, Interventional Radiology, St George's Hospital, London, UK

A Ross Naylor, MD FRCS Professor of Vascular Surgery, Leicester Royal Infirmary, Leicester, UK

Anthony Nicholson, MSc FRCR Consultant Vascular Radiologist, St James's University Hospital and Leeds General Infirmary, Leeds Hospital NHS Trust, Leeds, UK

Crispian Oates, MSc BSc MIPEM AVS Head of Regional Vascular Ultrasound, Northern Vascular Centre, Freeman Hospital, Newcastle-upon-Tyne, UK

Andrew Platts, FRCS FRCR Consultant Radiologist, The Royal Free Hospital, London, UK

Ted R Prins, MD Consultant Radiologist, University Hospital of Groningen, Groningen, The Netherlands

Shakeel Ahmed Qureshi, FRCP Consultant Paediatric Cardiologist, Guy's Hospital, London, UK

Aaron M Ranasinghe, MRCS Research Fellow, Cardiothoracic Surgery, Queen Elizabeth Hospital, University Hospital Birmingham NHS Trust, Birmingham, UK

Fergus Robertson, MRCP FRCR Specialist Registrar, Radiology, The Royal Free Hospital, London, UK

John Rose, FRCP FRCR Consultant Vascular Radiologist, Northern Vascular Centre, Freeman Hospital, Newcastle-upon-Tyne, UK

Peter C Rowlands, BMedSci MRCP(UK) FRCR Consultant Interventional Radiologist, Royal Liverpool University Hospital, Liverpool, UK

Geert Willem H Schurink, MD PhD Consultant Vascular Surgeon, University Hospital Maastricht, Maastricht, the Netherlands

Julian Scott, MD FRCS Reader in Vascular Surgery, Consultant Vascular Surgeon, St James's University Hospital, Leeds, UK

Paul S Sidhu, MRCP FRCR Consultant Radiologist and Honorary Consultant Neuroradiologist, Kings College Hospital and the National Hospital for Neurology and Neurosurgery, London, UK

Sriram Subramonia, MS FRCS Clinical and Research Fellow, Northern Vascular Centre, Freeman Hospital, Newcastle-upon-Tyne, UK

Peter R Taylor, MA MChir FRCS Consultant Vascular Surgeon, Guy's & St. Thomas' Hospital, London, UK

Ignace FJ Tielliu, MD Consultant Vascular Surgeon, University Hospital of Groningen, Groningen, The Netherlands

Steven Thomas, MRCP FRCR MSc Senior Lecturer Vascular Radiology, The Sheffield Vascular Institute, The Northern General Hospital, UK

Jos C van den Berg, MD PhD Interventional Radiologist, St. Antonius Hospital, Nieuwegein, The Netherlands

Jan JAM van den Dungen, MD PhD Consultant Vascular Surgeon, University Hospital of Groningen, Groningen, The Netherlands

Maarten J van der Laan, MD Resident Surgery, St. Antonius Hospital, Nieuwegein, The Netherlands

Eric LG Verhoeven, MD Consultant Vascular Surgeon, University Hospital of Groningen, Groningen, The Netherlands

Anthony F Watkinson, BSc MSc (Oxon) FRCS FRCR Consultant Radiologist, The Royal Devon and Exeter Hospital, Exeter, UK

Michael G Wyatt, MSc MD FRCS Consultant Vascular Surgeon, Northern Vascular Centre, Freeman Hospital, Newcastle-upon-Tyne, UK

Foreword

The co-operation of specialties to seek better outcomes for their patients is increasing, and opens new vistas which cut across traditional boundaries. In some countries such co-operation is rare and turf wars abound. The advance of technology is handicapped by the insular clinician determined to plough a lone furrow. We are delighted that in the United Kingdom such thinking is rare, and vascular intervention is performed in a spirit of co-operation rather than competition.

The Endovascular Forum is a biennial event sponsored jointly by both the Vascular Surgical Society of Great Britain and Ireland and the British Society of Interventional Radiology. This book has been written to support the meeting, and to encourage the interest of those who are unable to attend the event. Endoluminal treatment of vascular disease continues to develop at an ever-increasing pace. Vascular surgeons and interventional radiologists recognise the increasing importance of this field in their work. The manufacturers of the various devices are striving hard to improve the technology available to the clinicians. Patients know about minimally invasive options and will become more demanding about their use.

This book offers an instant snapshot of the most important current topics under discussion. We would like to congratulate all the authors and particularly the Editors, Mike Wyatt and Tony Watkinson, who have produced an excellent textbook in a very short space of time. Finally, our thanks to Nikki Bramhill of tfm Publishing Ltd. who continually defies the odds by producing very readable, user-friendly textbooks in record time with such good grace.

Anna-Maria Belli & Peter Taylor
Joint Chairpersons of the Endovascular Forum, Stratford, 2004

Chapter 1

Aortic stent grafts: development and current availability

Philip Davey, MRCS, Research Fellow, Vascular Surgery

Dominic Fay, FRCR, Specialist Registrar, Interventional Radiology

John Rose, FRCP FRCR, Consultant Vascular Radiologist

Michael G Wyatt, MSc MD FRCS, Consultant Vascular Surgeon

Northern Vascular Centre, Freeman Hospital, Newcastle-upon-Tyne, UK

Introduction

Since the first published case report in 1991 [1], it is estimated that over 25,000 patients worldwide have now received an aortic stent graft for the treatment of an abdominal aortic aneurysm (AAA) [2]. Initial enthusiasm for endovascular AAA repair (EVAR) was buoyed by the apparent early success of the minimally invasive technique, averting the need for conventional open surgery. Unfortunately, subsequent longer-term follow-up revealed the poor durability of the early devices, fuelling the debate over the role of EVAR in the management of AAA. The majority of late endograft failures have been attributed to inferior 'first-generation' technology [3] and the device manufacturers would suggest that sustained integrity can now be achieved as a result of the lessons learned from the earlier models. Notable commercial casualties include the Vanguard device (Boston Scientific, Natick, Massachusetts, USA) and more recently, the Ancure / EVT system (Guidant, Menlo Park, California, USA). The Vanguard was based on the Stentor (Mintec) system and although initial results were good, the high incidence of late device-related failures [4] led to its voluntary withdrawal. Despite initial concerns regarding metal fatigue and hook fractures, the Ancure / EVT system was associated with better long-term results [5]. However, this unique unsupported single piece device was taken off the market by Guidant because of expensive litigation following an FDA public health warning in 2001. These events reinforce the need for close follow-up after endovascular AAA repair and this account reviews the technological developments made in order to improve outcome in presently available aortic stent grafts.

Currently available aortic stent grafts

AneuRx® device

Pioneered by Dr Thomas J Fogarty in 1993, the AneuRx® stent graft system (Medtronic AVE, Santa Rosa, California, USA), was deployed into human subjects as part of US clinical trials in June 1996. Following review of the 1-year phase II results of these studies (AneuRx® compared to standard open surgical repair), FDA market approval was finally granted in September 1999.

The AneuRx® device is a self-expanding modular endograft designed for the treatment of infrarenal AAA. All components of the bifurcated system are

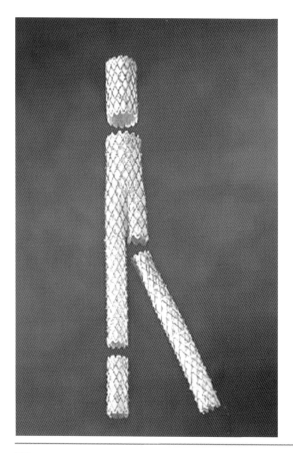

Figure 1. The AneuRx endograft.

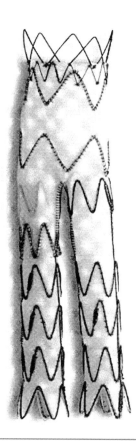

Figure 2. The Talent device.

composed of thin un-crimped woven polyester attached to a metal (nickel-titanium, 'nitinol') exoskeleton by individual polyester suturing (Figure 1). The nitinol-framed scaffold provides both radial and longitudinal structural support, with circulatory aneurysmal exclusion provided by its internal woven polyester conduit. A review of graft design in 1998 led to the original 5cm single-unit nitinol 'stiff-body' aortic bifurcation module being replaced (under FDA-approval) by the currently available 'flexible' aortic body composed of individual 1cm segmented nitinol rings joined end-to-end [6].

Following admission to the abdominal aorta under radiological control, AneuRx® stent deployment is achieved by gradual withdrawal of the Xpedient™ delivery catheter-covering sheath with handle (21 French for aortic bifurcation module; 16 French for iliac limbs). Radio-opaque orientation markers for exact positioning throughout the procedure facilitate graft assembly. The manufacturers currently advise

favourable morphological features including a neck length >10mm (maximal 45° angulation) and the generation of 'seal-zones' of ideally >15mm proximally and >25mm distally in the iliac arteries.

The six-year results of the three-phased (non-randomised) US AneuRx clinical trial have recently been published [7]. Between 1996-1999 a total of 1193 patients received the AneuRx® device at one of the 19 participating endovascular centres. The entire series 30-day mortality rate was 1.8% (22/1193), three of these deaths following subsequent aneurysm rupture. Protection from late (>30 days) aneurysm rupture was achieved in 99.2%, eight of the ten cases undergoing surgical conversion and an associated late rupture mortality of 50% (5/10). Earlier interim analysis has already shown significantly reduced post-stenting rupture risk with the introduction of the 'flexible' aortic module as opposed to the 'stiff-body' device [6]. Surgical conversion from stent graft repair was required in 53 patients during the study (11 intraoperative, four early and 38 late). The most common indications for conversion included endoleak with aneurysm enlargement (34%), rupture (21%), modular migration/displacement (21%) and access failure (13%). Kaplan-Meier survival analysis revealed a freedom from aneurysm-related death of 96.9% and an overall survival rate (accounting for all cause mortality) of 62.4% at four-year follow-up (n=291). Assessment of secondary outcome measures demonstrated at three years: rates of graft patency 98.2% (443/451), endoleak 14.0% (63/451) and device migration, 7.1% (32/449).

Talent LPS device

The Talent aortic stent graft system (Medtronic AVE, Santa Rosa, California, USA) was first introduced in December 1995 and has to date been deployed in over 13000 patients worldwide [8].

The device is a self-expanding modular system, composed of serpentine nitinol stents integrated into a woven polyester matrix (Figure 2). Since its original introduction, the graft has been modified with the use of a thinner, low profile graft fabric resulting in the Talent LPS. Columnar support is offered by its full-length uninterrupted nitinol spine to an otherwise flexible device that can adapt to moderate aorto-iliac angulations. This system is currently available as aorto-bi-iliac, tapered aorto-uni-iliac or aorto-aortic tube configurations. Proximal fixation of the Talent LPS endograft system may be assisted by use of a 15mm segment of uncovered bare metal attached to the aortic module and deployed trans-renally. At present, available device diameters are 16-36mm for the aortic body and 8-22mm for the iliac limbs. With this range of modular sizes, the recommended aneurysm morphology for treatment with the Talent LPS includes infrarenal neck >5mm long, 14-32mm diameter and <60° angulation, iliac artery diameter 8-18mm and 15mm long (landing-zone) and, a minimal external iliac diameter of 7mm for access [9].

Stent deployment is achieved by the coaxial sheath delivery system with internal pusher rod, managed under radiological control. A compliant polyurethane balloon is integrated into the delivery system and is located proximal to the top end of the device.

Following stent graft release, sequential balloon inflation during withdrawal is performed which improves both the modular connection and vessel wall seals.

There are several published reports of the results of endoluminal aneurysm repair with the Talent endoprosthesis [8-10]. In the largest of these studies, Faries et al enrolled 368 patients into a multicentre prospective trial to assess the Talent LPS. The 30-day mortality was 1.9% (7/368) with a primary technical success rate of 93.4% in the 366 patients who received a stent. Conversion to surgical repair was needed in four cases (1.1%), all with persistent type I endoleaks. There were two late aneurysm ruptures with death post-stenting (at 18 and 23 months), both cases not amenable to corrective endovascular intervention and unfit for surgical repair [8]. In a much smaller UK series of 38 patients, the Manchester group reported no early mortality but a slightly lower immediate aneurysm exclusion rate of 84% with use of the Talent device. One late death at three months was presumed to be aneurysm-related [10]. In their multicentre, prospective (non-randomised) trial, Criado et al compared 237 patients receiving the Talent LPS device with 126 open surgical controls. There was no significant difference in early mortality (0.8% stent, 0% surgery), but as expected, there was significantly reduced blood loss, transfusion requirement, critical care and total in-hospital stay in the endovascular limb of the study. Surgical conversion from stent was required in six cases (one intra-operative, five late) and none of the 26 late deaths (20 stent, six surgery) were regarded as aneurysm-related. Despite this, the investigators express concern at the presence of nitinol wire fractures found on plain x-ray follow-up in 11 patients. Although clinically 'inconsequential' at the time of the study, they allude to the evolution of the next generation of Talent devices ('Enhanced Talent LPS') that have already been shown to resist this metal fatigue in developmental bench testing.

Gore Excluder®

The Excluder® stent system (W. L. Gore and Associates, Flagstaff, Arizona, USA) was first implanted into human subjects in 1997 [11], and at the time of writing the Excluder® is still one of only three US-FDA approved endografts currently available for commercial use (Excluder®, AneuRx® and Zenith™).

The Excluder® is a self-expanding, bifurcated, two-component modular device composed of expanded polytetrafluoroethylene (ePTFE) lining an external support of thermo-sensitive nitinol. Strut design of the metal exoskeleton offers radial endograft support with an allowance for both longitudinal shortening and negotiation of any vessel tortuosity. At the proximal margin of the main stent body (termed 'trunk-ipsilateral' component) there are eight pairs of angled wire anchoring barbs to improve device fixation to the infra-renal neck and thus enhance columnar support. Attachment of the ePTFE fabric to the nitinol frame is by polyethylene tape, avoiding the need for sutures and hence suture holes on the luminal surface of the graft. Radio-opaque, gold band orientation markers are present at the proximal and distal ends of all modular components assisting device delivery. Aneurysm neck morphology favouring Excluder® stent repair includes a length >14mm which is not angulated more than 60°.

Modular component deployment of the Excluder® device is with Gore's innovative SIM-PULL system. The pre-loaded, non-sheathed delivery catheters are both extremely flexible and low profile (18 French introducer for trunk-ipsilateral component, 12 French for contralateral limb) and facilitate rapid and precise stent release. The delivery system contains two central channels, one for the guidewire and one for the deployment cord which is attached to a ePTFE sleeve enclosing the endograft. When the deployment string is pulled this sleeve is 'unzipped', thus permitting graft self-expansion and deployment.

The initial reports of endoluminal aneurysm repair with the Gore Excluder® were encouraging [12, 13]. Although both these studies were small (19 and 29 patients respectively), all devices were successfully deployed with no perioperative deaths. The post-stenting endoleak rate at one month was 17-39%, but the majority of these were self-limiting type II leaks (collateral flow). There were no late aneurysm-related deaths and no patients underwent surgical conversion. More recently, a larger multicentre (non-randomised), controlled clinical trial assessing the Excluder® versus open repair has been published [14].

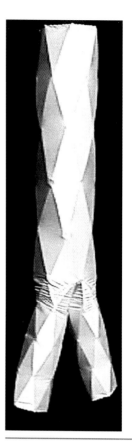

Figure 3. The PowerLink (Endologix) system.

Of the 334 patients recruited, 235 received the Excluder® device and 99 underwent open surgical repair. Comparative analysis revealed no difference in procedural mortality (0% control, 1% Excluder®), but significantly reduced blood loss, transfusion requirement, total in-hospital stay and incidence of major adverse events (14% versus 57%) in those patients receiving an endoprosthesis. At two-year follow-up, the Excluder® was associated with an endoleak rate of 20% and modular migration observed in 1%. Three cases required surgical conversion at 24, 28 and 29 months post-operatively, all performed for aneurysm expansion precipitated by endotension (n=2) and a type II leak in a patient who refused coil embolisation.

PowerLink (Endologix) device

The PowerLink system (Endologix Inc, Irvine, California, USA) is an innovative later-generation device, first introduced at European endovascular centres in 1999.

The device is a non-modular, unibody self-expanding bifurcated endograft. Its stainless steel chromium alloy ('conichrome') endoskeleton is created as a shaped single-wire body with a double spine in the absence of sutures or welds (Figure 3). This infrastructure is covered by a thin-walled ePTFE fabric that is only sutured to the metal frame at the ends of the device. Radial support is essentially achieved by graft over-sizing, whereas the long 'pre-bifurcation' body offers columnar stability and limited potential for distal migration. Proximal fixation with the PowerLink system may be infra- or supra-renal, the latter attained by means of a 2cm uncovered bare metal stent segment option. The device is available in two neck sizes of 25mm and 28mm, each with an incorporated limb diameter of 16mm.

The PowerLink stent is deployed using a novel delivery system. Surgical cut-down and exposure of only one vessel is required, contralateral access is obtained by a percutaneous approach and secured with a 9 French sheath. A 'contra-limb deployment wire' (attached to the middle of the cartridge containing the entire restrained device) is passed through the ipsilateral access site, pulled over the aortic bifurcation with a wire loop snare and then out through the 9 French sheath in the contralateral femoral artery. Following introduction of the delivery catheter into the aorta (via the exposed artery), the outer sheath that covers the entire device is retracted. This manoeuvre reveals the two limbs of the PowerLink, each covered by its own sleeve and with a wire attached to the contralateral limb. Next, the whole device is pulled caudally, moving the (constrained) device limbs into the iliac vessels and the stent bifurcation down to the aortic bifurcation. Distal to proximal deployment of the main-body is then initiated by pushing the retaining sheath off the leading end of the device in a cephalad direction. Prior to completion of main-body deployment, the contralateral limb is fully released by pulling the limb cover wire. After removal of this wire and limb cover, the device main-body and finally the ipsilateral limb, are deployed. Removal of the deployment catheter completes the aortic repair [15].

The intermediate results of a multicentre trial assessing the PowerLink device were published in 2002 [16]. Of the 118 patients recruited for this study, surgical conversion was required in four cases (3.3%, three intraoperative and one late). All devices were over-sized by 10-20% from pre-stenting CT measurements. Early mortality was 0.8% (1/118); this death was not stent-related. Nine late deaths were recorded, one of which was aneurysm-related following surgical conversion for a persistent proximal type I endoleak, despite previously attempted aortic cuff repair. Thirty-day endoleak rate was 5.9% (7/118) prompting secondary endovascular intervention in four cases (three type I and one type II). The remaining three type II leaks were managed expectantly with stable sac sizes observed at later follow-up. Distal device migration was reported in only one case (0.8%), and this did not require remedial intervention.

Lifepath

The Lifepath endograft (Edwards Lifesciences, Irvine, California, USA) has evolved from the adaptation of a first-generation prototype, the White-Yu GAD system [17].

The device is a balloon-expanding, modular and bifurcated system. An internal, wire-form endoskeleton is manufactured from 'elgiloy' (Elgiloy Ltd. Partnership, Elgin, Ill.), a stainless steel metal alloy of high chromium content that is covered in a full surgical-thickness woven polyester graft. Segmented fabric integration of the metal framework in circular fashion provides improved stent flexibility without loss of seal and the presence of external metallic crimping on the Lifepath further increases this stability. Unfortunately, early edition grafts fatigued easily and manifested as wire fractures, leading to the strengthened, currently available second-generation Lifepath device. The aortic body endograft component has a balloon-expandable trunk with two self-expanding legs and is available in neck sizes between 21-29mm. Tapered or straight iliac limbs are fully balloon-expandable, designed with a proximal 'docking' segment for superior inter-modular attachment. Favourable aneurysmal morphology for treatment with the Lifepath include an aortic neck diameter 19-27mm and length >14mm (angulation <60°) with native iliac vessels large enough to admit the delivery system (25 French ipsilateral main body and 19 French contralateral) and effect a non-aneurysmal 15mm landing-zone distally.

Lifepath delivery requires bilateral surgical cut-downs. Under fluoroscopic control, the 25 French main body sheath is advanced proximally over a stiff guidewire to the level of the lowest renal artery. Following confirmation of correct positioning by means of graft limb markers and angiography, the stent is unsheathed releasing the self-expandable short legs. The balloon is then slowly inflated with subsequent deployment of the remaining aortic body component. Bilateral iliac limb insertion (via 19 French access) is then performed in similar balloon-expandable fashion as above.

Carpenter et al have only just published the initial interim multicentre results of the Lifepath device [17].

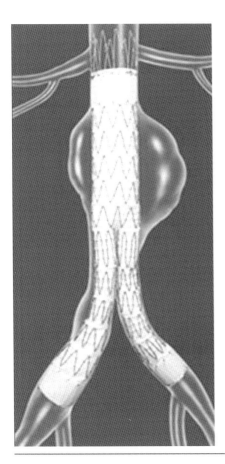

Figure 4. Zenith TriFab.

For the entire 227 patient series, successful device deployment was achieved in 98.7% (224/227). Surgical conversion was required in five cases (2.2%). Three of these operations were early (two aortic perforations, one refractory endoleak) and the other two performed at six months (persistent endoleak) and 12 months respectively (wire fracture, graft migration and endoleak). Perioperative mortality rate was 1.3% (three patients), one of which followed attempted open repair of endograft-associated aortic rupture. Of the 12 late fatalities within the study, none were reported as being aneurysm-related. Six-month endoleak rate was 5.9%, all except one case being of a collateral flow nature. There had been no graft thromboses or limb dislocations at the mean 11-month follow-up. Furthermore, comparison of the two generations of Lifepath revealed a significantly higher incidence of both wire fracture and migration (>10mm) in the earlier devices (n=79).

Zenith™

The Zenith™ AAA endograft (Cook Inc, Bloomington, Indianapolis, USA) has been under development since 1991. Originally, a prototype unsupported mono-iliac system, the device has now evolved into its current commercially available construction of a frame-supported, modular (three-piece, 'Tri-Fab') bifurcated endograft.

The Zenith™ system is constructed from a self-expanding stainless steel Z-stent skeletal framework with an integrated woven polyester (Dacron) conduit. Apart from the proximal and distal landing zones the metal scaffold resides on the external surface of the graft fabric, attached by multiple interrupted sutures providing a smooth interior surface for laminar blood flow (Figure 4). The main body component is designed so that the bifurcation into the iliac 'stumps' should be as close to the native aortic bifurcation as possible in order to minimise distal graft migration (currently available for lengths of 80-155mm). Secure proximal fixation is provided by the 22mm segment of uncovered trans-renal stent with the incorporated deployment of ten 5mm supra-renal anchoring barbs (orientated caudally) at graft implantation. Design of the bifurcated junctional area components is such that the ipsilateral (longer) stump extends 15mm into the common iliac artery in order to provide more stability at the junction with the ipsilateral limb. The contralateral (shorter) stump is deployed about 15mm above the aortic bifurcation where it will be docked with the proximal end of the contralateral limb. Radio-opaque markers at the trailing ends of both junctional areas facilitate docking of the limbs to the main stent body. A degree of main body and limb overlap may be finely adjusted during the procedure by 'tromboning' of the iliac components to correct any pre-operative calibration discrepancy [18]. Allowing for the recommended all-component over-sizing of 10-15%, suitable morphological features for treatment with the Zenith[TM] include an aortic neck length >10mm, diameter <28mm and angulation <80°. The common iliac arteries should ideally be >20mm in length and <22mm diameter at the landing zone sites for adequate distal fixation and the external iliacs >7mm for access [19].

Zenith[TM] stent implantation is with the H & L-B One-Shot[TM] Introducer System. The delivery technique is unusual in that deployment of the self-expanding main body is a two-staged process. Withdrawal of the delivery sheath under radiological control releases the central, covered segment of the main body endograft. After iliac limb docking and final manipulation of the stent into the correct position, the uncovered trans-renal bare metal Z stent at the leading end of the device can only be released from the nose cone after external removal of a safety wire.

Several multicentre studies assessing AAA repair with the Zenith[TM] stent have been recently published [19-21]. In the largest of these, Sternbergh reports the outcome in 351 patients receiving the TriFab device as part of a phase II FDA non-randomised clinical trial. At 12-month follow-up, caudal device migration (>5mm) was seen in 2.3% (6/261), although no patient required a remedial secondary intervention. The all-endoleak rate at one year was 8.2% (21/256), but the majority (n=16) of these were type II. There were no cases of early conversion, although five patients needed delayed open surgery with one aneurysm-related rupture. A similar high rate of technical success with the Zenith[TM] is reported by the UK investigators, with no early conversions and a perioperative mortality of 4.1% in a series of 269 patients [20]. Furthermore, mid-term follow-up (median 363 days) revealed the need for endovascular re-intervention in 19 patients and two late cases of aneurysm rupture.

Fortron LP (formerly Quantum LP)

Marketed by the Cordis Corporation (Johnson & Johnson, Miami, Florida, USA) and progressing from the Ariba Bifurcated Endovascular System ('ABES', Teramed, Maple Grove, Minneapolis, USA) [22], the recently renamed Fortron AAA endograft is one of the latest stents available (see Figure 5).

The Fortron stent is composed of a laser cut, electro-polished, seamless nitinol skeleton integrated into a woven polyester matrix. Numerous polyester point and blanket sutures attach the alloy frame to graft fabric. The main stent body is bifurcated with three distinct zones of nitinol configuration, which will be considered in turn. Proximal fixation is maximised by the widely spaced uncovered trans-renal nitinol

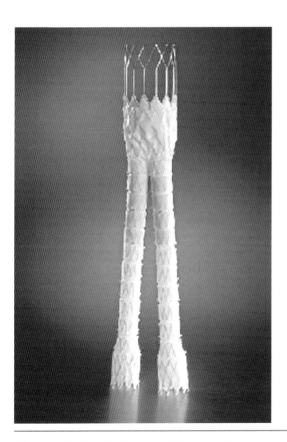

Figure 5. Cordis Fortron (Quantum).

segment, enhanced by six to eight distal (infra-renal) anchoring barbs. Stent bifurcation occurs within the next 3cm covered mid-graft aortic zone, translating finally into the terminal iliac stumps. Both of the 5cm stumps are constructed from sinusoidal 'Z-stent' nitinol that is pocketed within the endograft fabric for kink-resistant flexibility. The iliac limb components are polyester-covered seamless nitinol, with 2cm flared bell-bottom ends for distal fixation. Its unique telescoping iliac modular attachment system allows for a variable degree of component overlap (2-5cm), permitting on-table graft length adjustments of up to 3cm.

Each of the self-expanding modular components is pre-loaded in a single-platform, flexible delivery catheter system. Advancement of a screw-based handle retracts the outer sheath at 1mm intervals, thermally activating 'memory' nitinol graft expansion as the pre-cooled Fortron is exposed to body temperature. Both the aortic body and ipsilateral iliac limb are deployed through a 20 French delivery catheter with the contralateral limb requiring 17 French access.

To date there is only one small published feasibility study assessing the Cordis device [22]. Twenty-nine patients were entered into this study with successful primary endograft deployment in all but one case. This single initial deployment failure was attributed to technical error during delivery and was corrected by graft removal and re-introduction of a new device. At early follow-up (one month), there had been no deaths, no non-type II endoleaks and no surgical conversions. Type II endoleaks were found in 24% (7/29) but it is not reported whether or not they needed remedial secondary intervention. Of particular note in the three major adverse events (10.3%) reported, one patient developed ischaemic renal failure (confirmed by angiography) and required dialysis despite attempts at re-canalisation and reperfusion. Although the authors suggest that this probably occurred due to covered stent deployment too close to the renal artery ostia, the potential exacerbating role of the uncovered supra-renal segment is not discussed.

Recently, in a small number of cases (three), the delivery system of the Fortron AAA stent graft system has experienced a malfunction during deployment. According to the complaints submitted to Cordis, in each of these three cases (two contralateral and one ipsilateral), the leg prosthesis remained partially in the sheath after completion of rotation of the retraction knob of the handle. In each case, the physician elected to cut the sheath and complete the deployment manually. All deployments were eventually successful and patient safety was not compromised. Nevertheless, Cordis has decided to voluntarily withdraw the device (22.3.04) until the root cause of the deployment problem is determined and an appropriate corrective action is implemented.

Conclusions

Dramatic advances have been made in the development of the currently available aortic stent grafts. The problems of suspect long-term device durability seem to have been overcome and future evolution will probably focus more on designs (eg. fenestrated and branched endografts) to reduce the morphological criteria currently prohibiting this method of AAA repair. In addition, there is now much interest in applying endovascular principles in cases of ruptured AAA and specifically modified systems eg. Montefiore Endovascular Graft (MEG)/Vascular Innovation Graft (Vascular Innovation Inc., New York, USA) are currently under development for commercial use.

Despite these advances, there is still no level I evidence supporting the use of aortic stent grafts in the management of AAA. The results of several ongoing national multicentre randomised controlled studies (i.e. UK EVAR, Dutch DREAM and US OVER trials) are eagerly awaited and it is hoped that their publication will promote the continued use of aortic stent grafts in the management of AAA.

Summary

- Early aortic stent grafts were associated with poor long-term durability, which led to either device withdrawal or technical development and progression into the 'later generation' endografts.

- Improvements in system design include uncovered trans-renal fixation, proximal anchoring barbs, superior delivery techniques and the use of novel metal alloy infra-structure biomechanics.

- No level I evidence is currently available to support the use of aortic stent grafts in the management of either elective or emergency AAA. The results of ongoing randomised clinical trials are awaited.

- With the issue of unacceptable long-term durability apparently receding, the future of aortic stent grafts will probably focus more on developments to increase the availability of endovascular AAA repair eg. fenestrated and branched endografts.

- The need for improved management strategies in cases of ruptured AAA support an exciting key role for aortic stent graft technology that warrants further evaluation.

References

1. Parodi JC, Palmaz JC, Barone HD. Transfemoral intraluminal graft implantation for abdominal aortic aneurysms. *Ann Vasc Surg* 1991; 5: 491-499.

2. Jacobs TS, Won J, Gravereaux EC, *et al.* Mechanical failure of prosthetic human implants: a 10-year experience with aortic stent graft devices. *J Vasc Surg* 2003; 37: 16-26.

3. Alric P, Hinchliffe RJ, Wenham PW, *et al.* Lessons learned from the long-term follow-up of a first-generation aortic stent graft. *J Vasc Surg* 2003; 37: 367-73.

4. Holtham SJ, Rose JD, Jackson RW, *et al.* The Vanguard Endovascular Stent-graft: mid-term results from a single centre. *Eur J Vasc Endovasc Surg* 2004; 27: 311-18.

5. Moore WS, Matsumura JS, Makaroun M, *et al.* Five-year interim comparison of the Guidant bifurcated endograft with open repair of abdominal aortic aneurysm. *J Vasc Surg* 2003; 38: 46-55.

6. Zarins C, White R, Moll F, *et al.* The AneuRx stent graft: four-year results and worldwide experience 2000. *J Vasc Surg* 2001; 33: 135-145.

7. Zarins C. The US AneuRx Clinical Trial: 6-year clinical update 2002. *J Vasc Surg* 2003; 37: 904-908.

8. Faries PL, Brener BJ, Connelly TL, *et al.* A multicenter experience with the Talent endovascular graft for the treatment of abdominal aortic aneurysms. *J Vasc Surg* 2002; 35: 1123-28.

9. Criado FJ, Fairman RM, Becker GJ. Talent LPS AAA stent graft: results of pivotal clinical trial. *J Vasc Surg* 2003; 37: 709-715.

10. Cowie AG, Ashleigh RJ, England RE, *et al.* Endovascular aneurysm repair with the Talent stent-graft. *J Vasc Intervent Radiol* 2003; 14: 1011-16.

11. Pfammatter T, Mayer D, Pfiffner R, *et al.* Repair of abdominal aortic aneurysms with the Excluder bifurcated stent-graft. *J Cardiovasc Surg* 2003; 44: 549-52.

12. Bush RL, Najibi S, Lin PH, *et al.* Early experience with the bifurcated Excluder endoprosthesis for treatment of the abdominal aortic aneurysm. *J Vasc Surg* 2001; 34: 497-502.

13. Matsumura JS, Katzen BT, Hollier LH, *et al.* Update on the bifurcated Excluder endoprosthesis: Phase I results. *J Vasc Surg* 2001; 33: S150-153.

14. Matsumura J, Brewster D, Makaroun M, *et al.* A multicenter controlled clinical trial of open versus endovascular treatment of abdominal aortic aneurysm. *J Vasc Surg* 2003; 37: 262-271.

15. White RA. Clinical and design update on the development and testing of a one-piece, bifurcated, polytetra-fluoroethylene endovascular graft for abdominal aortic aneurysm exclusion: the Endologix device. *J Vasc Surg* 2001; 33: S154-156.

16. Carpenter JP. Multicenter trial of the PowerLink bifurcated system for endovascular aortic aneurysm repair. *J Vasc Surg* 2002; 36: 1129-37.

17. Carpenter JP, Anderson WN, Brewster DC, *et al.* Multicenter pivotal trial results of the Lifepath System for endovascular aortic aneurysm repair. *J Vasc Surg* 2004; 39: 34-43.

18. Greenberg RK, Lawrence-Brown M, Bhandari G, *et al.* An update of the Zenith endovascular graft for abdominal aortic aneurysms: initial implantation and mid-term follow-up data. *J Vasc Surg* 2001; 33: S157-164.

19. Abraham CZ, Chuter T, Reilly LM, *et al.* Abdominal aortic aneurysm repair with the Zenith stent graft: short to midterm results. *J Vasc Surg* 2002; 36: 217-225.

20.   Hinchliffe RJ, Goldberg J, MacSweeney STR. A UK multi-centre experience with a second-generation endovascular stent-graft: results from the Zenith Users Group. *Eur J Vasc Endovascular Surg* 2004; 27: 51-55.

21.   Sternbergh WC, Money SR, Greenberg R, *et al*. Influence of endograft oversizing on device migration, endoleak, aneurysm shrinkage and aortic neck dilation: results from the Zenith multicenter trial. *J Vasc Surg* 2004; 39: 20-26.

22.   Brener BJ, Faries PL, Connelly TL, *et al*. An in situ adjustable endovascular graft for the treatment of abdominal aortic aneurysms. *J Vasc Surg* 2002; 35: 114-119.

Chapter 2

Fenestrated and branched stent grafts: experience from a single centre

Eric LG Verhoeven, MD, Consultant Vascular Surgeon

Ted R Prins, MD, Consultant Radiologist

Ignace FJ Tielliu, MD, Consultant Vascular Surgeon

Jan JAM van den Dungen, MD PhD, Consultant Vascular Surgeon

University Hospital of Groningen, Groningen, The Netherlands

Introduction

It is now more than 10 years since Parodi reported the first endovascular procedures for abdominal aortic aneurysm repair, initially with tube-grafts, and later with bifurcated grafts [1]. For all devices presently in use, there are several anatomical requirements which make the aortic abdominal aneurysm (AAA) suitable for endovascular repair. One of these is a good proximal neck, consisting of a non-tapered cylindrical portion of at least 15mm below the renal arteries [2-4]. Several devices now employ a transrenal or suprarenal fixation, in order to enhance their stability in the proximal neck [5-9]. Nevertheless, as a general rule, patients with proximal necks shorter than 15mm are considered unsuitable for endovascular repair (see manufacturers' guidelines). An additional reason for concern is proximal neck dilatation after infrarenal endovascular aortic aneurysm repair (EVAR) [10-12].

These problems can be solved by using a customised stent graft design incorporating fenestrations (holes) for the aortic side-branches above such a short neck [13-15]. These allow for deployment of the stent graft above the renal arteries and possibly, the superior mesenteric artery, with the fenestrations and vessels lined up in order to maintain straight line patency. Because the technique of fenestrated aortic stent grafting is relatively new, there is very little data published to date in the literature. For this reason, the first part of this chapter will report the technique of fenestrated stent grafting and will report our own institution's early results.

Patients and methods

Between November 2001 and February 2004, 30 patients were accepted for fenestrated stent grafting. Of these 30 patients, 24 were operated on in Groningen, and six in another hospital by a local team in conjunction with one member of our team. All patients had proximal necks unsuitable for standard endovascular repair (Table 1). In addition, all patients had significant co-morbidity or a hostile abdomen precluding open abdominal repair. Contraindications to open surgery were cardiac in 13 patients, pulmonary in three and combined cardiopulmonary in six. Four patients had a hostile abdomen. The final group consisted of four patients who had type I endoleaks after previous stent grafting or open repair (anastomotic aneurysm), with a neck too short for normal cuff repair. Nineteen of the 30 patients were considered unsuitable for open repair. In each case

Table 1. Patient and fenestrated stent graft characteristics and procedural outcome.

Patient	Age	Sex (M;F)	ASA	AAA size* (mm)	Neck length (mm)	Anaesthesia (GA;EA;LA)	No. of side-branches Perf/Targ	Endoleak (type)	Serum creatinine change (µmol/l)	AAA size change (mm)
1	71	M	4	62	6	EA	2/2	-	No	-4
2	73	F	3	55	10	EA	2/2	-	No	-25
3	76	M	3	57	8	EA	3/4	-	92-125	-3
4	77	M	3	60	8	GA	3/3	-	No	-12
5	73	M	3	Type I (65)	4	GA	3/3	-	118-79	-4
6	60	M	3	55	7	EA	3/3	Type II (disappeared)	134-124	-23
7	75	M	3	Type I (55)	10	EA	1/1	Type I-Type II R/ laparotomy & stitching	125-112	-20
8	79	M	3	55	9	EA	2/2	Type II (IMA) R/coil embolisation	152-133	-5
9	66	M	2	55	6	EA	3/3	-	100-110	-27
10	66	M	3	Type I (55)	10	LA	2/2	-	94-178	-1
11	78	M	3	57	10	EA	2/2	-	No	-10
12	70	M	3	57	6	EA	2/2	-	No	-2
13	77	M	3	58	6	EA	3/3	-	No	-9
14	81	M	2	58	6	LA	3/3	-	No	-4
15	62	M	3	58	8	LA	2/2	-	No	-4
16	85	F	2	60	8	EA	3/3	-	104-115	-6
17	78	M	3	70	10	EA	3/3	-	No	-12
18	83	M	3	62	8	EA	3/3	-	No	-9
19	77	M	3	65	5	GA	3/3	-	No	-3
20	77	M	3	55	10	GA	2/3	-	-	-
21	80	M	3	78	10	EA	2/2	Type II (IMA)	No	+3
22	77	M	3	57	6	GA	2/2	-	No	-2
23	70	M	3	64	10	LA	2/2	-	75-91	-3
24	68	F	2	57	4	GA	3/3	-	No FU yet	No FU yet
25	79	M	4	Type I (64)	10	LA	1/1	-	No FU yet	No FU yet
26	78	M	3	62	5	EA	3/3	-	No FU yet	No FU yet
27	60	M	4	60	3	GA	3/3	-	No FU yet	No FU yet
28	72	M	3	66	4	GA	3/3	-	No FU yet	No FU yet
29	67	M	3	55	10	LA	3/3	-	No FU yet	No FU yet
30	76	F	2	55	4	GA	3/3	-	No FU yet	No FU yet

Abbreviations: M = male; F = female; ASA = American Society of Anesthesiologists Physical Status Classification; GA = general anaesthesia; EA = epidural anaesthesia; LA = local anaesthesia; Perf = perfused; Targ = targeted; IMA = inferior mesenteric artery; FU = follow-up.

Implantation technique

Patients were treated using various anaesthetic techniques according to the judgement of anaesthetist and surgeon, in conjunction with the patient. Nine patients were treated under general anaesthesia, 15 under epidural anaesthesia, and six under local anaesthesia (Table 1). Patients were prehydrated with a saline intravenous solution 12 hours before the procedure and renal output was carefully monitored. The complete deployment of the stent graft was only carried out following catheterisation of the side-branches and adjustment of the position using inflated balloons. Stenting of small fenestrations was routinely performed in order to secure the orifice of the side-branch and also to

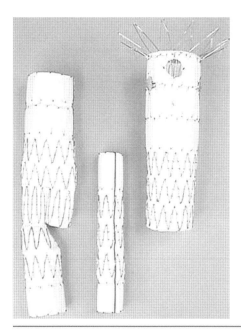

Figure 1. The Cook Zenith™ composite 3-part system consisting of a fenestrated tube, a bifurcated distal component, and a contra-lateral limb.

the indication for fenestrated endovascular repair was either an AAA of at least 55mm in diameter or a type I endoleak with a neck too short for standard proximal cuff treatment.

Stent graft configuration

Detailed evaluation of the proximal neck was obtained by spiral computerised tomography scanning with axial and perpendicular reconstructions. A calibrated angiogram was also performed. The stent graft used was a three-piece composite endoluminal prosthesis (Figure 1) based on the well-known Zenith™ system (William A. Cook Australia Pty. Ltd., Brisbane, Australia). The proximal tube graft was fitted with diameter reducing ties (Figure 2) to allow only partial deployment prior to catheterisation of the side-branches and final orientation of the stent graft.

Customisation of the stent grafts was based on each individual configuration. Three types of fenestrations were possible including scallops, large and small fenestrations (Figure 3).

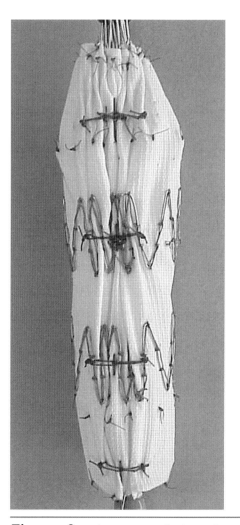

Figure 2. Diameter reducing ties facilitating repositioning of the graft during catheterisation.

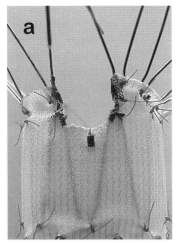

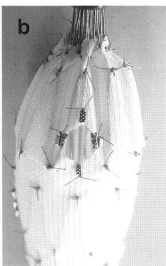

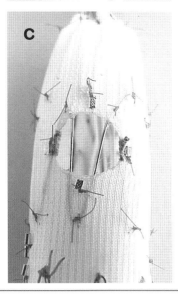

Figure 3. Different types of fenestrations including a scallop, a small fenestration, and a large fenestration.

match the fenestration with the ostium of that side-branch.

The procedure was completed with deployment of a bifurcated distal component and a contralateral limb. Finally, multiplanar completion angiography was carried out to confirm vessel patency and complete exclusion of the aneurysm.

Follow-up

All patients were followed-up with abdominal x-rays, duplex and CT scans at six weeks, six months, one year, and yearly thereafter. In addition, blood pressure as well as the renal function was monitored.

Results

Technical results

All endovascular procedures were successful and there were no conversions to open repair. One patient required aorto-uni-iliac conversion due to mis-positioning of the contralateral limb. Completion angiography showed complete exclusion of the aneurysm in 26 out of 30 patients (Table 1). There were four endoleaks, one a possible small proximal type I endoleak and three type II endoleaks. At the end of the procedure, 75 out of 77 targeted side-branches were patent. One accessory renal artery was noted to be occluded (patient number three) and there was doubt about a superior mesenteric artery (patient number 20). In total we used two large fenestrations, 35 small fenestrations, and 40 scallops for 19 superior mesenteric arteries, 56 renal arteries, and two accessory renal arteries. Stent placement was carried out in 33 of the 35 small fenestrations. The two small fenestrations not stented were for the main renal artery and an accessory renal artery, both on the left side in patient number three. Following stent graft deployment, the final angiogram showed good perfusion of the main renal artery, but occlusion of the accessory renal artery.

Mortality and morbidity

One patient died due to a mesenteric ischaemia (patient number 20). One day after the procedure, he

Table 2. Change in aneurysm diameter (mm) after fenestrated stent graft repair.

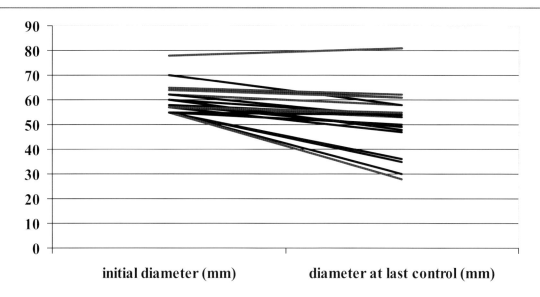

developed severe abdominal pain and was treated by laparotomy and a mesenteric bypass. Unfortunately, he died two days later and an autopsy was refused, prohibiting the final diagnosis (which could have included embolisation or covering of the mesenteric artery by the graft).

There were complications in seven patients. Patient number 13 suffered from cardiac decompensation, possibly related to a minor myocardial infarction, with subsequent pneumonia. Patient number 17 developed atrial fibrillation, which was treated with medication. Three patients (patient numbers one, five and seven), suffered from urinary tract complications (two urinary retentions and one infection). Patient number seven also developed a retroperitoneal haematoma, which was treated conservatively. Patient number 27 suffered from angina pectoris one day after the procedure and was treated successfully with medication. Finally, in patient number three, moderate perfusion of the left upper pole and poor perfusion of the left lower pole of the kidney was noted. A control spiral CT scan showed a well excluded aneurysm, with an occluded accessory renal artery and a severe stenosis of the left renal artery. We tried to catheterise the tight stenosis, but finally abandoned the attempt and lost the left kidney. This was despite the completion angiogram at the initial operation showing a good result.

Follow-up

The mean follow-up was 13 months (range 1-26). Except for the one renal problem already mentioned, spiral CT showed no other patency problems with the targeted vessels. In addition, no graft migration was demonstrated on plain abdominal films. Neither CT scans, nor duplex examinations, revealed any type I endoleak. The one possible small type I endoleak at completion angiography (patient number 7) was not demonstrated on the control CT scan, but a type II lumbar artery endoleak was diagnosed. Because the aneurysm continued to grow, a laparotomy was performed. This confirmed leakage from four patent lumbar arteries. These were sutured and the aneurysmal sac was wrapped around the device. One type II endoleak (patient number six) disappeared within six months with the aneurysm size decreasing. Two type II inferior mesenteric artery endoleaks were diagnosed and persisted. One was successfully treated by supra-selective embolisation and the second is currently awaiting the same procedure.

Renal function was carefully monitored. A serum creatinine increase was noted in five patients (including patient number three, who lost his left kidney) and in six patients the serum creatinine actually decreased. None of the patients required dialysis. The aneurysm diameter was carefully monitored (Table 2).

In four patients, the aneurysm disappeared completely. Only one patient has had their aneurysm increase in size, due to a patent inferior mesenteric artery. After successful embolisation, the aneurysm size quickly decreased to the original level. Patient number three, who lost his left kidney, died after eight months due to a metastasized adenocarcinoma (no primary tumour found). All remaining patients are alive and well.

Discussion

By customizing fenestrations and/or scallops for the renal arteries and, if required, the superior mesenteric artery, the proximal covered stent can be positioned in a more proximal and therefore straighter part of the aorta, thereby covering the full track of the proximal neck. This results in improved stent graft stability. Anderson [14] has shown this technique to be feasible, but it certainly requires adequate experience in both endovascular stent grafting and renal artery stenting. Our short follow-up, with a mean of 13 months, shows promising results. Many aneurysms diminished significantly in size, four of them disappeared completely and we did not see any proximal migration or a proximal type I endoleak. Longer follow-up is required to validate this technique and is the main reason why, at the time of writing, we reserve the technique for high-risk surgical patients.

Branched stent grafting

It would be fair to state that the fenestrated stent graft technique is becoming a real option for high-risk patients with a short neck. The grafts are now well established and with the standardisation of order forms, these devices are now widely available. Many different centres have used the technique and are now able to help others with their initial cases. More than 200 patients have been treated with fenestrated stent grafts worldwide, and all of the additional materials required for the procedure are readily available.

Branched stent grafting, however, is a newer technique and has only been used on rare occasions and just by a few people [16-18]. These branched stent grafts are highly experimental and not yet widely available.

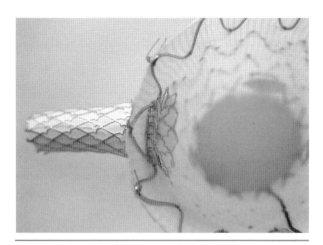

Figure 4. Example of a fenestrated graft provided with a covered Jostent®.

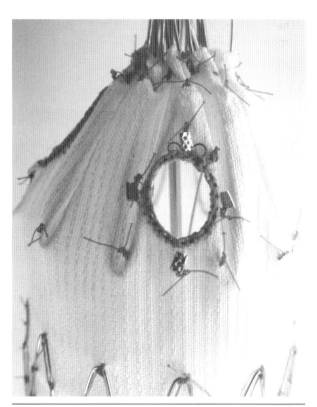

Figure 5. A fenestrated graft with a reinforced small fenestration.

The techniques for branched stent grafting can be divided into two categories. The first category derives from the fenestrated technique, but instead of using a non-covered stent to stabilize the small fenestrations, it is possible to use covered stents, like the Jostent® (previously JOMED GMBH, Germany; now ABBOT

Vascular, Redwood City, California, USA). This procedure has been successfully executed by Anderson in Adelaide, Australia and we have also used the technique for infrarenal aneurysms with necks too short to achieve sealing without a covered stent (Figure 4). In our view, the fenestrated technique with non-covered stents can be used for necks as short as about 4mm, but for juxta-renal aneurysms without a neck, a covered stent in a fenestrated graft may offer a better solution. At this moment in time, appropriate covered stents with enough flexibility to enter the fenestration and the renal artery, and with enough fixation and flaring possibilities to offer a good seal, are not available. Another option is to reinforce the fenestrations to enable a better seal and more security (Figure 5).

The second category involves grafts with incorporated side-branches, and to our knowledge, this has only been performed clinically by Chuter [16,18]. This technique requires meticulous positioning of the branched stent graft to allow catheterisation of all side-branches. Thereafter, a stent graft has to be introduced to seal both the branch of the stent graft and the targeted vessel. Problems of trackability, flexibility, and catheterising difficulties make the technique extremely difficult. In addition, paraplegia and thrombosis of side-branches is a real danger. We clearly need another few years of development, to warrant widespread use of this technique.

Acknowledgements

The development of the fenestrated technique has been made possible in co-operation with William Cook Australia, in conjunction with the endovascular teams of Perth, Adelaide, Frankfurt, Malmö, Cleveland, Liverpool, and Groningen. In Groningen, we greatly appreciated the possibility to join in with procedures performed both in Perth and Adelaide and to explore and discuss this technique.

Parts of this chapter have been published by the *European Journal of Vascular and Endovascular Surgery*: Verhoeven ELG, Prins TR, Tielliu IFJ, van den Dungen JJAM, Zeebregts CJAM, Hulsebos RG, van Andringa de Kempenaer MG, Oudkerk M, van Schilfgaarde R. Treatment of short-necked infrarenal aortic aneurysms with fenestrated stent grafts: short-term results. *Eur J Vasc Endovasc Surg* 2004; 27: 477-483.

Summary

◆ The treatment of short-necked aortic aneurysms with both fenestrated and branched stent grafts is feasible, but the technology is new and medium and long-term results are not yet available.

◆ Fenestrated stent grafts can be used to treat aortic necks as short as 4mm, whereas branched stent grafts should be used for the treatment of juxta-renal aneurysms.

◆ Following successful fenestrated stent grafting, the diameter of the aortic aneurysm does decrease in the absence of endoleak.

◆ Fenestrated stent grafting requires significant experience and these techniques are at present reserved for high-risk patients.

◆ Branched stent grafts are highly experimental and not yet widely available.

References

1. Parodi JC, Palmaz JC, Barone HD. Transfemoral intraluminal graft implantation for abdominal aortic aneurysms. *Ann Vasc Surg* 1991; 5: 491-499.

2. Schumacher H, Eckstein HH, Kallinowski F, *et al*. Morphometry and classification in abdominal aortic aneurysms: patient selection for endovascular and open surgery. *J Endovasc Surg* 1997; 4: 39-44.

3. Carpenter JP, Baum RA, Barker CF, *et al*. Impact of exclusion criteria on patient selection for endovascular abdominal aortic aneurysm repair. *J Vasc Surg* 2001; 34: 1050-1054.

4. Woodburn KR, Chant H, Davies JN, *et al*. Suitability for endovascular aneurysm repair in an unselected population. *Br J Surg* 2001; 88: 77-81.

5. Birch PC, Start RD, Whitebread T, *et al*. The effects of crossing porcine renal artery ostia with various endovascular stents. *Eur J Vasc Endovasc Surg* 1999; 17:185-190.

6. Bove P, Long G, Zelenock G, *et al*. Transrenal fixation of aortic stent-grafts for the treatment of infrarenal aortic aneurysmal disease. *J Vasc Surg* 2000; 32: 697-703.

7. Burks JA, Faries PL, Gravereaux EC, *et al*. Endovascular repair of abdominal aortic aneurysms: stent graft fixation across the visceral arteries. *J Vasc Surg* 2002; 35: 109-113.

8. Desgranges P, Kobeiter K, Coumbaras M, *et al*. Placement of fenestrated Palmaz stent across the renal arteries: feasibility and outcome in an animal study. *Eur J Vasc Endovasc Surg* 2000; 19: 406-412.

9. Malina M, Brunkwall J, Ivancev K, *et al*. Renal arteries covered by aortic stents: clinical experience from endovascular grafting of aortic aneurysms. *Eur J Vasc Endovasc Surg* 1997; 14: 109-13.

10. Makaroun MS, Deaton DH. Is proximal neck dilatation after endovascular aneurysm exclusion a cause for concern? *J Vasc Surg* 2001; 33: 39-45.

11. Prinsen M, Wever JJ, Mali WPTM, *et al*. Concerns for the durability of proximal aortic aneurysm endograft fixation from a two and three year longitudinal computed tomography angiography study. *J Vasc Surg* 2001; 33: 64-69.

12. Resch T, Ivancev K, Brunkwall J, *et al*. Midterm changes in aortic aneurysm morphology after endovascular repair. *J Endovasc Ther* 2000; 7: 279-285.

13. Stanley BM, Semmens JB, Lawrence-Brown MMD, *et al*. Fenestration in endovascular grafts for aortic aneurysm repair: new horizons for preserving blood flow in branch vessels. *J Endovasc Ther* 2001; 8: 16-24.

14. Anderson JL, Berce M, Hartley DE. Endoluminal aortic grafting with renal and superior mesenteric artery incorporation by graft fenestration. *J Endovasc Ther* 2001; 8: 3-15.

15. Browne TF, Hartley D, Purchas S, *et al*. A fenestrated covered suprarenal aortic stent. *Eur J Vasc Endovasc Surg* 1999; 18: 445-449.

16. Chuter TAM, Gordon RL, Reilly LM, *et al*. An endovascular system for thoracoabdominal aortic aneurysm repair. *J Endovasc Ther* 2001; 8: 25-33.

17. Inoue K, Hosokawa H, Iwase T, *et al*. Aortic arch reconstruction by a transluminally placed endovascular branched stent graft. *Circulation* 1999; 100: II316-II321.

18. Chuter TAM, Buck DG, Schneider DB, *et al*. Development of a branched stent-graft for endovascular repair of aortic arch aneurysms. *J Endovasc Ther* 2003; 10: 940-945.

Chapter 3

The endovascular treatment of ruptured abdominal aortic aneurysms

John Brennan, MD FRCS(Gen), Consultant Vascular Surgeon
Richard McWilliams, FRCS FRCR, Consultant Radiologist
Royal Liverpool & Broadgreen University Hospital, Liverpool, UK

Introduction

In the elective setting, endovascular aneurysm repair (EVAR) is now firmly established in many parts of the world and is currently the subject of two large randomised controlled trials in the UK (UK EVAR Trials I & II). It is hoped that data from these and other studies will help define the indications for the treatment of patients with an abdominal aortic aneurysm (AAA) with respect to EVAR for the next decade and beyond. Vast amounts have been written about EVAR since its inception in the early 1990s, but until recently, very little had been written with regard to emergency cases. This is perhaps unusual since it was inevitable from the start that the minimally invasive concept of EVAR would be applied to the emergency setting. Indeed, the first case report of successful stent grafting for a ruptured aortic aneurysm is now ten years old [1]. Intuitively one might imagine that the potential survival advantage for a patient undergoing EVAR for a ruptured aneurysm would be huge when compared with an identical case undergoing emergency open repair. This chapter aims to examine where things currently stand with regard to EVAR for ruptured aortic aneurysm and seeks to explain why its use in this setting has not flourished to anything like the extent of its role in elective repair.

Open surgery for ruptured abdominal aortic aneurysm

Very occasionally, one comes across a series reporting impressively low mortality following emergency open repair of ruptured aortic aneurysm, as low as 25% in one Dutch series [2]. These series are impressive, but most units recognise that in reality the perioperative mortality is much closer to 50%. This has not altered significantly in recent years despite perceived advances in both surgical and anaesthetic management [3,4]. A number of explanations have been forwarded to account for this apparent anomaly, such as the fact that older and sicker patients that might have been turned down previously are now offered surgery. However, this is not supported by evidence showing that, even when a selective policy is used, there is no improvement in mortality [5]. In fact, there is good evidence to show that the prime determinant of survival is the patient's preoperative fitness, as determined by specifically derived scoring systems, and that factors such as the skill of the medical team involved have frustratingly little impact [6].

It is against this background that the potential benefits of a minimally invasive approach appear very attractive.

EVAR for ruptured AAAs - preoperative considerations

Diagnosis and initial management

In conventional practice, the diagnosis of a leaking or ruptured aortic aneurysm is largely clinical and based on the classic triad of abdominal and/or back pain, collapse and documented hypotension. Once the diagnosis has been established, arrangements are made to transfer the patient to theatre as soon as possible for emergency open repair. The concept of permissive hypotension has been introduced in order to prevent aggressive fluid resuscitation until aortic control has been obtained. Whilst it is now deemed acceptable to maintain a systolic blood pressure as low as even 50mmHg [7], this should only be tolerated for as short a time period as is absolutely necessary.

If one is to consider EVAR, this initial phase is likely to be extended by the need for some form of imaging (which will also confirm the diagnosis). This should determine whether or not the case is anatomically suitable for stent graft placement.

Imaging for anatomical suitability

Most of the centres reporting their experience of EVAR in the emergency setting have used contrast-enhanced spiral computed tomography (CT) for decision-making [8]. This inevitably introduces a delay into the process and is dependent on fairly rapid access to good quality CT, which will vary in different centres and relies on the patient remaining haemodynamically stable. While the scan itself may take as little as a few minutes, there are inevitably going to be other procedural delays which extend the preoperative phase, especially outside normal working hours. Resch et al reported a mean duration of symptoms prior to undergoing EVAR in emergency cases of 12 hours compared with <1 hour for a contemporaneous group undergoing open repair [9]. Strict adherence to such a policy means that there would inevitably be a small number of deaths directly attributable to the delay if applied to allcomers. This must be weighed against the undeniable advantage of obtaining a CT, since there is virtual consensus that it is currently the best means of determining whether or not a case is suitable for EVAR.

A potential alternative, described by the Montefiore group [7], is to transfer the patient directly to the operating theatre as for open repair and perform on-table angiography after gaining access via a 5 French sheath in the right brachial artery. The decision to proceed with EVAR is based on angiographic findings. In an unstable patient (systolic BP <50mmHg), a 40mm intra-aortic occlusion balloon can be inflated in the supracoeliac aorta, although this necessitates exchange to a 14 French sheath. The disadvantages of angiography alone are that it will not necessarily confirm the presence of rupture and can give misleading information with regard to aortic dimensions due to its inability to demonstrate intraluminal thrombus. It has been suggested that intravascular ultrasound (IVUS) may have a role in this situation as an adjunct to on-table angiography [10].

What constitutes suitability for EVAR?

Aneurysm morphology

In elective programs patient suitability for EVAR has increased steadily as a result of development of stent graft technology and interventionalists' natural tendency to stretch initial, conservative limits with regard to aneurysm morphology. Is the same applicable in the emergency setting?

Not surprisingly, the most important factor to consider is the infrarenal neck, which should be at least 10mm long with a maximum diameter of no more than 30mm. This assumes that devices with a diameter of 34-36mm are available, enabling a 15-20% oversize, and that some form of suprarenal fixation will be used.

Iliac artery anatomy was more of a problem in the early days of EVAR, both elective and emergency, but a lot of issues with regard to access through tortuous vessels have been resolved by the use of very stiff wires and improved delivery systems. The issue of common iliac artery aneurysms (CIAA) remains, however, especially if bilateral. Since the majority of CIAAs extend down to the common iliac bifurcation, it is standard practice in an elective case to embolise the internal iliac artery and extend the stent graft limb into the external iliac. In the presence of bilateral CIAA most centres would be very reluctant to deliberately occlude both internal iliac arteries. Yilmaz *et al* [11] reported two deaths due to colonic ischaemia in two patients undergoing EVAR for ruptured AAAs in whom both internal iliacs were deliberately covered in order to exclude bilateral CIAAs. It would seem wise to conclude that bilateral internal iliac occlusion is poorly tolerated in the emergency setting.

There is clear indication in the published series to date that the perceived advantages of the minimally invasive approach have led centres to adopt more liberal criteria in terms of applying EVAR in emergency cases. Rose *et al* [12] retrospectively reviewed 46 CT scans with confirmed ruptured AAAs and concluded that only 20% were suitable for EVAR, which is in distinct contrast to the high suitability rates of 58-81% reported by others[11,13,14]. Not surprisingly, the main exclusion criteria were short and/or wide necks and it would seem that criteria created for the elective setting are not adhered to quite as strictly. There are concerns that this more relaxed approach may not only result in higher rates of complications during graft deployment (eg. proximal endoleak), but also of intermediate complications requiring secondary intervention. Lachat *et al* reported that seven of their 20 cases had some form of reintervention during a median follow-up of 19 months [13].

Patient inclusion
The majority of patients presenting with a ruptured AAA tend to be relatively stable for a short while at least, but the duration of this window of opportunity is unpredictable. Emergency EVAR has, in the main, been confined to patients with a contained rupture, who are haemodynamically stable and thus able to tolerate the inevitable logistical delays. This would seem to exclude those patients who are haemodynamically unstable at presentation from even being considered. The concept of fluoroscopically-guided placement of a supracoeliac aortic occlusion balloon as described above, however, suggests that even this group can be managed by EVAR, if appropriate arrangements are in place.

A second group to consider are those patients whom the surgical team would ordinarily turn down for open repair due to its perceived futility in the face of severe co-morbidities. A number of reports identify patients who would in normal circumstances be turned down for open repair, but who subsequently undergo successful EVAR and survive. In the series from Nottingham, eight out of their total of 20 cases had been declined open surgery [15]. Also, Greenberg *et al* describe three patients turned down for open repair who underwent successful EVAR [16]. There seems to exist therefore, the potential to extend treatment beyond established parameters, which is an almost inevitable consequence of any radical therapeutic advance.

A final group to consider is those with an acute, symptomatic aneurysm without documented rupture. Ordinarily, patients presenting acutely would undergo urgent repair, preferably on the next available elective list, but often more urgently. This is known to be a high-risk group, however, with a mortality of up to 20%. In their series Yilmaz *et al* included seven cases with symptomatic non-ruptured aneurysm, all undergoing successful EVAR with no mortality [11].

Intraoperative considerations

Technique of aneurysm exclusion

Modular bifurcated devices

The overwhelming majority of elective EVAR procedures are performed using commercially available modular bifurcated systems. Since most experience has been gained with these, it would seem logical to apply this expertise to emergency cases. An important factor to consider, however, is the length of time required to successfully exclude the aneurysm and arrest the potential for further haemorrhage. The rate-limiting step with a bifurcated device is often the time taken to cannulate the contralateral stump and this is an area of potential concern. The series from Zurich [13], Ulm [14] and Rotterdam [17], in which commercially available modular bifurcated systems were largely used, suggest that the experience gained from a large elective EVAR programme is crucial in enabling the device to be deployed safely and rapidly.

The Zurich group described a technique of aortic balloon control used as an adjunct to deployment of a bifurcated system. Access was obtained transfemorally and the balloon inflated in the suprarenal aorta over a stiff guidewire. Once the main body segment of the device had been deployed, the balloon was removed and then reinflated within the main body (aortic 'neck') in order to maintain aortic control and prevent prolonged renal/visceral ischaemia. This manoeuvre was only necessary in three out of their 21 cases, in one as an emergency in order to achieve control prior to any intervention and in the other two at a later point in the procedure.

Aortomonoiliac devices

The alternative strategy of aneurysm exclusion is to use an aortomonoiliac graft configuration. This necessitates some means of occlusion of the contralateral common iliac artery and a femorofemoral crossover bypass in order to perfuse the contralateral leg. The perceived advantages of this approach are the technical simplicity, speed of deployment, and the fact that a greater proportion of cases are treatable. The initial reports, however, described time-consuming construction and sterilisation of custom-made devices in theatre, although this is no longer advocated. The Montefiore group still use a custom-made device but these are prepared and sterilised in advance [7].

More recent reports describe the use of modular 2-piece systems [11]. The proximal component of both devices has a bare stent to enable suprarenal fixation. A second component is then introduced and the two pieces overlapped, as required, depending on the length of the aneurysm and the segment of iliac artery selected for distal sealing. Yilmaz et al report that using a stock of eight components (four proximal and four distal), 21 out of a prospective cohort of 26 were potential candidates for EVAR. They have since modified the design to include a 'bell-bottomed' limb to accommodate ectatic common iliac arteries, thus minimising the need to exclude the internal iliac artery, but experience with this modification is not reported.

The attractive features of speed and simplicity of deployment of the aortomonoiliac configuration, however, must be set against the adjunctive procedures necessary. While occlusion of the contralateral common iliac artery is usually achieved

by endovascular means, the femorofemoral bypass is undeniably surgical.

Type of anaesthesia

This is particularly relevant where ruptured AAAs are concerned, since induction of general anaesthetic (GA) is often associated with dramatic haemodynamic deterioration in patients undergoing open repair, due to a loss of abdominal tone and reversal of compensatory vasoconstriction mechanisms. This raises the question of whether local anaesthetic (LA) should be considered, given the relatively minimally invasive nature of the surgery necessary to deploy the device. It is, however, interesting to note that although the feasibility of performing EVAR under LA and intravenous sedation in elective cases has been described, the overwhelming majority of procedures worldwide are still performed under GA. It is perhaps for this reason that most of the reported experience of emergency EVAR involves GA rather than LA. Only Lachat et al set out to use LA (in combination with remifentanyl) as the anaesthetic technique of choice [13]. In their series, the majority of deployments were achieved successfully without the need for GA, with only five out of 21 requiring intubation. Others have been less successful with LA, reporting patient discomfort as the main indication for converting to GA [8].

Patient outcomes

The driving force behind emergency EVAR is the desire to reduce the formidable risk profile of open repair. Given the fact that the patient has by definition sustained a major physiological insult at the time of presentation, it is not surprising that emergency EVAR is not as benign as its elective sister procedure.

Mortality

The reported mortality varies from 0% to 45% (Table 1) and thus covers the range from undeniably superior to frustratingly equivalent when compared with open repair. The zero mortality reported by van Sambeek et al [17] must be seen in context in that it was a small

Table 1. Published series of EVAR for ruptured AAAs.

Centre	No. cases	Study period	Mortality (%)
Nottingham	20	6yrs	45
Montefiore	20	6yrs	10
Eindhoven	17	30 months	24
Zurich	21	3yrs	9.5
Ulm	21	6yrs	12.5
Malmo	21	5yrs	19
Rotterdam	6	7 months	0

series of six cases and during the study period six equivalent patients underwent emergency open repair and all survived. There is then a cluster of five series with mortality ranging from 9.5% to 24% which seems to be a truer reflection of what might be achievable. The 45% mortality reported by Hinchcliffe et al [15] inevitably gives pause for thought and is worthy of closer critical evaluation. In general, there were a higher number of complications relating to graft delivery and deployment, and this is a reflection of the fact that their program commenced in 1994 at a time when custom-made devices were being constructed in theatre. Conversion to open repair was undertaken in four (failure to deliver the device in three, persistent proximal endoleak in one), of whom three died. Renal failure was seen in six and was fatal in four, one patient died following massive haemorrhage from stress ulceration and one patient died of sepsis following small bowel perforation during the femorofemoral crossover bypass. The overriding take home message from this series is the potentially formidable learning curve that was encountered. In spite of all this, the mortality was in fact equivalent to the lower end of the range for open repair. The more recently compiled series suggest that a number of the issues raised in Nottingham, UK have already been addressed.

Morbidity

Compared with the complication profile of patients surviving open surgery for a ruptured AAA, successful EVAR appears to be well tolerated. Little reference is made with regard to the cardiopulmonary complications, which are very common after open repair. It is not clear whether these problems are simply not seen, which is unlikely, or just that they are not as significant an issue after EVAR.

More reference is made with regard to renal failure [8]. This is also an issue after open repair where it is associated with a high mortality. Deterioration in renal function following EVAR can be due to coverage of one or both renal arteries with the stent graft as described by Hinchcliffe et al [15], but is also related to the effect of large doses of non-ionic contrast medium in the presence of haemodynamic compromise. Lachat et al [13] reported renal impairment in 28%, although only two out of six required renal replacement therapy.

Another potential area of concern is that of abdominal compartment syndrome (ACS), which is increasingly recognised as a major source of complications following emergency open repair. There is perhaps a reluctance to consider drainage of intra- or retroperitoneal haematoma following successful EVAR but it may occasionally be necessary and should at least be considered [8]. Lachat et al reported two cases in whom ACS was managed by ventilation and haemofiltration without drainage of haematoma.

The principal complication specific to EVAR is that of endoleak. Continued perfusion of the aneurysm in the presence of a rupture is of major concern. The reported incidence following EVAR for a ruptured AAA is small. Proximal Type I endoleak is potentially the most serious and a range of different strategies have been employed to deal with it, including immediate open conversion [15], banding of the aortic neck at laporotomy [11] and secondary endovascular intervention [13]. Type II endoleak is less commonly seen and does not appear to be a significant issue [8].

Logistical considerations

The small number of reports which are reviewed in this chapter are from centres with large elective EVAR programmes. This degree of experience is clearly crucial. At least two describe how emergency EVAR was introduced cautiously and that encouraging early results led to formalisation and expansion of the programme. In spite of this, the largest series amount to 21 cases each accumulated over three to five years [13,14]. In Eindhoven, 17 ruptured AAAs and seven acute, symptomatic AAAs were recruited in two years [11].

If it were just the technical aspects of the procedure that needed to be resolved, there would no doubt be many more centres reporting their experience. That this is not the case, points to other factors being responsible. Foremost among these are the complex logistical factors involved in the setting up of an emergency programme and then the more specific factors pertaining to each individual case.

Personnel

For emergency open repair, the principal requirements are an available operating theatre, trained theatre staff, an anaesthetist and a vascular surgeon. Hospitals accepting cases of ruptured AAAs are familiar with the urgency of the situation and have appropriate systems in place to activate the appropriate personnel. Emergency EVAR necessitates extending the requirements for experienced personnel within a short time frame.

Most elective EVAR procedures in the UK are performed jointly by an interventional radiologist and a vascular surgeon, with varying levels of input from each. In an emergency, it would therefore be necessary to call on both. Whilst vascular surgeons are familiar with the unpredictable and fickle nature of the beast that is a ruptured AAA, and will always be available, there are concerns currently about the ability of most interventional departments to support such a programme, especially outside normal working hours.

This issue has been addressed in Eindhoven by the development of an on-call rota involving endovascular specialists drawn from a pool of vascular surgeons and interventional radiologists, such that only one is required. Such a set-up can only exist where there is a sufficient number of enthusiastic, appropriately trained individuals.

There is also a need for experienced radiography personnel to perform an urgent CT scan and then to operate fluoroscopic imaging during the procedure. Again, this would probably need to be in addition to the normal radiography on-call service in a speciality that already has recruitment difficulties in the UK.

Equipment and venue

Elective EVAR can be equally well performed in an intervention suite or an operating theatre depending on local circumstances. In an emergency, however, the patient is best managed in an operating theatre environment from the anaesthetic point of view and in case of the need for urgent surgical intervention. The ideal set-up would be a true, theatre-grade intervention suite, but this is a luxury available to very few.

As far as stent grafts are concerned, there would need to be an available stock of component parts able to deal with most cases. Given the urgency of the situation and the fact that reasonably generous oversizing seems to cause little in the way of problems, it would probably be possible to have an appropriate stock with a relatively small number of components, depending on which configuration is opted for. It would also be necessary to have appropriate stock of all the various consumables (wires, sheaths, catheters etc.), required during EVAR immediately available.

Should there be a randomised trial?

In the current clamour for evidence to support any new initiative or change in practice, the randomised controlled trial (RCT) is considered almost mandatory. Indeed, vascular surgical practice is notable for the number of RCTs which have been successfully carried out and which have helped shape patient management. It is, therefore, reasonable to consider whether or not there should be a RCT comparing EVAR with open repair for ruptured AAAs.

With regard to endovascular repair of ruptured aortic aneurysms, the results from enthusiastic centres all carry the same message; EVAR is feasible and warrants further evaluation. The critical end-point to consider is perioperative mortality and it would seem reasonable to expect a potential halving in mortality from 50% down to 25%. The major difficulty facing a RCT is going to be recruitment of sufficient centres (and cases) to make it a viable proposition. Whatever sample size the statisticians deduce would be necessary in order to produce a meaningful result, a large number of centres would need to be involved. Given that each centre would need to overcome the formidable logistical issues involved in establishing an emergency EVAR programme and then surmount their individual learning curves, a RCT seems to be a laudable, but unachievable goal. The slow recruitment of cases reported from undeniably enthusiastic centres suggests that this is a formidable hurdle. Even if a trial were carried out and a convincing advantage were demonstrated in favour of EVAR, it is debatable whether or not it would become widely adopted because of the logistical problems already alluded to.

Conclusions

There is no doubt that EVAR is a feasible proposition for patients presenting with a ruptured AAA. There are a limited number of small series which suggest that EVAR may produce a significant reduction in the mortality observed following emergency open repair, but there are no randomised controlled studies to support this proposition.

There are a number of major logistical difficulties which must be overcome in order to establish an effective emergency EVAR programme and it is this aspect which has prevented more widespread application. It is likely that emergency EVAR will continue to be offered in those centres with the necessary enthusiasm, equipment and expertise required. More convincing data to support a significant survival advantage are going to be necessary in order to persuade other centres and health purchasers to make the investments required to establish their own programmes.

Summary

◆ EVAR for ruptured AAA is logistically complex but feasible.

◆ Urgent CT scan is the imaging modality of choice to determine suitability for EVAR.

◆ A relatively high proportion of cases (up to 80%) may be anatomically suitable.

◆ Both modular bifurcated and aortomonoiliac configurations have been used successfully.

◆ A mortality rate in the region of 10-25% might be reasonably expected.

◆ A RCT comparing EVAR with open repair for ruptured AAA is unlikely due to logistical issues and recruitment difficulties.

References

1. Yusuf SW, Whitaker SC, Chuter TA, Wenham PW, Hopkinson BR. Emergency endovascular repair of leaking aortic aneurysm. *Lancet* 1994; 344: 1645.

2. van Dongen HP, Leusink JA, Moll FL, *et al*. Ruptured abdominal aortic aneurysms: factors influencing postoperative mortality and long-term survival. *Eur J Vasc Endovasc Surg* 1998; 15: 62-66.

3. Berridge DC, Chamberlain J, Guy AJ, *et al*. Prospective audit of abdominal aortic aneurysm surgery in the northern region from 1988 to 1992. *Br J Surg* 1995; 82: 906-910.

4. Bradbury AW, Makhdoomi KR, Adam DJ, *et al*. Twelve-year experience of the management of ruptured abdominal aortic aneurysm. *Br J Surg* 1997; 84: 1705-1707.

5. Basnyat PS, Biffin AHB, Moseley LG, *et al*. Mortality from ruptured abdominal aortic aneurysm in Wales. *Br J Surg* 1999; 86: 765-770.

6. Neary WD, Crow P, Foy C, *et al*. Comparison of POSSUM scoring and the Hardman Index in selection of patients for repair of ruptured abdominal aortic aneurysm. *Br J Surg* 2003; 90: 421- 425.

7. Ohki T, Veith FJ. Endovascular grafts and other image-guided catheter-based adjuncts to improve the treatment of ruptured aortoiliac aneurysms. *Ann Surg* 2000; 232: 466-479.

8. Hinchcliffe RJ, Braithwaite BD, Hopkinson BR. The endovascular management of ruptured abdominal aortic aneurysms. *Eur J Vasc Endovasc Surg* 2003; 25: 191-201.

9. Resch T, Malina M, Lindblad B, *et al*. Endovascular repair of ruptured abdominal aortic aneurysms: logistics and short-term results. *J Endovasc Ther* 2003; 10: 440-446.

10. van Essen J, Gussenhoven EJ, van der Lugt A, *et al*. Accurate assessment of abdominal aortic aneurysm with intravascular ultrasound: validation with computed tomographic angiography. *J Vasc Surg* 1999; 29: 631-638.

11. Yilmaz N, Peppelenbosch N, Cuypers PWM, *et al*. Emergency treatment of symptomatic or ruptured abdominal aortic aneurysms: The role of endovascular repair. *J Endovasc Ther* 2002; 9: 449-457.

12. Rose DFG, Davidson IR, Hinchcliffe RJ, *et al*. Anatomical suitability of ruptured abdominal aortic aneurysms for endovascular repair. *J Endovasc Ther* 2003; 10: 453-457.

13. Lachat ML, Pfammatter Th, Witzke HJ, *et al*. Endovascular repair with bifurcated stent-grafts under local anaesthesia to improve outcome of ruptured aortoiliac aneurysms. *Eur J Vasc Endovasc Surg* 2002; 23: 528-536.

14. Scharrer-Pamler R, Kotsis T, Kapfer X, *et al*. Endovascular stent-graft repair of ruptured aortic aneurysms. *J Endovasc Ther* 2003; 10: 447-452.

15. Hinchcliffe RJ, Yusuf SW, Macierewicz JA, *et al*. Endovascular repair of ruptured abdominal aortic aneurysm - a challenge to open repair? Results of a single-centre experience in 20 patients. *Eur J Vasc Endovasc Surg* 2001; 22: 528-534.

16. Greenberg RK, Srivastava SD, Ouriel K, *et al*. An endoluminal method of haemorrhage control and repair of ruptured abdominal aortic aneurysms. *J Endovasc Ther* 2000; 7: 1-7.

17. Van Sambeek MRHM, van Dijk LC, Hendriks JM, *et al*. Endovascular versus conventional open repair of acute abdominal aortic aneurysm: feasibility and preliminary results. *J Endovasc Ther* 2002; 9: 443-448.

Chapter 4

Overview of the current European randomised aortic stent graft trials

Louise C Brown, MSc, EVAR Trials Manager

Roger M Greenhalgh, MA MD FRCS MChir, Professor of Surgery

Imperial College of Science, Technology & Medicine

Charing Cross Hospital, London, UK

Introduction

In the early 1990s Parodi, Palmaz and Barone in Argentina [1] and Volodos in the Ukraine introduced EndoVascular Aneurysm Repair (EVAR). These pioneers used custom-made stent graft systems beginning with a repair to lie entirely within the abdominal aorta (aorto-aortic graft). Subsequently, it was shown that the aorto-aortic endovascular grafts were applicable in less than 10% of patients and bifurcation systems were developed which enable a greater proportion of aneurysms to be managed by an EVAR method [2]. 'In-house systems' were introduced in the UK in Nottingham [3] and Leicester [4]. However, during the last five years there has been a move towards commercially available systems as technological improvements have made them a more viable choice of treatment.

Originally, the EVAR technique was developed for use in patients who were considered unfit for conventional open repair surgery. However, as endovascular technology has progressed EVAR devices have been selected over open repair as an alternative, less invasive treatment for fit patients. However, the efficacy of EVAR against standard management for Abdominal Aortic Aneurysm (AAA) in fit and unfit patients has yet to be proven and a number of randomised controlled trials have been undertaken to investigate whether EVAR could become an alternative or better treatment for AAA. There are currently four European randomised trials in progress, namely the UK EndoVascular Aneurysm Repair (EVAR) trials 1 and 2, the Dutch Randomised Endovascular Aneurysm Management (DREAM) trial and the French Aneurysme Chirurgie de l'aorte contre Endoprothese (ACE) trial. In the USA, the Open Versus Endovascular Repair (OVER) trial has also started and has recently randomised its 200th patient. The first results from two of these European trials are expected later this year and an overview of the European trial methodologies is given here.

European registries and open audit

The UK Registry for Endovascular Treatment of Aneurysms (RETA)

The National RETA Registry, based at the Northern General Hospital in Sheffield, UK was initiated in January 1996 to audit 'in-house' and commercially available EVAR systems deployed within the UK [5]. It is a voluntary audit that includes both prospective and retrospective EVAR cases and currently holds data on more than 1600 EVAR deployments across the UK. RETA audit reports are produced annually on behalf of the Vascular Surgical Society of Great Britain & Ireland and the British Society of Interventional Radiology and these have provided invaluable data on the performance of EVAR devices over the last seven years. However, it is important to appreciate that national registries are voluntary and are also audited in an 'open' fashion and this can lead to selection bias problems.

EUROSTAR

The EUROSTAR project was launched in 1996 to audit prospectively the performance of endovascular aneurysm repair across 102 centres in 17 European countries [6]. This Registry is also voluntary. However, the data are collected prospectively which reduces the extent of selection bias providing good follow-up data are collected. It is the largest registry of EVAR devices in Europe with over 4500 cases of EVAR being followed for durability, graft performance and secondary intervention procedures.

European randomised trials in progress

The UK EndoVascular Aneurysm Repair (EVAR) trials 1 and 2
Lead applicant - Professor RM Greenhalgh (UK)

Objectives

The EndoVascular Aneurysm Repair (EVAR) trials started recruitment on 1st September 1999 and aim to assess the efficacy of endovascular aneurysm repair in the treatment of abdominal aortic aneurysm. EVAR is currently being used both in fit and unfit for open repair patients and the goal of the EVAR trials is to evaluate the mortality, quality of life, durability and cost-effectiveness associated with EVAR, open repair and best medical therapy in fit and unfit patients with AAA diameters ≥5.5cm.

Materials and methods

Summary of trial design

A full design and methodology paper has previously been published [7]. In summary, male and female patients aged at least 60 years with an AAA diameter measuring at least 5.5cm on a Computed Tomography (CT) scan are assessed for anatomical suitability for EVAR. Suitable patients are offered entry either into EVAR trial 1 if they are considered fit for conventional open repair or EVAR trial 2 if they are considered unfit. EVAR 1 randomly allocates patients to EVAR or open repair and EVAR 2 randomly allocates patients to EVAR with best medical treatment or best medical treatment alone. Target recruitment is 900 patients in EVAR trial 1 and 280 patients in EVAR trial 2.

Eligibility of participating centres

In order to ensure that participating centres have the necessary experience in performing EVAR, the Trial Management Committee has set some eligibility criteria for participation in the trials. Each centre needs to have performed at least 20 EVAR procedures and these must be submitted to the RETA Registry for audit. RETA then informs the EVAR Trial Management Committee when a UK hospital has met these requirements. At the start of the trials in September 1999, only 13 centres met the eligibility requirements for participation but there are now 41 centres recruiting patients across England, Wales, Scotland and Northern Ireland.

Generalisability and the EVAR study

It is of particular importance that patients found to be unsuitable for an EVAR device are recorded. Numbers of unsuitable patients are logged and reasons for unsuitability are recorded in order to determine what proportion of AAA patients are anatomically suitable for an EVAR device at the national level. Thus, all patients registered for assessment of anatomical suitability for an EVAR device form the EVAR study and trial patients are drawn from this pool of AAA patients if they are found to be suitable for an EVAR device. Each trained regional centre also acts as a specialist centre in its own area. In many cases it has been possible for surrounding non-vascular specialist hospitals to support recruitment by referring vascular patients believed to be suitable for the EVAR trials to that regional centre. If anatomically suitable for EVAR and agreeable to randomisation, the patient receives treatment at the regional centre. Thus *all* EVAR, OR, best medical treatment and follow-up is performed at the regional centre.

Entry criteria for patients entering EVAR trial 1

◆ Males or females aged at least 60 years.
◆ An aneurysm diameter measuring ≥5.5cm according to a CT scan.
◆ Aneurysm anatomically suitable for an EVAR device.
◆ Patient considered fit for conventional open repair.
◆ Signed informed consent.

Entry criteria for patients entering EVAR trial 2

◆ Males or females aged at least 55 years.
◆ An aneurysm diameter measuring ≥5.5cm according to a CT scan.
◆ Aneurysm anatomically suitable for an EVAR device.
◆ Patient considered unfit for conventional open repair. This excludes patients who are unsuitable for an open repair on the grounds of hostile abdomen who would otherwise be anaesthetically fit for an open repair.
◆ Signed informed consent.

Choice of EVAR device

Participating centres are free to decide which commercial or 'in-house' device to use, although the use of commercially available devices is favoured. These all carry the CE mark and are therefore freely available on the market and have undergone certain checks before being released. It is assumed that each centre will take the time to discuss the evidence for the safety of each device with the company. The anatomical suitability of EVAR devices will therefore be very centre-specific depending on the number of devices that they choose to use in that hospital. It is not feasible for the trial protocol to intrude on the choice of device at each centre and this has been left as a pragmatic decision for the participating clinicians.

Fitness for surgery

Recommended cardiac, respiratory and renal fitness guidelines are provided for all participating clinicians and baseline data will be used to assess fitness of randomised patients at the final analysis. These guidelines should provide some conformity of fitness classification for EVAR trial 1 or 2. Furthermore, randomisation is stratified by centre and this should ensure that any differences in assignment of fitness status between centres should not lead to any considerable differences between randomised groups.

Randomisation

Randomisation is performed for each trial using 50:50 ratio randomly permuted block sizes constructed by the STATA statistical software package. Randomisation is stratified by centre and is only performed when all necessary baseline data have been received at the Trial Management Office based at Charing Cross Hospital in London. Centres are encouraged to perform surgery within a month of randomisation.

Outcome measures

The primary endpoint for both trials is all-cause mortality.

All-cause mortality for EVAR trial 1

Data from the UK Small Aneurysm Trial [8,9] (UKSAT) were used to estimate mortality rates for the EVAR trials power calculations. The UKSAT ran from 1991 until the first publication of results in November 1998 and was a randomised controlled trial which allocated patients with small aneurysms measuring between 4.0 and 5.5cm on ultrasound to either regular ultrasound surveillance or early elective surgery. No survival benefit was gained by offering early surgery and it was concluded that surveillance was a safe management option for patients with a small AAA. Patients randomised to early open repair in the UKSAT experienced an annual all-cause mortality of 7.1%. In the EVAR trials, patients are undergoing AAA repair for larger aneurysms and we have assumed an annual mortality rate of 7.5%. If EVAR can reduce this mortality to 5% per year then EVAR might be justified as a viable treatment alternative for AAA. By 31st December 2003, 1082 patients had been recruited into EVAR trial 1 and these will be followed until April 2005 accumulating an average follow-up of 3.33

years per patient. This produces 90% power at the 5% significance level to detect a difference in annual mortality of 7.5% versus 5%.

All-cause mortality for EVAR trial 2

Patients with a large AAA considered unfit for open repair in the UK Small Aneurysm Study were followed-up for AAA growth and rupture and were shown to have an annual all-cause mortality of 25%. The RETA Registry has shown that patients considered unfit for open repair who have been treated with EVAR have an annual all-cause mortality of 15%. By 31st December 2003, 338 patients had been recruited into EVAR trial 2 and these will be followed until April 2005 accumulating an average follow-up of 3.33 years per patient. This produces 90% power at the 5% significance level to detect a difference in annual mortality of 25% versus 15%.

30-day operative mortality

From The UK Small Aneurysm Trial data, 30-day operative mortality was calculated for patients who were randomised to surveillance but whose aortic aneurysm subsequently grew to >5.5cm when surgery was performed (n=191). Eleven were dead at 30 days leading to a 30-day operative mortality of 5.8% [95% CI 2.9-10.1%]. Power calculations for 30-day operative mortality in EVAR trial 1 based on 90% power at the 5% significance level using 6% in one treatment arm versus 2% in the other arm indicate that 552 patients would be required in each arm leading to a total of 1104 patients to detect this difference should it exist.

Graft durability

The incidence of endoleaks and rupture from EVAR devices and rupture of grafts in patients who have undergone an open repair is being monitored. The long-term durability of open repair procedures is being scrutinised as well as EVAR device performance, as follow-up of patients in the UK Small Aneurysm Trial detected a number of AAA ruptures as the cause of death in patients who were known to have had an open repair. CT scans are being performed annually to record the sac and anastomosis diameter measurements in open repair patients. Endoleaks in EVAR patients are classified according to an amended version of the Geoffrey White (Sydney, Australia) classification [10]. Incidence

of graft migration, rupture, anastomotic aneurysm, thrombosis, stenosis and infection is also being monitored.

Health Related Quality of Life (HRQL)

Generic and specific HRQL measurements are being collected for all patients in both EVAR trial 1 and 2. The generic assessment includes the EuroQol-5D questionnaire [11], the Short-Form 36 scores [12] and the State-Trait Anxiety Index. The Patient Generated Index (PGI) [13] has been selected to assess any changes in specific HRQL.

Economic evaluation

The overall aim of the analysis will be to estimate the cost-effectiveness of alternative treatment strategies for patients with abdominal aortic aneurysm. The economic analysis will carry out two comparisons:-

◆ EVAR versus open repair in patients fit for open repair.
◆ EVAR plus best medical management versus best medical management alone in unfit patients.

Cost data are being collected for all procedures and subsequent interventions associated with the AAA. The primary outcome measure for the economic analysis will be the Quality-Adjusted Life Year (QALY), calculated using patients' replies to the EuroQol-5D questionnaire administered at baseline, one month, three months and annually thereafter.

Follow-up

All trial patients are flagged for mortality at the Office for National Statistics (ONS). Full HRQL data are collected at one, three and 12 months following treatment and cost evaluation is based on operation costs, secondary interventions during the course of follow-up and annual EuroQol-5D questionnaires. The incidence of adverse events is also being collected and these have been defined as tender AAA, ruptured AAA, conversion to open repair, myocardial infarction, stroke, renal failure and amputation. CT scans are used for assessment of growth rates, persistent endoleaks and durability that may vary with stent graft type. Centres are encouraged to provide data from as many CT scans as possible but the minimum requirement for CT scan follow-up is at one and three months post EVAR procedure for EVAR patients and then annual CT scans for all randomised patients in each arm of both trials. Centres are free to utilise any additional imaging modality beyond a CT scan if it is felt appropriate. However, data are not collected for any additional imaging as the CT scan form can be used to record any problems that have been identified with the AAA or graft.

Trial management structure

Data Monitoring & Ethics Committee (DMEC)

This Committee is chaired by Professor Philip Poole-Wilson (Professor of Cardiology, National Heart & Lung Institute) and includes two representatives of the Vascular Surgical Society of Great Britain & Ireland (VSSGBI) and also, two representatives of the British Society of Interventional Radiology (BSIR) as agreed with their councils. There is also independent statistical representation on the Committee. If required, the Medical Devices Agency (MDA) will attend on matters concerning device performance. The Committee is completely confidential and is the only Committee to see any of the trial data before the final analysis. Audit of the data is 'closed' as well as being device, operator and centre-specific. Information from EVAR procedures elsewhere can be fed into the DMEC and the manufacturer can feed in details of product modification. The performance of devices will be scrutinised using 'tracker trial' methodology [14].

Trial Steering Committee (TSC)

This meets as required but generally once per year and is chaired by Professor Richard Lilford (Professor of Clinical Epidemiology, University of Birmingham). Surgical and radiological input is supplied by two operators from the participating centres and the Committee is generally concerned with trial progress and funding issues and liaises between the Data Monitoring & Ethical Committee and the Trial Management Committee.

Trial Management Committee (TMC)

This is concerned with the day-to-day running of the EVAR trials and is chaired by the lead applicant,

Professor Roger Greenhalgh. It relates to both the DMEC and Trial Steering Committee and includes specialists who advise on good clinical trial practice in terms of data management and statistics, HRQL, health economics, best medical practice and EVAR performance. There is also one nominated surgeon and radiologist who serve on this Committee to represent the participating trialists.

Regional Trial Participants Committee (RTPC)

This includes each trial co-ordinator and a surgical and radiological representative of each participating centre. It can be requested at any time by trial centres, training centres or the trial co-ordinating centre whenever the need arises and is used as a feedback forum for all the centre participants. It usually meets at the annual meetings of the Vascular Surgical Society of Great Britain and Ireland and the British Society of Interventional Radiology.

Recruitment and progress

Planned trial recruitment closed on the 31st December 2003 by which time 4803 patients had been registered into the EVAR study. Suitable patients have been drawn from this pool of EVAR study registrations and recruitment targets have been surpassed in both trials with 1082 patients randomised into EVAR trial 1 and 338 patients randomised into EVAR trial 2. Patients who do not enter the trials are excluded for various reasons including unsuitability for an EVAR device, AAA <5.5cm on CT scan, refusals for entry into either trial or refusals for any CT scan or further treatment. Recruitment rates vary considerably between the 41 centres with some hospitals more enthusiastic about EVAR trial 2 than others.

Timing of results and publication

A common dilemma in any trial is when to publish results. In the EVAR trials, patients need to be followed for a minimum of one year in order to accrue sufficient patient years of follow-up and also, to allow assessment of costs and quality of life after one year of treatment. It is anticipated that the last few patients will have their operations performed by the end of March 2004 and they will then be followed until March 2005 when the data analysis will commence. It is expected that full results of the trials will be available in mid 2005. Therefore, the problem arises on how to treat new aneurysm patients in the intervening 18 months from close of recruitment at the end of 2003 until release of full results in 2005. The four EVAR trials committees debated various options and are all in agreement that randomisation should be allowed to continue during this intervening period for those centres who wish to wait until full results become available. Therefore, the trials will continue randomising according to the same protocol and these additional patients will form part of a long-term durability analysis that aims to follow all the trial patients for a minimum of four years and possibly until death. It has also been decided that a separate analysis on early 30-day operative outcome should be published in 2004 to coincide with the November Annual General Meetings of the Vascular Surgical Society of Great Britain & Ireland (VSSGBI) and the British Society of Interventional Radiology (BSIR). Once these data are released into the public domain it is felt that equipoise will be lost and randomisation will therefore cease when these early 30-day results are released. A full schedule of the trial milestones is given in Figure 1.

The Dutch Randomised Endovascular Aneurysm Management (DREAM) trial. Lead applicant - Professor JD Blankensteijn (Netherlands)

Objectives

The DREAM Trial is a multicentred randomised study that started recruitment in February 2001 and aims to compare the performance and cost-effectiveness of endovascular aneurysm repair with conventional open repair in patients suitable for both treatment modalities. The primary outcome is combined mortality and morbidity within 30 days of the AAA operation.

Materials and methods

Summary of trial design

A full design and methodology paper has already been published [15]. In summary, eligible patients from participating centres with AAAs anatomically suitable for EVAR measuring at least 5.0cm who are being

considered for elective aneurysm repair, are randomised to either receive standard open repair or EVAR. Recruitment began in February 2001 and the target is a total of 400 patients over three years. The primary outcome is combined 30-day mortality and morbidity but data on costs and quality of life are also being collected and early quality of life outcome data have already been published [16].

Eligibility of participating centres

The participating centres are required to comply with the guidelines issued by the Endovascular Safety Committee of the Dutch Society for Vascular Surgery and the Dutch Society for Radiology. Essentially, each centre needs to have performed at least 20 EVAR cases and are also required to have an annual volume of at least 30 conventional AAA repairs and 50 endovascular procedures, eg. EVAR or percutaneous transluminal angioplasty. In some cases, patients are referred from non-EVAR hospitals to a DREAM trial centre for randomisation. If these patients are randomised to open repair, the referring centre are able to perform this procedure at their hospital whilst patients randomised to an EVAR device must have their EVAR performed at the DREAM trial centre.

Entry criteria for patients entering the DREAM trial

A fuller list of inclusion and exclusion criteria are given in the methodology paper [15] but the most important criteria are given here.

Inclusion criteria

◆ Non-symptomatic infrarenal AAA for which intervention is indicated.
◆ An aneurysm diameter measuring ≥5.0cm.
◆ Adequate infrarenal neck.
◆ Adequate anatomical aorto-iliac configuration for device selected.
◆ Life expectancy of at least two years.
◆ Signed informed consent.

Exclusion criteria

◆ Ruptured AAA or symptomatic AAA requiring emergency surgery.
◆ Maximum AAA diameter <5.0cm.
◆ Juxtarenal or suprarenal AAA.
◆ Inflammatory AAA.
◆ Neck or aorto-iliac anatomy unsuitable for EVAR.
◆ Anatomical variations, eg. horseshoe kidney or arteries requiring reimplantation.

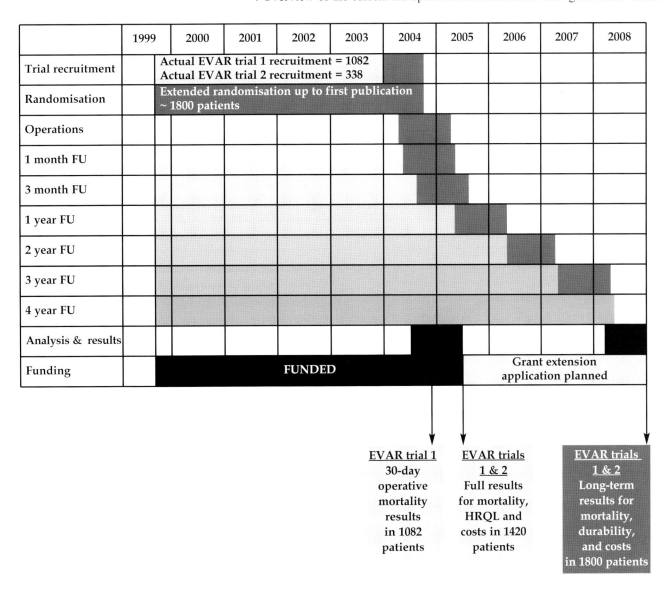

Figure 1. Milestones for EVAR trials recruitment, follow-up and publication.

◆ Administration of contrast agent not possible.
◆ Life expectancy less than two years.
◆ Active infection present, transplant patients, presence of connective tissue disease.

Choice of EVAR devices

The DREAM trial allows the use of all EVAR devices that are approved and available on the market and requirements are consistent with the European CE mark, Preliminary Market Approval (PMA) or United States Food and Drug Administration (FDA). Any shape of device is allowed including extender limbs, cuffs and suprarenal fixation.

Randomisation

A telephone randomisation service is available for centres to call and this allocates patients using a 50:50 ratio and is stratified by centre.

Outcome measures

Mortality and morbidity

The primary endpoint for the DREAM trial is combined perioperative mortality and morbidity. All moderate and severe complications are independently assessed at 30 days and combined into one primary outcome. Power calculations based on 80% power at the 5% significance level have indicated that 400 patients (200 in each arm) are required to detect a difference in the 30-day incidence of combined mortality or morbidity of 20% in the open repair arm versus 10% in the EVAR arm. It was anticipated that this number should be recruited in three years.

Health Related Quality of Life (HRQL)

Generic HRQL measurements are being collected using the EuroQol-5D questionnaire [11] and the Short-Form 36 [12] as well as a short questionnaire on sexual function.

Economic evaluation

Cost-effectiveness data are being collected in terms of operative mortality, early and late complications, overall mortality and quality of life and these will be used to compare the two arms of the trial in terms of quality-adjusted life years gained. Short-term results are to be analysed within 30-day and 6-month timeframes and mid-term results are to be analysed within a 2-year time frame. As follow-up beyond two years is limited, it is expected that the long-term results will be modelled using a Markov Monte Carlo simulation model. In addition to the direct costs of each procedure, indirect costs will also be collected to account for losses in production and loss of paid and unpaid labour.

Follow-up

All patients are followed at one month for early outcome data. Further analysis will be undertaken one year after inclusion of the last patient when the majority of patients will have been followed for between 18 and 30 months.

Trial management structure

Site and Device Selection Committee (SDSC)

This Committee ballots potential participating centres and physicians and oversees the application of the guidelines issued by the Endovascular Safety Committee of the Dutch Society for Vascular Surgery and the Dutch Society for Radiology.

Trial Steering Committee (TSC)

A surgeon and a radiologist from each participating centre stand on this Committee. The main responsibility of the TSC is trial monitoring but it also compiles reports on the progress of the trial and performs interim analyses whenever required and these are presented to the Data Monitoring & Ethics Committee (DMEC).

Data Monitoring & Ethical Committee (DMEC)

This Committee monitors the ethical aspects of the trial and ensures that it is conducted safely and in the best interests of the participating patients. Information is sourced from reports written by the Trial Steering Committee.

Continuous sequential safety monitoring

EVAR is a developing technology and there have already been a number of safety alerts issued and various devices have already been withdrawn from the market. For this reason, the DREAM trial investigators have decided to use continuous sequential safety analysis to monitor the outcomes of the trial. Monitoring of clinical trials is complex, particularly when controversial new treatments are under scrutiny and the decision to stop a trial is based on many factors. The concept of continuous safety monitoring allows an interim analysis to be performed at any time during the accumulation of data, yet the overall alpha significance level is maintained (usually set at p=0.05). This differs from grouped sequential monitoring in that the interim analyses are triggered by the occurrence of a pre-determined 'serious event' rather than *apriori* agreed fixed timepoints when sufficient events or patient years of follow-up have been accrued. For this trial, if during the course of follow-up a primary outcome event occurs, i.e. serious morbidity or mortality, graft infection or AAA rupture, the Trial Steering Committee performs a blinded survival analysis of the results and presents a report to the DMEC for advice. The number of interim analyses is accounted for by using an alpha spending function that adjusts the significance level at each interim analysis according to the number of events or amount of follow-up that have been accrued up to that time and the number of interim analyses that have previously been performed. Stopping rules have been selected that allow the Steering Committee to take action if an interim analysis shows a hazard ratio between the groups of >2.0 or <0.5.

Recruitment and progress

The DREAM trial website at http://www.endovascular.nl/dream/ provides updates on trial recruitment and by December 2003, 351 patients had been randomised into the DREAM trial from 29 centres with 178 allocated to open repair and 173 to EVAR. It is expected that the 400 patient target will be reached in early 2004 with the 30-day results anticipated sometime during 2004.

The first DREAM trial publication of results was released in February 2004 [16] and reported the results of a comparison between open repair and EVAR in terms of quality of life at three weeks, six weeks, three, six and 12 months. The analysis was performed on a subset of 153 patients who were randomised between February 2001 and August 2002 and followed for at least one year. The analysis indicated a small but significant advantage in quality of life in the early postoperative period (three weeks) following an EVAR compared to an open repair. However, after six and 12 months this benefit was reversed with evidence to suggest a significant improvement in open repair patients compared to EVAR patients in terms of the SF-36 general health domain and the EuroQol.

The Aneurysme Chirurgie de l'aorte contre Endoprothese (ACE) trial
Lead applicant - Professor JP Becquemin (France)

Objectives

The ACE trial is a french multicentred randomised study that aims to compare the performance of endovascular aneurysm repair with conventional open repair in patients suitable for both treatment modalities. Limited information was available for the ACE trial, as start-up problems have delayed publication of a methodology paper on the trial protocol. Essentially, patients eligible for the trial are

randomised to conventional open repair or EVAR and the protocol is understood to be similar to the UK EVAR trials with patients followed for mortality and complication rates.

Eligibility criteria for participating centres

Training criteria demand that trial operators have participated in at least 10-15 stent graft deployments and collaboration must exist between surgeons and radiologists at each centre. It is also a requirement that the operating or radiology suite complies with french recommendations for endovascular procedures.

Choice of EVAR device

Centres are free to choose which EVAR device they wish to treat patients but limitations in financial reimbursement for grafts has meant that only a few manufacturers are eligible to obtain private funding and this has marred recruitment, despite some charitable money being made available for centres to get started.

Outcome measures

The primary outcome is combined mortality and complications following the AAA operation. Target recruitment is for 600 patients with 300 in each arm.

Recruitment and progress

Unfortunately, the ACE trial suffered delays in starting recruitment due to issues relating to financing of the EVAR grafts. However, it finally started entering patients towards the end of 2003 with 15 centres participating. Latest recruitment figures show that 55 patients have been randomised across 32 centres and recruitment has recently started increasing. It is expected that a further five centres will join the trials and the investigators are hopeful that recruitment will be completed in about three years from 2004.

Summary

◆ **EVAR trial 1 (UK)** Between September 1999 and December 2003 a total of 1082 patients with an AAA at least 5.5cm in diameter that was suitable for an EVAR device and who were considered fit for open repair were randomised to either open repair or EVAR. Patients will be followed until March 2005 and results on all-cause mortality, quality of life, durability and cost-effectiveness are expected for publication in mid-2005. Results on 30-day operative mortality are expected in November 2004.

◆ **EVAR trial 2 (UK)** Between September 1999 and December 2003 a total of 338 patients with an AAA at least 5.5cm in diameter that was suitable for an EVAR device and who were considered unfit for open repair were randomised to either EVAR with best medical therapy or best medical therapy alone. Patients will be followed until March 2005 and results on all-cause mortality, quality of life, durability and cost-effectiveness are expected for publication in mid-2005.

◆ **DREAM trial (Netherlands)** Between February 2001 and early 2004 a target of approximately 400 patients with an AAA at least 5.0cm in diameter that is suitable for an EVAR device and who are considered fit for open repair will have been randomised to either open repair or EVAR. The primary endpoint is combined 30-day mortality and morbidity and full results are expected in 2004.

◆ **ACE trial (France)** The ACE trial began recruitment towards the end of 2003 and plans to recruit 600 patients over three years. Patients are randomly allocated to receive open repair or EVAR and a combined outcome of mortality and complication rates will be analysed.

References

1. Parodi JC, Palma JC, Barone HD. Transfermoral intraluminal graft implantation for abdominal aortic aneurysm. *Ann Vasc Surg* 1991; 5: 491-497.
2. Andrews SM, Cuming R, MacSweeney ST, *et al.* Assessment of feasibility for endovascular prosthetic tube correction of aortic aneurysm. *Br J Surg* 1995; 7: 917.
3. Yusef SW, Baker DM, Hind RE, *et al.* Endoluminal transfemoral abdominal aortic aneurysm repair with aorto-uni-iliac graft and femorofemoral bypass. *Br J Surg* 1995; 82: 916.
4. Nasim A, Thompson MM, Sayers RD, *et al.* Endovascular repair of abdominal aortic aneurysm: an initial experience. *Br J Surg* 1996; 83: 516-519.
5. Thomas SM, Gaines PA, Beard JD on behalf of VSSGBI and BSIR. Short term (30 day) outcome of endovascular treatment of abdominal aortic aneurysms: results from the prospective Registry of Endovascular Treatment of Aneurysms (RETA). *Eur J Vasc Endovasc Surg* 2001; 21: 57-64.
6. Harris PL. The need for clinical trials of endovascular abdominal aortic aneurysms stent/graft repair: the Eurostar Project. *J Endovasc Surg* 1997; 4: 72-77.
7. Brown LC, Epstein D, Manca A, Beard JD, Powell JT, Greenhalgh RM. The UK EndoVascular Aneurysm Repair (EVAR) Trials: design methodology and progess. *Eur J Vasc Endovasc Surg* 2004; 27: 372-381.
8. The UK Small Aneurysm Trial Participants. Results for randomised controlled trial of early elective surgery or ultrasonographic surveillance for small abdominal aortic aneurysms. *Lancet* 1998; 352: 1649-1660.
9. The UK Small Aneurysm Trial Participants. Long-term outcomes of immediate repair compared with surveillance of small aortic aneurysms. *N Engl J Med* 2002; 346(19): 1445-1452.
10. White GH, May J. Failure of endovascular repair of abdominal aortic aneurysms: endoleak, adverse events and grading of technical difficulty. In: *The Durability of Vascular and Endovascular Surgery.* RM Greenhalgh, Ed. WB Saunders, London, 1999.
11. The EuroQol Group. EuroQol - a new facility for the measurement of health-related quality of life. *Health Policy* 1990; 16: 199-208.
12. Ware JE, Sherbourne CD. The MOS 36-item short-form health survey (SF-36): conceptual framework and item selection. *Medical Care* 1992; 30: 473-483.
13. Ruta DA, Garratt AM, Leng M, *et al.* A new approach to the measurement of quality of life - the Patient-Generated Index. *Medical Care* 1994; 11: 1109-1126.
14. Lilford RJ, Braunholtz DA, Greenhalgh RM, *et al.* Trials and fast changing technologies: the case for tracker studies. *BMJ* 2000; 320: 43-46.
15. Prinssen M, Buskens E, Blankensteijn JD. The Dutch Randomised Endovascular Aneurysm Management (DREAM) Trial. Background, design and methods. *J Cardiovasc Surg* 2002; 43(3): 379-384.
16. Prinssen M, Buskens E, Blankensteijn JD. Quality of life after Endovascular and open AAA repair. Results of a randomised trial. *Eur J Vasc Endovasc Surg* 2004; 27: 121-127.

Chapter 5

The RETA database:
what have we learned?

Steven Thomas, MRCP FRCR MSc, Senior Lecturer Vascular Radiology
Jonathan Beard, ChM FRCS, Consultant Vascular Surgeon
The Sheffield Vascular Institute, The Northern General Hospital, UK

Introduction

The Registry for Endovascular Treatment of Aneurysms (RETA) was established to collect data on endovascular abdominal aortic aneurysm repair (EVAR) from United Kingdom (UK) centres, as this new approach to the treatment of abdominal aortic aneurysms (AAAs) was introduced into UK practice. Since its inception on the 1st of January 1996 [1] a total of 1684 cases have been submitted to the Registry. With the start of the UK EVAR trials in 1999, the majority of EVARs have been performed within these trials. The cases submitted to RETA are now cases performed outside of the trials. These are predominately those performed early in a centre's experience, to allow entry into the EVAR trials. This means that the full RETA dataset is less representative of current UK practice. However, follow-up of the first 1000 cases submitted is valuable as a measure of long-term outcome for those cases treated early in UK practice. This is now the main aim of the Registry.

This chapter briefly presents data on short-term outcomes (these have been published elsewhere [1]), but concentrates on EVAR durability and late patient outcome. Follow-up is not yet complete with the aim to follow patients for at least five years following their procedure. The available dataset is also incomplete because of the problems of voluntary data submission, though our aim is to maximise the amount and quality of the follow-up data for the first 1000 patients submitted to RETA before publication of the EVAR trial results. This will involve continued support from submitting centres with the provision of data as it is requested from the co-ordinating centre in Sheffield, UK.

Statistical analysis

Analysis was performed using the SPSS® for Windows™ statistical software. Patients are divided into subgroups defined by stent graft type, fitness for open repair and aneurysm diameter. The 'stent graft type' group was further divided into those with an aorto-uni-iliac stent graft and cross-over graft (AUIC) and those with an aortic tube or bifurcated stent graft (AT/BI). Patients corresponding to the American Society of Anaesthesiology (ASA) grade I-III, were deemed 'fit' for open repair and those corresponding to ASA IV-V, were deemed 'unfit'. Patients with hostile abdomens or other contraindications to open repair, but ASA I-III were included in the 'fit' group.

Table 1. Immediate outcome.

	All cases	AT/BI	AUIC
Aneurysm excluded No complication	769/996 (77.2%)	566/733 (77.2%) (OR 1.13 [95% CI: 0.79-1.6] p=0.5)	203/263 (77.2%)
Additional endovascular procedures	110/996 (11%)	94/733 (12.8%) (OR 0.42 [95% CI: 0.24-0.75] p=0.003)	16/263 (6.1%)
Additional surgical procedures	52/996 (5.2%)	40/733 (5.5%) (OR 0.67 [95% CI: 0.33- 1.37] p=0.27)	12/263 (4.6%)
Conversion to open repair	33/996 (3.3%)	13/733 (1.8%) (OR 5.03 [95% CI: 2.3- 10.8] p=0.0001)	20/263 (7.6%)

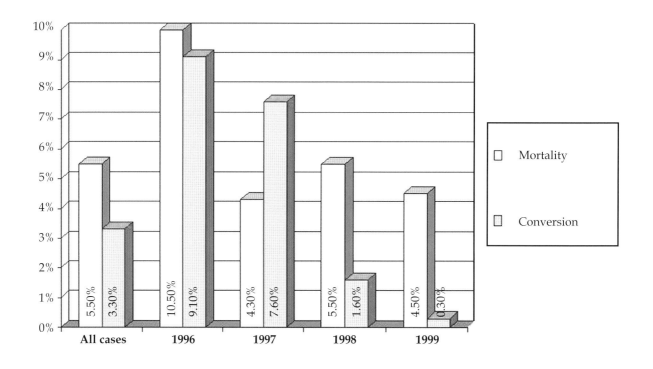

Figure 1. Fall in 30-day conversion and mortality rates by year.

Subgroups of 'small' AAA <6cm diameter and 'large' AAA >6cm were analysed separately.

Statistical analysis was performed using the Chi-squared test of independence (for categorical data) and t-tests (for continuous data). Logistic regression was used to compare differences in outcomes adjusting for available confounders for defined subgroups. Results are presented as odds ratios (OR). These represent the increased (or decreased) odds (with 95% confidence intervals) of an outcome in the first compared to the second group. Kaplan-Meier analysis was used for the analysis of long-term outcomes.

Short-term (30-day) results

Between 1st January 1996 and 3rd March 2000, 1000 cases were submitted to the Registry from 41 centres. The number of cases per centre ranged from 2-143 (median 16). The number of centres and cases increased each year until the EVAR trial began. The indication for repair was elective asymptomatic abdominal aortic aneurysm (AAA) in 83.2%, elective symptomatic in 13.5%, acute non-rupture in 1.6% and stable rupture in 1.4%.

Overall, 3.2% of patients received an AT, 26.3% an AUIC and 70.2% a BI (missing data n=3). There were relatively few ATs in the Registry and their use fell out of favour in the first two years because of distal endoleaks. AUICs built 'in-house' were the commonest stent graft used at the beginning of the Registry but these have now been superseded by commercially available and CE marked devices. The increase in the proportion of BI stent grafts is also reflected in the fact that more than 60% of endovascular repairs were performed in the operating theatre when the Registry commenced, but by 1998, more than 60% were undertaken in the radiology suite. The proportion of patients having the procedure under loco-regional anaesthesia also increased.

The median aneurysm diameter was 6cm (range 2.5-15) with a median infra-renal neck length of 2.4cm. Overall, 42% were classified as large (>6cm). There were significantly more large aneurysms in the AUIC group (132/253, 52.3%) compared to the

AT/BI group (288/735, 39.7%), OR 1.65, 95% CI 1.24-2.2, p<0.001. Patients with larger aneurysms were also more unfit (95/559, 17% vs 125/420, 29.8%, OR 2.1, 95% CI 1.5-2.8, p<0.001).

A total of 22.7% patients were considered unfit for open repair (missing data n=3). Of the fit patients, 67 (8.8%) were considered fit but unsuitable for open repair. There was a significantly higher proportion of unfit patients in the AUIC group (96/263, 36.5%) compared to the AT/BI group (130/174, 17.7%). The increased odds of being unfit in the AUIC group was 2.67 [95% CI 1.95-3.65], p<0.001.

The median age of the patients was 73 years (range 44-93) with a male: female ratio of 9:1. There was no difference in age between those treated with an AUIC and those treated with an AT/BI respectively (72 vs 73 years). Nor was there any difference in age between fit and unfit patients (72 vs 72 years). Patients with small aneurysms were younger than those with large aneurysms and this difference, though small, reached statistical significance (72 vs 73 years respectively [95% CI 0.4-2.2], p=0.006).

Overall, 77.2% of endovascular repairs resulted in successful exclusion of the aneurysm, without complications, by the end of the procedure (missing data n=4). The success rate was the same for both stent graft types (Table 1). Additional endovascular procedures were required significantly more often in the AT/BI group (p=0.003). However, conversion to open repair occurred more frequently in the AUIC group (p=0.001). The overall conversion rate was 3.3%, but this fell significantly from 13/143 (9.1%) in 1996 to 1/335 (0.3%) in 1999 (p=0.002) (Figure 1). Mortality following immediate conversion was 30%, but rose to 66.7% for unfit patients.

Post-procedure complications within 30 days occurred in 27.8% of cases (Table 2). There were significantly more complications in the AUIC group (p=0.006). At 30 days, 90.4% of aneurysms had been successfully excluded, 6.1% had persistent endoleaks and 5.8% had died. There were significantly more deaths in the AUIC group, (33/263, 12.5% vs 24/726, 3.3%, OR 2.6, [95% CI 1.18-5.86], p=0.018). There were also significantly more deaths in unfit patients (33/223, 14.8% vs 25/769,

Table 2. Post-procedure complications (30 days).

	All cases	AT/BI	AUIC
Any complication	272/976 (27.8%)	175/716 (24.4%) (OR 1.57 [95% CI: 1.1- 2.1] p=0.006)	97/268 (37.3%)
Technical complication	55/976 (5.6%)	31/716 (4.3%) (OR 2.1 [95%CI: 1.16-3.7] p=0.013)	24/268 (9.2%)
Wound complication	78/976 (8%)	55/716 (7.7%) (OR 1.1 [95% CI: 0.6-1.8] p=0.84)	23/268 (8.8%)
Renal failure	40/976 (4.1%)	21/716 (2.9%) (OR 2.1 [95% CI: 1.07-4.2] p=0.03)	19/268 (7.3%)
Colonic ischaemia	6/976 (0.6%)	4/716 (0.6%) (OR 1.1 [95% CI: 0.18-6.7] p=0.9)	2/268 (0.8%)
Other medical complication	147/976 (15.1%)	92/716 (12.8%) (OR 1.5 [95% CI: 1.01-2.22] p=0.045)	55/268 (21.2%)

3.3%, OR 4.9, [95% CI 2-12], p<0.001). The higher mortality rate in the AUIC group remained significant even after adjusting for available confounding influences such as the higher proportion of unfit patients within this subgroup (Figure 2). The mortality rate halved from 15/143 (10.5%) in 1996 to 15/335 (4.5%) in 1999, but this failed to achieve significance (Figure 3). The mortality rate in women was significantly higher than men (p=0.01). Persistent endoleaks and mortality were significantly higher in those with larger aneurysms (p<0.0001 and p=0.0046 respectively). The median length of stay was longer for patients in the AUIC group (mean eight vs five days, p=0.001, after adjusting for confounders).

Fate of primary endoleaks

Endoleaks [2] were identified in 142 cases either during the primary procedure or at 30-day follow-up. Proximal anastomotic (PA) type I endoleaks [2] at the end of the primary procedure were the most commonly reported and occurred in 47 cases (Figure 3). Most (45/47) were identified immediately post-procedure and two at 30-day follow-up. Most had urgent treatment, either immediately the endoleak was identified or within a few days. Of the 47 endoleaks, nine were converted to OR immediately (three deaths) and two were converted later (both survived). Six had operative banding, but this was only successful in two cases (three deaths). Proximal cuffs were successful in 9/10 cases (one death at three months due to rupture from a persistent leak). In three patients a second stent graft repaired the leak and PTA was successful in 2/5 cases. Twelve patients had no immediate treatment and three died of rupture at ten days, 16 days and four months. Overall, 14 patients had a persistent PA endoleak, with or without treatment and four (28%) subsequently died of rupture within one year. Operative repair was attempted in 17 cases, resulting in six deaths (mortality rate 35%).

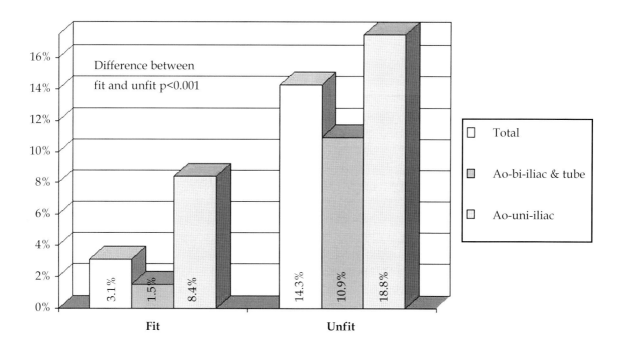

Figure 2. Comparison of 30-day mortality rates for patients deemed fit or unfit for open repair, by graft type (AUIC vs AT/BI).

Collateral (type II) endoleaks [3] were the next most common endoleak reported and occurred in 42 cases (35 visible immediately and nine within 30 days). Twenty of these had occluded spontaneously by 30 days. At one year, five of the remaining patients had been treated and six had spontaneously occluded. One patient with an apparently sealed collateral endoleak and an excluded aneurysm on follow-up CT died of AAA rupture ten months post-procedure.

Distal anastomotic (DA) type I endoleaks at the end of the primary procedure occurred in 28 cases (21 detected immediately and seven within 30 days). Of these, ten spontaneously sealed, one had an open repair, two were embolised and two were stented within 30 days. Of the 12 persistent DA endoleaks, four were treated within one year and there were no procedural or rupture-related deaths.

Occluder endoleaks occurred in three cases. Two had occluded spontaneously within 30 days and one was successfully banded.

Midgraft (type III) endoleaks occurred in 13 cases. Nine were successfully excluded with another covered stent within 30 days. Three of four persistent midgraft endoleaks had spontaneously occluded within one year. No site was stated for nine endoleaks.

Late results (up to 5 years)

The return rates for requested follow-up have been reasonable at 87% at one year and 77%, 65%, 52% and 51% at two, three, four and five years respectively.

Mortality in the first year post-procedure was 11%, with most deaths due to cardiac disease or malignancy, i.e. unrelated to graft complications. Six deaths were related to AAA rupture, three of which had a primary proximal type I endoleak (see above). One other had a secondary DA type I endoleak, the other two cases had apparently excluded aneurysms

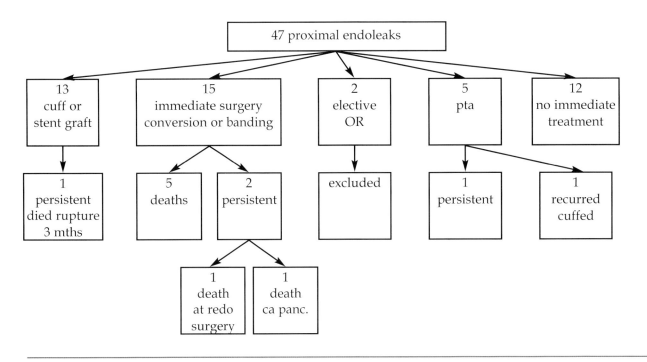

Figure 3. Fate of primary proximal anastomotic type I endoleaks.

at follow-up CT scanning. The mortality rates were 10%, 7%, 10% and 8%, at two, three, four and five years post-procedure respectively. Again, most deaths were not related to graft complications, although five other fatal ruptures were reported. One other patient ruptured with an associated secondary proximal endoleak, and survived open repair. One patient died following surgery for a secondary endoleak, and two patients died as a result of overwhelming sepsis and infected stent grafts. The cumulative risk of rupture was 2% at the 5-year follow-up point.

Overall, 255 complications related to the device or aneurysm were reported, occurring in 12.8%, 14.2%, 14.8%, 16.1% and 18%, at one, two, three, four, and five year follow-up intervals respectively. Fifty-four percent (n=139) of these were secondary endoleaks or graft migration, with secondary collateral (type II) endoleaks the most common problem reported. Many collateral endoleaks were not treated, but other types of endoleak and proximal graft migration were usually successfully treated using endovasular techniques, such as embolisation or further stent grafts.

Graft or limb occlusions and/or kinks were the next most common problem accounting for 18% (n=45) of device or AAA complications. Limb or graft occlusion often required a surgical bypass procedure. Increasing size of the sac remnant with no endoleak was also reported in a number of cases, although most cases were kept under close observation, conversion to OR was reported in 25% (n=5/20) of cases. During later years of follow-up, graft distortion and suture breaks were widely reported, though most did not require treatment as they were not necessarily associated with endoleak or graft migration. Follow-up of secondary complications and their treatment suggests that of those patients treated for secondary complications, only about 30% survive with no further problems, with many problems persisting or recurring.

Using Kaplan-Meier analysis the cumulative freedom from endoleak was 88.1%, 81.5%, 75.6% and 72% and the cumulative freedom from secondary procedure rates were 89.4%, 80.8%, 68.2%, 59.8% at one, two, three and four years of follow-up respectively (Figure 4).

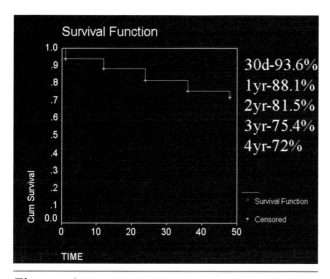

Figure 4. Cumulative freedom from endoleak obtained using Kaplan-Meier analysis.

Discussion

The 30-day results of EVAR are encouraging, but not clearly better than those reported for open repair. This must be tempered with the fact that these are early results with nearly 25% of patients considered unfit for open repair and another 25% receiving AUIC stent grafts that were fabricated in-house, due to an initial lack of commercially available alternatives. The mortality rate of a group more comparable to those being offered open repair, i.e. fit patients treated with AT/BI stent grafts, was only 1.5%, which is impressive compared to a mortality rate of 6% in the UK small aneurysm trial [4]. The fall in conversion rates and mortality with time also reflects advances in stent graft design, better patient selection and possibly reflects improved mentoring of new centres.

RETA shows that larger aneurysms have worse 30-day outcomes with fewer large aneurysms excluded and a higher mortality. This is important, particularly for unfit patients who tend to present when their aneurysms are larger. This may be related to these aneurysms being more technically challenging, though there was no increase in the rate of technical complications in larger aneurysms, but there was a trend towards an increased need for conversion to open repair. It may be that the larger aneurysms had wider necks and available stent grafts were

undersized, but these data were not collected in the Registry.

It is recognised that AUIC devices can be used to treat a larger proportion of aneurysms [5] and we have shown that those treated with it tend to be older, more unfit and to have larger aneurysms. Comparisons with the AT/BI group remain difficult in the context of a registry because these differences confound direct comparison of the two groups. Conversions to open repair and technical complications were more frequent in the AUIC group and even after adjustment for available confounding influences, the morbidity and mortality rates were higher for those treated with AUIC devices. Also, after adjustment, patients treated with an AUIC device had a significantly longer hospital stay. This is probably related to the surgical cross-over graft that is required for this type of device.

The mortality rate post-procedure was about 10% per annum, fairly typical for patients with arterial disease. Most deaths at follow-up were unrelated to stent graft complications and were mostly due to cardiac disease or malignancy. Between 30 days and one year, six ruptures (1%) were reported. Of these, three had primary proximal perigraft endoleaks that had persisted despite attempts at endovascular treatment and one had a documented secondary endoleak. The annual rupture rate was about 1% per year in the first couple of years post-procedure, giving a cumulative risk of rupture of 2% at five years post-procedure. All but one rupture was fatal, and proximal endoleaks, if not corrected, were particularly associated with a poor outcome, emphasising the need to correct these endoleaks whenever possible. It should be noted that two deaths were attributed to systemic sepsis thought to be secondary to stent graft infection. With the move towards deployment of stent grafts in the radiology suite, this underlines the importance of theatre-quality asepsis.

There was an overall primary endoleak rate of over 14% (142 endoleaks). Of these, the most common were endoleaks from the proximal anastomosis or from collaterals. Of the 14 persistent proximal endoleaks at 30 days, 28% lead to AAA rupture during follow-up. This appears to justify an aggressive approach to treatment of proximal anastomotic endoleaks, when they occur. However, surgical treatment of this group of patients resulted in perioperative mortality in 35%, and the mortality rate of converting patients deemed unfit was 66.7%. This suggests that unfit patients must be counselled about the poor chances of survival, should endovascular repair fail and conversion become necessary. This mortality from conversion to open repair is higher than that reported in other series [6]. Patients did better if an endovascular treatment such as cuffing was feasible. However, if conversion is necessary, and it can be deferred for a few days, such an approach seems sensible to allow recovery from the primary procedure and related nephrotoxicity. Nevertheless, undue delay should be avoided. Other primary endoleaks had a more benign course with a reasonable chance of sealing spontaneously, though one patient with an apparently sealed collateral endoleak and an excluded aneurysm at follow-up, died of AAA rupture ten months post-procedure. Other ruptures with no obvious endoleak have also been reported, and this probably accounts for the conversion to OR of cases with increasing size of the AAA sac, but no identifiable endoleak. The Eurostar Registry has also found similar associations between collateral endoleaks and continued aneurysm expansion, and the risk of rupture with an increasing size of the AAA sac [7]. More frequent surveillance and/or intervention is therefore warranted in such cases.

Most of the uncertainty surrounding EVAR relates to the long-term complications of the procedure. It is therefore vital that the durability of the devices and the long-term outcomes of these cases are subjected to rigorous assessment. In this cohort, reported complications related to the aneurysm or device occurred at a rate of approximately 15% per annum. Many of these were secondary endoleaks, and often these could be successfully treated using endovascular techniques. However, follow-up of these secondary problems suggest that many recur or persist, and only about 30% of patients survive with no further problems. Therefore, although most complications can be treated successfully, continued long-term surveillance is required. The cost of this surveillance, and subsequent treatment, may outweigh the short-term benefits of EVAR, but only a long-term cost analysis as part of the EVAR trials would confirm this. Also, a large proportion of the stent grafts in the Registry were first generation devices that were fabricated in-house or second-generation devices that have been withdrawn, due to failure of structural integrity, or superseded by devices with improvements in design. It remains to be seen whether third-generation devices suffer from the same problems. The initial data suggests that they may be better in this respect [8].

As a first step, registries can be of value in the assessment of new treatments. Organisations such as the UK National Institute for Clinical Excellence (NICE) will often accept that, in the absence of formal trials, registries can act as a means of assessment of new treatments or technologies. In the case of EVAR, NICE specifically recommends that all patients undergoing EVAR should either be treated as part of a randomised trial or entered into one of the existing registries [9]. However, it is important to understand the limitations of Registry data as presented here. The only way to eliminate confounding and obtain clear results when comparing interventions, is to use randomisation. As data submission to many registries is voluntary there is a risk of bias in the data submitted and it is often not possible to ascertain the amount and characteristics of data not submitted. The results presented represent the best estimates within the limitations of the data collected. If these problems are borne in mind, then registry data can provide useful insight into the results of new treatments, and can be used in planning trials and to generate hypotheses to be tested. Indeed, results from RETA have been used in the planning of the EVAR trials and as an audit tool to assess centres for trial entry. The outcomes from the randomised trials will provide more definitive results of EVAR in fit and unfit patients. However, continued follow-up of the 1000 patients within the RETA cohort remains vital. The duration of follow-up is a long way ahead of the randomised trials. The collection and analysis of data from this and similar registries should facilitate the early identification, quantification and correction of device-related problems.

Acknowledgements

All participating centres for their data submission and provision of follow-up data.

Financial support has been provided by the BSIR and VSSGBI and by the following device companies:- BARD UK Ltd, WL Gore (UK) Ltd, Medtronic Ltd, Cook (UK) Ltd, Boston Scientific Ltd and Cordis (UK).

Summary

◆ Short-term outcomes (30 days): 90.4% of aneurysms were successfully excluded, 6.1% had persistent endoleaks and 5.8% had died.

◆ Conversion rates and mortality fell with time reflecting better patient selection, advances in stent graft design, and possibly, improved mentoring of new centres.

◆ A higher mortality rate in the AUIC group remained significant after adjusting for the higher proportion of unfit patients.

◆ Most deaths at follow-up were unrelated to the stent graft or aneurysm. Persistent proximal endoleak was associated with significant mortality both from attempted open repair or from rupture if untreated.

◆ Complications related to the aneurysm or device occurred at a rate of approximately 15% per annum. Many of these complications were secondary endoleaks, many of which could be successfully treated by endovascular technique.

◆ Long-term costs of stent graft surveillance, and secondary treatment, may outweigh the short-term benefits of EVAR.

References

1. Thomas SM, Gaines PA, Beard JD, on behalf of the Vascular Surgical Society of Great Britain & Ireland and the British Society of Interventional Radiology. Short-term outcome of endovascular treatment of abdominal aortic aneurysms: results from the prospective Registry of Endovascular Treatment of Abdominal Aortic Aneurysms (RETA). *Eur J Vasc Endovasc Surg* 2001; 21: 57-64

2. White GH, May J, Waugh RC, Chaufour X, Yu W. Type III and type IV endoleak: toward a complete definition of blood flow in the sac after endoluminal AAA repair. *J Endovasc Surg* 1998; 5: 305-309.

3. White GH, May J, Waugh RC, Yu W. Type I and Type II endoleaks: a more useful classification for reporting results of endoluminal AAA repair [letter]. *J Endovasc Surg* 1998; 5: 189-191.

4. The UK small aneurysm trial participants. Mortality results for randomised controlled trial of early elective surgery or ultrasonographic surveillance for small abdominal aortic aneurysms. *Lancet* 1998; 352: 1649-1655.

5. Armon MP, Hopkinson BR. How much does an aorto-uni-iliac stent-graft increase the endovascular options for abdominal aortic aneurysm repair? In: *Indications in vascular and endovascular surgery*. Greenhalgh RM, Ed. Saunders, London, 1998: 221-227.

6. May J, White GH, Yu W, Waugh R, Stephen M, Sieunarine K, *et al*. Conversion from endoluminal to open repair of abdominal aortic aneurysms: a hazardous procedure. *Eur J Vasc Endovasc Surg* 1997; 14(1): 4-11.

7. Van Marrewijk C, Buth J, Harris PL, Norgren L, Nevelsteen A, Wyatt MG. Significance of endoleaks after endovascular repair of abdominal aortic aneurysms. The EUROSTAR experience. *J Vasc Surg* 2002; 35: 461-473.

8. Bove PG, Long GW, Zelenock GB, *et al*. Transrenal fixation of aortic stent-grafts for the treatment of infrarenal aortic aneurysmal disease. *J Vasc Surg* 2000; 32: 697-703.

9. Interventional procedure overview of stent-graft placement in the abdominal aortic aneurysm. National Institute for Clinical Excellence, 2003. http://www.nice.org.uk/ip026overview.

Chapter 6

The case for laparoscopic assisted aortic surgery

Andreas M Lazaris, MD, Research Fellow, Vascular Surgery

Jeremy S Crane, MRCS, Research Fellow, Vascular Surgery

Nick J Cheshire, MD MRCS, Consultant Vascular Surgeon

Regional Vascular Unit, St Mary's Hospital, London, UK

Open repair

Abdominal aortic surgery has advanced dramatically over the past 50 years as a result of improvements in anaesthesia and surgical techniques. Conventional open surgery with a transperitoneal approach is the standard treatment for abdominal aortic aneurysms (AAAs). Similarly, aortobifemoral bypass grafting has proved to be a time-honoured operation for patients with symptomatic aortoiliac occlusive disease.

Overall, the morbidity and mortality rate for elective abdominal aortic aneurysm repair is now routinely between 3% and 5% [1]. Complications are usually due to the extent of the incision and the dissection required to repair the aneurysm. These factors contribute directly to respiratory impairment, which in turn leads to atelectasis and occasionally pneumonia, large fluid shifts, prolonged postoperative ileus, and significant postoperative pain. Complications such as haemorrhage, renal failure and infection, are related to the surgical invasiveness of the procedure [2].

In 1980, Williams *et al* reported an AAA repair technique that used the extraperitoneal approach [3], and which has since been shown to have the advantage of avoiding intestinal manipulation, and thus ileus. Recently, however, it has become evident that a postoperative bulge in the abdominal wall occurs in the long-term, probably because of the extensive muscle division and injury to the intercostal nerves [4].

Numerous physiologic alterations occur that are virtually coincident with surgical tissue injury and proportional to its extent. Concentrations of circulating neuroendocrine mediators rise significantly and remain elevated for a prolonged period of time after the procedure. Riles and associates documented rapid elevations in plasma epinephrine and norepinephrine levels during open aneurysm resection and suggested a link between these stress mediators and postoperative myocardial ischaemia [5]. This link between the neuroendocrine response to surgery strengthens the relationship between tissue injury and adverse outcome.

Endovascular repair

In the 1990s, endovascular repair was developed. Transluminally placed endovascular grafts have played an important role in AAA repair. This technique is now widely used with the continuing developments made to stent grafts, sheaths and delivery systems markedly improving the mortality and primary success rates of the procedure.

The treatment of vascular disease using a percutaneous approach is associated with less tissue trauma. There is a growing body of data regarding a reduction of the neuroendocrine response associated with this form of aneurysm repair. Thompson and associates documented greater rises in plasma catecholamine concentrations, more significant changes in cardiovascular parameters, and greater alterations in acid-base status in patients undergoing open aneurysm resection compared with those having aortic stent graft replacement [6]. Such studies suggest that these reductions in stress mediators may result in a decreased cardiac mortality and support the use of an aortic stent graft.

However, several drawbacks and limitations are associated with this method of aortic aneurysm repair. There is an anatomical limitation to the feasibility of this procedure. In patients with a short or angulated proximal aneurysmal neck, or with a small, diseased or tortuous access route, endovascular repair may be inappropriate. Furthermore, after more than a decade of development, application and evaluation of aortic stents, unpredicted shortcomings are still being observed. Access route injury, fabric holes, degradation of the metal exoskeleton or fixation sites, endoleaks, and slippage, represent some of the more vexing unforeseen problems with this technology. Many of the patients who have sustained such complications have been treated with open surgery, thereby eliminating the benefits of a percutaneous approach.

Recently, the late results of 2464 stent graft patients were reported by the EUROSTAR (European Collaborators on Stent/graft Techniques for Aortic Aneurysm Repair) collaborators [7]. Although the surgical mortality rate was low at approximately 3%, late complications associated with endoleaks were still crucial problems. Fourteen patients had a confirmed aneurysm rupture related to endoleaks or graft migration and nine of these patients died. Furthermore, 41 patients with endoleaks, graft migration or graft kinking underwent late conversion

to open repair with a perioperative mortality rate of 24.4% (10/41).

Endovascular repair is the only aneurysmal exclusion technique that does not require suturing. Consequently, there is concern regarding the durability of the anchoring sites between the arterial wall and the metal stents/barbs/hooks. Endovascular stent grafting might be less invasive, but its reliability remains in doubt and the stability of the very thin-walled stent grafts is unclear.

Laparoscopic repair

During the past decade, laparoscopic techniques have been applied to nearly every aspect of abdominal surgery. The use of minimally invasive techniques is associated with a reduced neuroendocrine response. Comparison between open and laparoscopic cholecystectomy have documented a blunting of the stress response with the minimally invasive procedure [8]. Since these operations are otherwise the same, the reduction in the level and duration of stress mediators has been attributed to the smaller incisions of the laparoscopic procedure. The postoperative alterations in respiratory mechanics have been observed to be less severe after laparoscopy than after laparotomy, which reflects in a lower incidence of postoperative pulmonary complications [9]. Therefore, minimally invasive procedures, like percutaneous interventions, minimise the postoperative stress response and these technologies may be complementary.

A less invasive procedure for abdominal aorta operations is desirable. Laparoscopically assisted aortic surgery could have the clinical advantages of better visualisation of the aneurysm neck, less bowel manipulation, avoidance of hypothermia, early removal of nasogastric suction and shorter period of intensive care and hospitalisation.

History of laparoscopic assisted aortic surgery

A gynaecologist, K. Semm, performed the first laparoscopic appendectomy in 1982, initiating a revolutionary development in general surgery [10]. Just a few years after their development in the early 1990s, laparoscopic cholecystectomy, fundoplication, and hernia repair are now routinely performed using laparoscopic techniques.

Similar progress did not occur in vascular surgery. In 1993, Dion *et al* were the first to describe a laparoscopy-assisted aortobifemoral bypass [11]. They dissected the infrarenal aorta under video control, and performed the anastomosis conventionally through an 8cm midline incision. A similar approach was used by Berens and Herde [12], who performed four procedures on aorto-iliac vessels in a gasless laparoscopic technique. Nevertheless, a 4cm working incision was still required. Indeed, the first totally laparoscopic aortobifemoral bypass was reported by Dion *et al* [13], who performed the procedure using a retroperitoneal approach.

The first report with regard to laparoscopically assisted AAA repair was by Chen *et al* in 1995 [14]. They described a case of a 6cm infrarenal AAA which they dissected under video control. A standard aneurysmorraphy using a PTFE tube graft was subsequently performed through a 10cm mini-laparotomy. In 1999, Jobe and associates described a totally laparoscopic abdominal aneurysm repair [15]. The aneurysm was first excluded using an endoscopic stapling device, and an aortobi-iliac reconstruction was performed. However, the first totally laparoscopic aneurysm repair without exclusion of the aneurysm was described by Dion in 2001 [16]. Previously in 2000, Arous *et al* [17] had described the use of the hand-assisted laparoscopic techniques for aortobifemoral grafts. This involved insertion of the surgeon's hand into the abdominal cavity together with the laparoscopic instruments. This method was also performed by Kolvenbach *et al* [18, 19] in the treatment of abdominal aortic aneurysm disease.

Techniques of laparoscopic assisted aortic surgery

The main philosophy in laparoscopic assisted aortic surgery is the same as with all laparoscopic procedures. This involves intervention with tiny instruments introduced into the abdominal cavity through the abdominal wall and guided by a magnifying camera, following the same steps as in an open procedure. However, due to the complexity of the procedures, the position of the aorta within the deep retroperitoneal space, and the increased risks associated with accurate dissection, various different techniques have been described.

Retroperitoneal laparoscopic aorta dissection followed by open retroperitoneal aneurysm resection [20, 21] or aortobifemoral grafting

This technique involves the creation of a retroperitoneal space using a distension balloon system. This is inserted to bluntly dissect the retroperitoneal space. Subsequently, the balloon is exchanged for a laparoscope which is placed into the retroperitoneal space through a trocar. Carbon dioxide is then insufflated to allow visualisation of the retroperitoneal structures. After identification of the left iliopsoas muscle and the left ureter, the left common iliac artery, the abdominal aorta and the left renal vein can be identified. The inferior mesenteric artery is identified and divided to make the subsequent dissection easier. The lumbar arteries can also be divided outside the aorta and proximal control can be obtained endoscopically with a tape passed around the infrarenal aorta. A peritoneal apron-like shield can be created by fixation of the left side of the peritoneum to the right abdominal wall [21]. This procedure prevents the intestines from entering the surgical field. After the aortic dissection is completed, a small supra-umbilical mini-laparotomy is done which allows access to the retroperitoneum and through which an open resection of the aneurysm, or the proximal anastomosis of an aortobifemoral graft is performed.

Intraperitoneal laparoscopic aorta dissection followed by open aneurysm resection [22] or aortobifemoral grafting

The peritoneal cavity is entered through a small (around 1cm) supra-umbilical incision. A modified Glassman viscera retainer 'fish' (Adept-Med) is then inserted directly into the peritoneal cavity. A pneumoperitoneum is obtained, and under direct visualisation, several further trocars are inserted. These ports are used for either dissection, small bowel retraction, or suction. The 'fish' is used to expose the aorta and to keep the small bowel away from it. The retroperitoneum is opened at the level of the duodenum and aortic dissection is carried out on the anterior, medial, and lateral surfaces of the aorta down to the vertebral bodies. On completion of the aorta dissection, the 'fish' is moved inferiorly, and the common iliac arteries are dissected in a similar fashion. At the end of the laparoscopic dissection, the trocars are removed and a short periumbilical incision is made. The iliac vessels and aorta are controlled and a standard repair is performed through this incision, using standard open instruments.

Totally laparoscopic abdominal aneurysm repair [16] or aortobifemoral bypass grafting [11, 23]

According to this technique, dissection, proximal anastomosis, and peritoneum closure are performed using laparoscopic techniques. The procedure can be done transperitoneally [23] or retroperitoneally [13].

In the transperitoneal approach, after induction of the pneumoperitoneum, the greater omentum and the small bowel are shifted in the upper abdomen. Only a small incision, around 5cm long, is required to open the retroperitoneum, after which the aorta is dissected. Particular attention is required in identifying and closing lumbar branches to avoid disturbing bleeding. After proximal and distal clearance, an arteriotomy is performed. A vascular graft is introduced into the abdomen via one of the trocars and an end-to-side (aortobifemoral) or an end-to-end (aneurysm) anastomosis is performed using a continuous running suture.

Hand-assisted laparoscopic abdominal aorta dissection [17-19, 24]

The main purpose of this technique is to perform a hand-assisted laparoscopic abdominal aorta dissection and then complete the proximal

anastomosis in a conventional way through a small abdominal incision (5-7cm only) (Figure 1). The hand is introduced through an airtight seal into the laparoscopic field with the maintenance of the pneumoperitoneum. The Hand-Port System [17, 19] (Smith and Nephew, Andover, Massachusetts, USA) has been used for this purpose. The vascular surgeon's non-dominant hand is used to provide exposure of the aorta and retraction of the small bowel during the laparoscopic portion of the procedure. (Figure 2). Repositioning the hand facilitates critical dissection around the duodenum, left renal vein, lateral aortic attachments and the common iliac arteries in the case of an aneurysm [19].

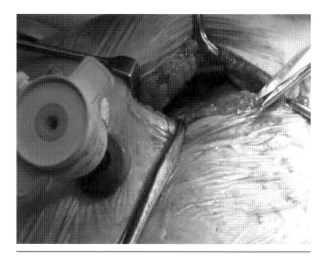

Figure 1. 5-7cm paramedian incision.

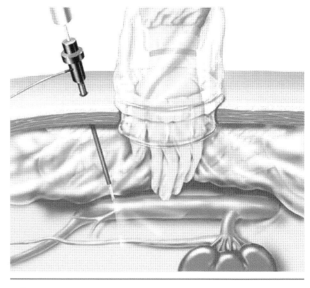

Figure 2. Dissection using the Hand-Port.

This technique maintains the principles of minimally invasive surgery, whilst providing a number of significant advantages. Insertion of the surgeon's hand into the peritoneal cavity during laparoscopy allows for tactile feedback while the unique intrinsic hand has the ability to function as a blunt dissector, grasper, or retractor. After dissection is completed, the protector device is removed and a conventional retractor (i.e. Omnitract, St Paul, Minneapolis, USA), is inserted. An open aorta aneurysm repair or the proximal anastomosis of an aortobifemoral graft can then be performed in a conventional way. In patients with iliac artery aneurysms, the distal anastomosis is performed to the common iliac artery. If, for technical reasons, this cannot be accomplished, two oblique incisions are made above the inguinal ligament, the common iliac artery occluded using a stapler, and an anastomosis performed to the external iliac artery. When this is not feasible, a laparoscopic approach with conventional instruments and a gasless technique can be used [18, 19].

Benefits and limitations of laparoscopic surgery

Laparoscopic assisted surgery is a relatively new methodology for the surgical treatment of aortic disease, which at the moment remains at an experimental stage. The overall world experience with this technique is still small and both benefits and limitations have been described.

Benefits

The clinical benefits of laparoscopic aortic surgery include reduced pain, early gastrointestinal motility, lower infection rates, potentially reduced cardiopulmonary complications, and reduced surgical trauma [25]. Barbera and associates [23] have reported a comfortable postoperative course in most patients. Mobilisation and oral feeding were started soon after the operation and were well tolerated. A quicker postoperative recovery and shorter hospitalisation [20, 23] are also associated with laparoscopic surgery.

The long-term outcome after laparoscopy assisted AAA repair can be expected to be the same as that of the standard open repair, as the concept of the operation is not changed. However, laparoscopy assisted graft replacement via a mini-incision might be more durable than endoluminal stenting techniques with their associated risk of endoleak [20].

The laparoscopic approach allows for magnification, better visualisation and results in good haemostasis and safer dissection [20]. In addition, minimal blood losses are experienced compared to open procedures [19, 23].

With hand-assisted laparoscopic surgery (HALS), aortic reconstructive procedures can be performed using a mini-laparotomy only. The mini-incision permits the surgeon to use a wider array of instruments [26]. The surgeon can use conventional clamps and more efficient suction devices or needle holders without fear of compromising the operative cavity [19]. As a hybrid procedure, HALS expands the armamentarium of the vascular surgeon who is perhaps less experienced in advanced laparoscopic techniques [19]. The hand represents the best-known intestinal retractor until now, and the ability to use the hand for retraction in laparoscopic AAA surgery can be performed with much greater confidence than in total laparoscopic aortic operations [23]. In addition, the learning curve for vascular surgeons who want to set up a laparoscopic aortic program is considerably less steep with HALS compared with a total laparoscopic approach [19].

HALS could provide access in complex cases to implement conventional operative instruments or techniques in situations where limited laparoscopic instrumentation is available. The approach is feasible and offers many potential advantages over either a purely laparoscopic approach or the conventional open approach. The operative hand facilitates the laparoscopic dissection of the aorta offering more control and the potential for increased safety and speed. In addition, access through the base retractor at the level of the infrarenal aorta allows performance of the anastomosis in an open fashion, avoiding potentially difficult, tedious, and time-consuming intracorporeal suturing.

Perhaps, the most important benefit is the performance of the operation without the need to eviscerate the small intestine in order to facilitate adequate exposure. This results in a reduced incidence of postoperative ileus and allows for earlier resumption of diet. The reduced postoperative stay and shorter time to complete recovery after hand-assisted laparoscopic aortic surgery appear to offer a significant advantage over conventional surgery (Figure 3).

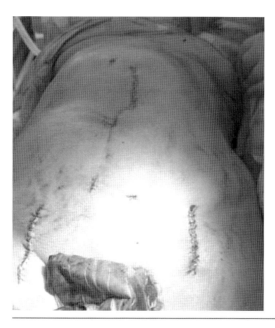

Figure 3. Closure after aortobifemoral grafting.

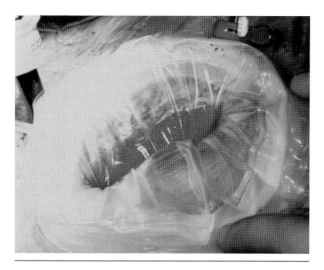

Figure 4. Hand port entry site.

Limitations

Advanced laparoscopic surgery can be difficult. Additionally, the sense of tactile feedback and the intrinsic ability of the operator's hand to function as a blunt dissector, grasper, or retractor is lost with conventional laparoscopy [17]. A potentially valuable adjunct is that of hand-assisted laparoscopic surgery, in which the hand is introduced into the laparoscopic field whilst a pneumoperitoneum is maintained [26] (Figure 4).

Advanced laparoscopic surgery can be time-consuming. Almost all laparoscopic vascular procedures require longer surgery times than open surgery, but a trend toward faster procedures has been recorded [23]. However, just as for laparoscopic cholecystectomy or hernia repair, we expect further shortening of operating times as experience grows.

The need for *ex-vivo* model training is of major importance in laparoscopic surgery. Training in laparoscopic suture techniques using a pelvitrainer and porcine models are essential for the surgeon to achieve good technical skills.

Laparoscopic assisted aortic surgery requires a team commitment involving both an experienced vascular surgeon and a surgeon with advanced laparoscopic expertise. Like any other new intervention, it requires a certain learning curve to perform these procedures safely and efficiently. In addition, technical challenges such as the obese patient, extensive infrarenal atherosclerotic aortic disease, previous abdominal surgery, and the ability to alter hand and trocar configurations, need to be addressed as experience with this technique expands.

A specific problem might be the effect of the pneumoperitoneum on the circulation, especially that of the bowel, and on the cardiopulmonary function. Cases with cardiac or pulmonary diseases are not suitable because insufflation to the abdominal cavity with carbon dioxide can lead to deterioration of the cardiopulmonary system. Laparoscopic techniques cannot be considered feasible for patients that have a contraindication to laparoscopy, such as severe obesity or previous surgery via a midline incision [22].

The method's efficiency and safety regarding suprarenal aortic dissection and extensive iliac exposure is not proven. Therefore, laparoscopic assisted aortic surgery may not be possible in patients with aneurysms involving the perirenal aorta or the iliac vessels [22].

Technical difficulties involved in laparoscopic aortic dissection include mainly the retention of the small bowel away from the operative field, and the control of lumbar arteries. Various retraction devices, such as fan retractors and polypropylene mesh grafts have been used [23], but not always with good results. Tilting the table in a steep Trendelenburg's position, shifting the small bowel into the upper abdomen, and avoiding the anaesthetic nitrous oxide, which evokes significant dilatation of bowel loops [23], are methods proposed to impove the situation. In addition, as specific laparoscopic techniques (especially the retroperitoneal laparoscopic dissection), require specific positioning of the patient on the operation table, an emergency conversion of the laparoscopic approach into an open procedure might be a problem especially if a change of patient position is required

Conclusions

Laparoscopic procedures performed on the aorta and the iliac arteries should be considered experimental. They should be carried out under an experimental protocol. Before attempting these procedures, the surgeon would be well advised to attend formal didactic courses and hands-on animal workshops that are readily available. In addition, the vascular surgeon could request the assistance of a general surgeon with a solid experience in laparoscopy for his first clinical procedures [16]. Careful patient selection is mandatory when developing this technique. Growing experience and technological progress may in the future broaden the spectrum of laparoscopic procedures on vessels in order to reduce tissue trauma and at the same time still apply the already established, well worked principles of vascular surgery.

It is still necessary to evaluate the safety of laparoscopic assisted aortic surgery. The world experience with minimally invasive vascular surgery remains small. Therefore, further randomised trials are needed to define the role of the laparoscopic approach in vascular surgery. Similarly, follow-up examinations of the study groups are needed to describe the durability of the presented procedures. With its acceptance, minimally invasive vascular surgery should show the same benefits that accompany minimally invasive surgery in other patient groups.

Laparoscopic vascular surgery must not be introduced into the clinical arena based only on the assumption that it is feasible. Clearly, it is a technically challenging procedure with a steep learning curve that requires specialised instrumentation and sophisticated laparoscopic suturing capability. However, with continued investigation, including prospective randomised trials, laparoscopic treatment of aortic aneurysms and aorto-iliac disease may become a standard option of treatment.

Summary

◆ Laparoscopic assisted aortic surgery offers the clinical benefits of minimal invasive procedures, without changing the philosophy of conventional repair. Thus, a similar long-term outcome to standard open repair is expected.

◆ Laparoscopic assisted aortic surgery has a steep learning curve. There is need for extensive model training with hands-on animal workshops and didactic courses. Assistance of a general surgeon with solid experience in laparoscopy is necessary, initially.

◆ Hand-assisted laparoscopic aortic surgery is an innovative technique utilising a moderately difficult laparoscopic procedure to perform a conventional, well-established operation.

◆ Randomised studies comparing laparoscopic assisted aortic surgery with standard open procedures and endovascular open repair are necessary to evaluate the safety and durability of this method.

References

1. DeBakey M, McCollum C. Surgical treatment of non-ruptured infrarenal and juxtarenal abdominal aortic aneurysms. In: *Current therapy in vascular surgery.* Ernst C, Stanley J, Eds. B.C Decker Inc., Philadelphia, 1991: 261-264.

2. Blankensteijn JD. Mortality and morbidity rates after conventional abdominal aortic aneurysm repair. *Semin Interv Cardiol* 2000; 5: 7-13.

3. Williams GM, Ricotta J, Zinner M, Burdick J. The extended retroperitoneal approach for treatment of extensive atherosclerosis of the aorta and renal vessels. *Surgery* 1980; 88: 846-855.

4. Gardner GP, Josephs LG, Rosca M, *et al.* The retroperitoneal incision. An evaluation of postoperative flank 'bulge'. *Arch Surg* 1994; 129: 753-756.

5. Riles TS, Fisher FS, Schaefer S, *et al.* Plasma catecholamine concentrations during abdominal aortic aneurysm surgery: the link to perioperative myocardial ischemia. *Ann Vasc Surg* 1993; 7: 213-219.

6. Thompson JP, Boyle JR, Thompson MM, *et al.* Cardiovascular and catecholamine responses during endovascular and conventional abdominal aortic aneurysm repair. *Eur J Vasc Endovasc Surg* 1999; 17: 326-333.

7. Harris PL, Vallabhaneni SR, Desgranges P, *et al.* Incidence and risk factors of late rupture, conversion, and death after endovascular repair of infrarenal aortic aneurysms: the EUROSTAR experience. European Collaborators on Stent/graft techniques for aortic aneurysm repair. *J Vasc Surg* 2000; 32: 739-749.

8. Glaser F, Sannwald GA, Buhr HJ, *et al.* General stress response to conventional and laparoscopic cholecystectomy. *Ann Surg* 1995; 221: 372-380.

9. Kimberley NA, Kirkpatrick SM, Watters JM. Alterations in respiratory mechanics after laparoscopic and open surgical procedures. *Can J Surg* 1996; 39: 312-316.

10. Semm K. Endoscopic appendectomy. *Endoscopy* 1983; 15: 59-64.

11. Dion YM, Katkhouda N, Rouleau C, Aucoin A. Laparoscopy-assisted aortobifemoral bypass. *Surg Laparosc Endosc* 1993; 3: 425-429.

12. Berens ES, Herde JR. Laparoscopic vascular surgery: Four case reports. *J Vasc Surg* 1995; 22: 73-79.

13. Dion YM, Gracia CR, Demalsy YC. Laparoscopic aortic surgery [letter]. *J Vasc Surg* 1996; 23: 539.

14. Chen MH, Murphy EA, Halpern V, *et al.* Laparoscopic-assisted abdominal aortic aneurysm repair. *Surg Endosc* 1995; 9: 905-907.

15. Jobe BA, Duncan W, Swanstrom LL. Totally laparoscopic abdominal aortic aneurysm repair. *Surg Endosc* 1999; 13: 77-79.

16. Dion YM, Gracia CR, Ben El Kadi HH. Totally laparoscopic abdominal aortic aneurysm repair. *J Vasc Surg* 2001; 33: 181-185.

17. Arous EJ, Nelson PR, Yood SM, *et al.* Hand-assisted laparoscopic aortobifemoral bypass grafting. *J Vasc Surg* 2000; 31: 1142-1148.

18. Kolvenbach R. Hand-assisted laparoscopic abdominal aortic aneurysm repair. *Semin Laparosc Surg* 2001; 8: 168-177.

19. Kolvenbach R, Cheshire N, Pinter L, *et al.* Laparoscopy-assisted aneurysm resection as a minimal invasive alternative in patients unsuitable for endovascular surgery. *J Vasc Surg* 2001; 34: 216-221.

20. Matsumoto Y, Nishimori H, Yamada H, *et al.* Laparoscopy-assisted abdominal aortic aneurysm repair: first case reports from Japan. *Circ J* 2003; 67: 99-101.

21. Dion YM, Gracia CR. A new technique for laparoscopic aortobifemoral grafting in occlusive aortoiliac disease. *J Vasc Surg* 1997; 26: 685-692.

22. Kline RG, D'Angelo AJ, Chen MH, *et al.* Laparoscopically assisted abdominal aortic aneurysm repair: first 20 cases. *J Vasc Surg* 1998; 27: 81-87; discussion 88.

23. Barbera L, Mumme A, Metin S, *et al.* Operative results and outcome of twenty-four totally laparoscopic vascular procedures for aortoiliac occlusive disease. *J Vasc Surg* 1998; 28: 136-142.

24. Kelly JJ, Kercher KW, Gallagher RN, *et al.* Hand-assisted laparoscopic aortobifemoral bypass versus open bypass for occlusive disease. *J Laparoendosc Adv Surg Tech A* 2002; 12: 339-343.

25. Kolvenbach R, Deling O, Schwierz E, Landers B. Reducing the operative trauma in aortoiliac reconstructions-a prospective study to evaluate the role of video-assisted vascular surgery. *Eur J Vasc Endovasc Surg* 1998; 15: 483-488.

26. Litwin DE, Darzi A, Jakimowicz J, *et al.* Hand-assisted laparoscopic surgery (HALS) with the HandPort system: initial experience with 68 patients. *Ann Surg* 2000; 231: 715-723.

Chapter 7

Training and evaluation in aorto-iliac endovascular procedures

Anthony Nicholson, MSc FRCR, Consultant Vascular Radiologist
St James's University Hospital and Leeds General Infirmary, Leeds Hospital NHS Trust, Leeds, UK

Julian Scott, MD FRCS, Reader in Vascular Surgery, Consultant Vascular Surgeon
St James's University Hospital, Leeds, UK

Introduction

The proposed changes to medical training will result in a significant reduction in hours worked. It is estimated that before Calman the average time spent between SHO and Consultant post was 30,000 hours, which is likely to fall to 6,000, based upon the reforms recommended by the Chief Medical Officer [1]. The acquisition of new skills, from house jobs to the end of Basic Surgical Training is almost non-existent, with one third of orthopaedic trainees not receiving any formal teaching in theatre or outpatients [2]. At the present time it is recognised that specialist registrars require more time to perform operative procedures. The recent attentions of Dr Foster have focused the minds of the surgical community on outcomes for major index procedures. There are currently no incentives for newly appointed, let alone established consultants, to allow junior trainees to undertake major surgery. Adverse outcome, no matter the cause, will be attributed to the consultant and Trust. Finally, all Trusts, lead clinicians and individual consultants are forced to address the issues surrounding waiting lists. Training does limit the number of cases that can be potentially treated and the costs of providing additional theatre time (270 extra days per year) amount to £1.3 million [3].

Forty years ago Charles Dotter performed the first angioplasty. Although this was performed in the superficial femoral artery it was not long before the same procedure was performed for an iliac stenosis. The treatment of superficial femoral artery occlusive disease remains controversial. By contrast, the results in the aorto-iliac arteries have been such that endovascular procedures when possible, are now the treatment of choice. Aorto-iliac interventions have moved on from angioplasty of aorto-iliac stenoses to stenting of aorto-iliac occlusions and aneurysms. Each stage in the development of these treatment modalities has required different thought processes and a changing requirement for pre- and post-procedural clinical imaging.

Endovascular practitioners have also been presented with a changing pattern of early, intermediate and long-term problems. These are often treated by endovascular means but occasionally, open surgery is required. The increasing complexity of aorto-iliac intervention requires practitioners to be competent and experienced. This has been accepted by both the Vascular Surgical Society of Great Britain and Ireland (VSSGBI) and the Royal College of Radiology. They have stated that any practitioner who wishes to practice endovascular radiology as an endovascular specialist should undergo training that involves 'the equivalent of a one-year full-time fellowship in a recognised vascular radiology training unit. Trainees should be required to perform the core number of procedures specified for sub-speciality training in vascular interventional radiology' [4]. In addition, practitioners 'will have to satisfy the training recommendations outlined in the regulations of ionising radiation' [5]. In the new SAC curriculum in general surgery, it has been agreed that vascular surgeons in training will be allowed time off to fulfill the above criteria. Further proposed changes to training in vascular surgery will enable specialist registrars to gain a greater understanding in all aspects of interventional radiology and vascular ultrasound.

There are those that think that the physical act of inserting a stent or stent graft into the aorto-iliac system should be all that needs to be taught and evaluated. If this were true then endovascular procedures would be akin to a ploy by an American football team. The technician who arrives to insert the stent graft might be likened to a field goal kicker. An analogy closer to home would suggest that a practitioner trained to laparoscopically remove gallbladders should not have the skills to convert a laparoscopic procedure to an open procedure if things went wrong, and would be able to perform fundoplications and myomectomies simply because he had basic laparoscopic skills.

Clearly, this approach is unlikely to succeed and the future training of endovascular specialists, be they from vascular surgery or interventional radiology, must be based upon a curriculum, which provides a template for the specific learning process involved in aorto-iliac endovascular procedures. It defines the necessary knowledge, skills and attitudes, the standards to be achieved and can be assessed by an external body. The curriculum is currently being developed by a process of:-

◆ needs assessment;
◆ setting a clear aim and goals;
◆ brainstorming ideas;
◆ classifying ideas into themes;
◆ identifying incremental learning blocks;
◆ identification of constraints;
◆ production of formal lists;
◆ identifying the methods of assessment;
◆ timetables;
◆ publication;

◆ implementation; and
◆ evaluation.

Domains of learning

Four domains of learning have been identified: knowledge, skills, attitudes and social behaviour. Each has components which progress from simple to complex cognitive activity or hierarchies.

The hierarchy of knowledge is composed of the following: 'memory', 'understanding', 'application', 'synthesis' and 'evaluation'. It is relatively easy to define basic knowledge and can be tested by multiple choice questions. By contrast, evaluation requires logical thought combined with experience and judgement, all of which are difficult to define.

The hierarchy of skills consists of 'awareness', 'knows what', 'shows how', 'does' and 'mastery'. For the purpose of this chapter, the trainee is 'aware' that an iliac angioplasty is a possible intervention. They are aware of what is involved such as the use of the Seldinger technique and can show how the procedure is undertaken. 'Does' reflects an ability to undertake the majority of cases and 'mastery' relates to the complex intervention and or complication such as maldeployement of a stent with distal embolisation.

The hierarchy of attitude consists of 'receives', 'responds', 'values', 'arranges' and 'acts'. It is difficult to measure but represents an important element in training.

The social domain reflects the ability of the individual to work within a team, to communicate effectively and also the ability to undertake specific tasks, all of which are important for future professional development.

Teaching a skill

The old adage of see one, do one, teach one, is defunct, particularly in the eyes of the law. Training should follow the principles laid down in Training the Trainers. In particular, skill teaching should be based upon the four-step approach:-

1. Trainer does run through at normal speed without a commentary.

2. Trainer talks through and trainer does.
3. Trainee talks through and trainer does.
4. Trainee talks through and trainee does.

Clearly, this approach will take some time to achieve in the case of an aorto-iliac intervention, but the task can be split up into many different component parts, eg. access to the artery. Over time the trainee will acquire the skill through drill, repetition and practice. In this approach, the trainee/trainer should have access to a dedicated list of comparable cases, so that the individual skills can be acquired rapidly. In the case of a more experienced trainee, a modified approach can be used with effect:-

◆ Trainer demonstrates in real time with no particular explanations.
◆ Discussion between trainee and trainer, highlighting any significant areas of difference from previous training (i.e. wires, catheters and balloons).
◆ Decision is made to revert to steps 2-4 or to proceed straight to stage 4 and allow the trainee to carry out the procedure, discussing the important steps with the trainer.

At all stages the trainee should be asked to reflect upon the performance either verbally or through diaries. Critiquing is a useful tool and provides positive feedback:-

◆ Ask the trainee what went well.
◆ Ask the other trainee/radiographer/nurse what went well.
◆ Ask the trainee what could be improved.
◆ Ask the other trainee/radiographer/nurse what could be improved.

This approach has a lot to commend it and should become a useful tool in the training of endovascular practitioners within a limited time frame.

The learning cycle

There are four stages in the process of achieving mastery of aorto-iliac intervention (Figure 1). In the first stage, the trainee is aware of the principles of the technique, but not of all the exact details and may have a false belief that they could undertake the procedure. The trainee is described as unconsciously incompetent.

Given an opportunity to undertake the procedure, the trainee will concentrate specifically on access to the blood stream via needle, wire and sheath. This method allows introduction of catheters, further guidewires, angioplasty balloons, stents and other devices and instruments. This is normally done using an imaging technique, usually real time fluoroscopy which provides a two-dimensional image of the operating region and the instrument. At this point, they should recognise the complexity of the task and move towards a stage of conscious incompetence. At this stage, the trainee should be highly motivated to learn the new skill, which will require repeated exposure under varying levels of supervision. It sounds simple, but there are problems. These relate to the catheter as a long, flexible tool, difficult to manoeuvre in the desired direction. Friction with the vessel wall hinders movement of the catheter and there is poor force feedback from the catheter tip resulting in unknown forces at that site. The lack of direct vision causes a loss of depth perception. The trainee will move into the stage of conscious competence. With further exposure to increasingly more difficult cases, the trainee will achieve mastery and become unconsciously competent.

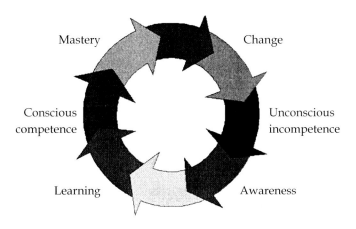

Figure 1. The learning cycle.

The development of competence

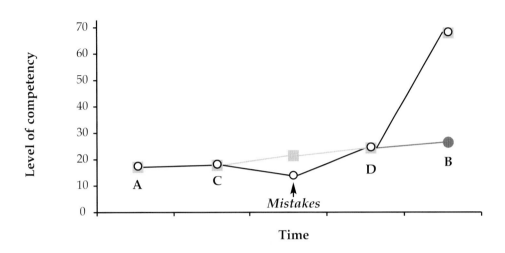

Figure 2. Competency versus time.

In the case of aorto-iliac interventions, the learning process can be represented in Figure 2. Prior to aortic stent grafting, established consultants (trainers) were acquiring competence in routine aorto-iliac angioplasty/stenting (line A-B). At point C, endovascular aneurysm surgery became a treatment option. Each consultant was forced into learning the new skill or rejecting it, and to continue on the line to B. At this point, those that decided to learn the endovascular aneurysm procedure, moved back into a stage of consciously incompetent and became a trainee again. Mistakes occurred during this time frame and were related to the degree of change in the technique. The provision of training courses and one-to-one supervision by experts and industry, led to the development of new competencies and so the consultant moved back into the consciously competent stage (D). The level of support was slowly withdrawn and by gaining more experience most consultants moved back into a stage of unconscious competence, thereby completing the learning cycle. The rapidity at which existing consultants acquired the new skills reinforces the old adage that one retains 5% of what is heard, 10% of what is seen, and 90% of knowledge that is put into action.

In the past, interventional radiologists obtained their first basic training skills during diagnostic angiographic procedures. However, this traditional method of training is rapidly disappearing. The advent of vascular ultrasound, Magnetic Resonance and Computed Tomographic angiography means that now and in the future we need to develop new training methods. The primary goal of training is to improve procedural efficiency and to reduce errors. From the man machine literature it is known that errors can be classified according to the cognitive level of behaviour. Future training methods should take into account these levels of behaviour to yield maximum effectiveness.

Rasmussen's model

Rasmussen's model of human behaviour distinguishes three different levels of behaviour: skill, rule and knowledge-based [6].

Skill-based

Skill-based behaviour represents sensory motor performance during acts or activities that are carried out without conscious control. These actions are performed as smooth, automated and highly integrated patterns. An example might be guiding the tip of a catheter through a blood vessel. To determine the desired movement of the tip and its location, the vessel anatomy and the target vessel must be known. An experienced interventionalist can move the catheter without conscious control via the actions of his hands. To move the catheter into a side branch, the curved catheter tip can be rotated by turning the catheter at the proximal end outside the patient. The forces needed to move and turn the catheter are very much dependent on anatomy and the varying friction with the vessel wall. Because visual feedback is obtained via a 2D x-ray image, manipulation of the tip can be hampered and therefore, focused training is required to achieve these skills at this behavioural level, i.e. moving from conscious competence to unconscious competence by training and repeated experience.

Rule-based

Rule-based behaviour is the next level for processing information. Here, task execution in familiar work situations is controlled by stored rules. These rules may have been derived empirically on previous occasions, perhaps communicated from someone else's know-how as an instruction, or from a cookbook recipe. Rules may on occasion be prepared by conscious problem-solving and planning. A good example would be the choice to change one catheter for another with a different shape or to use a special type of guidewire. Such decisions may be based on previous experience. The differences between skill-based and rule-based behaviour are not strict. Training may result in a transition from task execution on a rule-based behaviour level to a more efficient skill-based behaviour level.

Knowledge-based

Knowledge-based behaviour occurs when faced with unfamiliar situations in which no rules or skills are available from previous encounters. At this point, the control of performance must move to a higher conceptual level that is goal-controlled and knowledge-based. Interpretation of 2D images, variations in anatomy and pathology, and complications during intervention, may require creativity and decision-making at the knowledge-based behaviour level.

All three levels of behaviour occur in interventional vascular radiology. Psychomotor skills are needed at the skill-based behaviour level, operation protocol determines the rule-based behaviour, and dealing with complications and variations requires knowledge-based behaviour. At all stages information is being gathered and Rasmussen categorises this information as signals, signs and symbols. Signals are defined as the sensory information obtained during skill-based behaviour such that the visual information from the catheter tip on a monitor is used as a continuous signal to control the catheter through the blood vessel. As most procedures consist of a series of steps or actions at the rule-based behaviour level, signs are constantly being sought. These can be used to select or modify rules and to generate new rules in unfamiliar situations. Symbols occur at the knowledge-based behaviour level and allow us to form concepts providing the basis for reasoning and planning.

With this information to hand, an efficient training programme should reduce the number of errors at skill, rule and knowledge-based levels. Generically, errors occur when a planned sequence of mental or physical activities fails to achieve their intended outcome when such failures cannot be attributed to the intervention of some chance factor. They can be due to slips resulting from some failure in execution or lapses resulting from some forgotten stage of an action sequence. Slips are observable, but lapses are not. Both are execution failures at the skill-based behaviour level. Mistakes are deficiencies or failures in judgement or the inferential process involved in the selection of an object during the specification of the means to achieve it, irrespective of whether or not the actions directed by this decision scheme go according to plan. Mistakes are planning failures that arise at the rule-based or knowledge-based behaviour level. Put more simply, if the intention is not appropriate, this is a mistake. If the action is not what was intended, this is a slip.

Clinical example of slips and lapses

A good example of an error at the skill-based level might be an error in catheter manipulation. Due to friction, forces at the catheter tip are not always fed back to the operator. This may result in the operator producing high forces at the tip on the vessel wall. In addition, due to the flexibility of the tip, movements of the hand do not always agree with movements of the tip. This may result in unintended movements. Also, visual information from the treated area, being two-dimensional, may lead to misinterpretation with further unintended movements of the tip.

Clinical example of a mistake

At the rule-based level, errors may occur during PTA of an iliac artery. To cross an iliac lesion, continuous fluoroscopy should be applied and all deviations of the guidewire should be noticed. After crossing the lesion the catheter position should be checked and heparin given. An appropriate stent should be selected followed by an appropriate balloon. Following this, angiography should be performed and the stent inserted and dilated. Omitting any one of these steps is a mistake at the rule-based behaviour level and may result in an adverse event. During the procedure an unexpected event may occur. As stated, this may be due to variations in anatomy or pathology. A great deal of knowledge and experience is required to avoid mistakes at this time and errors might occur at the knowledge-based behaviour level.

Sources of error

Errors can be divided into latent and active (Figure 3). Latent errors are removed from the direct control of the trainee/trainer and relate to many factors including organisational issues, communication processes and deficiencies within the training scheme. In active errors, the trainee/trainer are at fault. When all the loopholes in the system (organisation/line management/individual/team) line up, this results in a failure of clinical decision-making.

Errors and the impact upon training

This is probably the most difficult part of any training programme to get right. It is therefore essential that the trainee be exposed to varying levels of complexity. In this way the slips and lapses associated with skill behaviour would have been overcome during the early part of training. In the latter stages, the trainees should be exposed to more complex problems, in an appropriate institutional environment, which allows them the opportunity to formulate an adequate and achievable plan of action. Effective training therefore, involves the acquisition of appropriate levels of skill, rule and knowledge-based behaviour. In addition, the trainer must be aware of the level that the trainee is able to progress towards, i.e. identifying their needs should be a constant monitoring process.

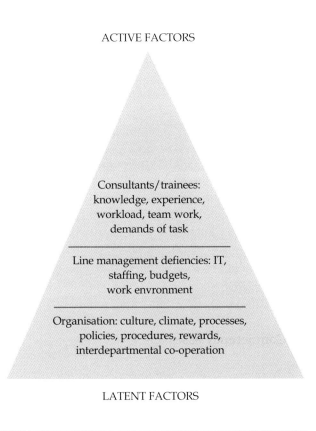

ACTIVE FACTORS

Consultants/trainees: knowledge, experience, workload, team work, demands of task

Line management defiencies: IT, staffing, budgets, work envronment

Organisation: culture, climate, processes, policies, procedures, rewards, interdepartmental co-operation

LATENT FACTORS

Figure 3. Latent and active errors.

Training schemes

From the discussion above, it is obvious that any training scheme has to be effective, i.e. it should meet its objective, and be efficient, i.e. cost and time should be minimised. Rasmussen's framework of human behaviour has been applied previously to laparoscopic training [7]. This can also be applied to vascular interventional radiology training in order to increase safety and decrease errors. Training objectives should define the level of competence a trainee is expected to have at every stage of training. The training needs should be determined by the difference between the initial level of competence and the required level on completion. The means whereby this is achieved are provided by the tools and methods used to fulfil the training programme.

Issues in training

Part versus task

A large number of vascular interventions are long and complex. This raises the issue of part versus whole task training. Although this has been covered in training a skill, part task training is best used when individual elements are difficult, eg. how to access an acute aortic bifurcation, whilst the organisation of the iliac angioplasty is straightforward. Whole task is best undertaken when the interrelationship between the task elements is complex. Having completed a task of procedure it is important to critique the performance. In the case of simulators one may have access to additional feedback including times, force and range of movements.

Competency assessment

Overall competence can be assessed using global assessment and task-specific sheets (see Appendix). The latter relates to procedural knowledge, whereas psychomotor skills can be evaluated by comprehensive assessments. The elements of the tools used have to be validated in terms of reliability, content, construct, concurrence and prediction.

Validity

Reliability can be assessed by test-retest and by internal consistency within multiple observers. Content measures whether or not the simulation is appropriate for the task to be trained. Construct validity is a measure of quality in the sense that an expert surgeon performs better than a trainee on the simulator. Concurrent validity looks at the performance of the assessment against current gold standard methods of assessment. Finally, predictive validity looks at the simulator's ability to predict the performance in the clinical setting and possibly to identify which doctors might make good surgeons.

Live case training

This provides the best case scenario. However, many training programmes are fixated on numbers of cases as a measure of 'competency'. At the present time, trainees and trainers fail to maximise the benefit of this important resource. Time should be set aside to review case selection, issues of consent and communication with patients and staff. In aorto-iliac interventions, the procedure should be digitally recorded and be made available for the trainee and trainer. Specific assessment tools can be used including task-specific check lists, global rating objective structured assessments of technical skills (OSATS) along with clinical outcome indicators and logbooks. Finally, the trainee as part of ongoing reflection and portfolio documentation, should use the video/digital recording. However, the recent spotlight of Dr Foster has forced many junior consultants away from teaching, as poor results may be misinterpreted and lead to prolonged periods of garden leave.

Training on animals is one obvious solution but in many countries this has met with growing public resistance. Furthermore, it is very expensive and only large animals can really simulate the live patient experience. In the UK, the use of animals for training is banned (Cruelty to Animals Act 1876 and the Protection of Animals Act 1911).

Simulators and models

Training on simulators and models does not have these problems and would appear at first sight to be a good alternative. However, the effectiveness and efficiency of virtual reality trainers and models in interventional radiology has not been fully evaluated at this time. There has been some experience in surgery but at the present time, they require further development to become a reliable assessment tool. In aviation, the human behaviour models discussed have been implemented to develop and evaluate new training methods. The problem in interventional radiology, however, is that realistic force feedback from contact of the catheter tip to the vessel wall to the hands of the interventionist is very difficult to achieve. Haptic feedback, which attempts to reproduce the resistance of a guidewire/catheter, is some way off the real thing. Training of rule-based behaviour can be achieved with VR simulators and through books, publications and workshop courses. Training in knowledge-based behaviour is much more complex to realise and at the moment, cannot be incorporated into virtual reality or model training systems of interventional radiology. There are, however, virtual operating room simulators which assess technical competency along with communication, teamworking and efficiency [8]. Further work is required to expand the technology into the area of aorto-iliac endovascular interventions. Presently, the only available method of knowledge-based training is with patients in a secure and well-supervised training programme. This will be the case until full-scale interventional simulators are developed that can provide such knowledge-based skills to be learnt. These will have to be accurate anatomic models with variants of both anatomy and pathology. They will need to reproduce vessel wall dynamics and the interaction of wall with instrument. Somehow they will have to generate a series of random unfamiliar events. Such simulators will be vastly expensive and their effectiveness difficult to evaluate.

Evaluation

Over the last decade there have been large scale technological advances in interventional radiology. Evaluation is required to translate these advances into improved patient outcomes. However, evaluation is time-consuming and requires a dedicated session (programmed activity [PA]) in all the job plans of new consultant trainers. Evaluation is based upon the collection of data (assessment), which is

subsequently interpreted. Valued judgements are made about progress and the impact upon the patient. As such it is important in the overall development of an individual practitioner but should be incorporated into the ongoing curriculum development which is led by the British Society of Interventional Radiology (BSIR) and the VSSGBI. Several common areas should be evaluated. These should include:-

◆ What was the intended learning outcome(s)?
◆ Was it appropriate?
◆ Was it achievable?
◆ How efficient and effective was the process?

However, at the time of writing there are no performance measures available to either the BSIR or VSSGBI. Consequently, training effectiveness can only be measured by time action analysis or observations in the angio lab [9-10]. These only assess the efficiency of actions by the time they take, the number of actions they require or the radiation dose they produce. Whilst useful and probably the only tool available at the present time, they only assess at the skill-based behaviour level. Evaluations that measure performance and the effect of training at rule and knowledge-based behaviour levels are urgently required and should be developed in conjunction with the curriculum.

Who should evaluate?

In the case of aorto-iliac interventions it is important for both vascular radiologists and surgeons to have input into the process. Failure to do so will lead to problems of ownership and overall commitment to the process. We have already seen differential agendas and so the future must be based upon debate and agreed solutions. In general terms this is met by a steering group, which provides cross-sectional representation of the interested parties and so determines the: remit, boundaries, time scales, methodologies and nature of the evaluations. This approach will enable teachers, specialist registrars and institutions to be evaluated, which ultimately leads to the objectives being met, with an effective use of resources and a quality assured competent-based training scheme which attracts the best candidates. Finally, the process will include an external assessor who in this case could be either the respective Royal Colleges or the Postgraduate Medical Education and Training Board (PMETB).

When to evaluate?

This should be undertaken before, during and after the completion of the curriculum. The use of informal and formal feedback should be used. Longer-term evaluation should be used to demonstrate that the desired learned behaviour has been achieved.

How to evaluate?

These methods should be agreed at the outset of the curriculum and usually consist of observation, oral and written assessments.

To date, little attention has been paid to the evaluation of training methods in interventional radiology. Work place assessments, which are often task-orientated, require 75% decision-making and 25% technical dexterity. However, they can be evaluated using logbooks, outcome audits and peer review. A number of tools have been developed including objective structured assessments of technical skills (OSATS), objective structured clinical examination (OSCE), and objective structured long examination record (OSLER). The Royal College of Surgeons of England has further developed the use of simulated standardised patients (OSCE/OSLER). They have used actors in the assessment of communication skills for both the giving and taking of information. In the case of OSATS, they consist of a global checklist (end product assessment) and have been developed to have validity and reliability. In the UK, Jonathon Beard (Sheffield Vascular Institute) has undertaken extensive work in this field and an example of the VSSGBI carotid endarterectomy OSATS is seen in the appendix.

Appendix

Task-specific checklist Initial puncture	Not done or incorrect (0)	Done correctly (1)	Instruction or help required
1. Selects puncture site appropriate to the target stenosis/occlusion			
2. Uses pulse, fluoroscopy, anatomical landmarks or ultrasound appropriate to gaining arterial access			
3. Uses approved and effective LA technique			
4. Uses beveled or Seldinger needle correctly at a correct angle			
5. Punctures artery within 5 attempts			
6. Selects non-hydrophilic guidewire			
7 Checks that lead end of wire is floppy before insertion			
8. Uses appropriate force to pass guidewire into artery			
9. Uses contrast appropriately to delineate position and anatomy			
10. Records image on DVI			

Sub Score (MAX 10)

Task-specific checklist Catheterisation	Not done or incorrect (0)	Done correctly (1)	Instruction or help required
1. Displays appropriate dexterity in wire passage			
2. Cleans wire with wet gauze or sponge at each exchange			
3. Chooses appropriate sheath/catheter			
4. Uses fluoroscopy correctly			
5. Displays awareness and knowledge of anatomy in wire positioning			
6. Observes ALARA principle			
7. Uses exchange wire of appropriate length			

Sub Score (MAX 7)

Task-specific checklist Crossing lesion	Not done or incorrect (0)	Done correctly (1)	Instruction or help required
1. Selects appropriate catheter			
2. Obtains angiogram in an appropriate projection			
3. Uses heparin in appropriate dose and at an appropriate time.			
4. Uses road map/fluoro fade appropriately			
5. Selects wire/catheter combination most suitable to cross the target lesion			
6. Manipulation of catheter wire combination to demonstrate understanding of interaction			
7. Demonstrates appropriate response to catheter tip forces			
8. Obtains angiogram having crossed lesion			
9. Uses transcatheter pressure measurements on either side of the target lesion			
10. Uses vasodilators appropriately and displays understanding of limitations of pressure gradient measurements			

Sub Score (MAX 10)

Task-specific checklist Treating target lesion	Not done or incorrect (0)	Done correctly (1)	Instruction or help required
1. Chooses balloon appropriate to target lesion			
2. Positions balloon appropriately			
3. Inflates balloon to correct pressure using correct inflation device			
4. Correct use of screening while inflating balloon			
5. Fully deflates balloon before removal			
6. Manipulates balloon withdrawal leaving wire *in situ* across target lesion			
7. Uses angiography and pressure gradients to assess result			
8. Uses information obtained to finish procedure, re PTA or stent as appropriate			
9. Chooses balloon mounted or self-expanding stent as appropriate to lesion.			
10. Rechecks angio and pressures			

Sub Score (MAX 10)

Task-specific checklist End of procedure	Not done or incorrect (0)	Done correctly (1)	Instruction or help required

1. Checks run-off to foot by angiography
2. Removes pigtail catheters over straight wire
3. Decides on digital pressure, or sealing device as appropriate to the size of the sheath used and the patient's body habitus and anticoagulant state
4. If using digital pressure recognises the importance of back bleeding and arterial puncture position
5. Presses for appropriate time
6. Checks pulses
7. Checks image status and gives instructions about image record
8. Makes sure antiplatelets prescribed appropriately
9. Gives appropriate instructions to ward
10. Arranges imaging follow-up as appropriate

Sub Score (MAX 10)

Summary

◆   From this theoretical discussion about training, it should be obvious that if training is really going to equip practitioners at the skill, rule and knowledge-based levels it cannot be geared to learning just one trick such as the insertion of an iliac stent! It is not acceptable in the man machine industry and it cannot be acceptable in medicine.

◆   Training should provide focused and directed experience in order to accelerate the learning curve, optimise results and reduce error. Not surprisingly, endovascular training will require significant resources both in terms of time and money.

◆   Skilled trainers need to be identified and resourced accordingly.

◆   The development of dedicated courses, access to skills laboratory and dedicated training lists are essential prerequisites for a successful training programme and the creation of competent endovascular practitioners of the future.

◆   Despite all these ideals, the harsh reality is that the training time will be severely curtailed.

◆   We need to think hard about the future provision of training in endovascular therapies, in particular the move to a more centralised service based upon large consultant groups of 10-12 people. Within these groups there should be the facility to incorporate vascular radiologists and surgeons into a new breed of endovascular practitioners.

References

1.   Donaldson L. Unfinished Business: proposals for reform of the senior house officer grade. NHS consultation paper. Department of Health, London, August 2002.

2.   British Orthopaedic Association. Education and Training for SHOs: a snapshot of the moment and recommendations for the future. British Orthopaedic Association, London, July 2002.

3.   Crofts TJ, Griffiths JM, Sharma S, Wygrala J, Aitken RJ. Surgical Training an objective assessment of recent changes for a single health board. *BMJ* 1997; 314: 814.

4.   Training in Interventional Vascular Radiology. Proposal by the VSSGBI/RCR Liaison Group, 2001. (Obtainable from the Vascular Surgical Society of Great Britain and Ireland at the Royal College of Surgeons of England, London WC2A 3PE, UK. www.vssgbi.org).

5.   Statutory Instrument No. 1059. The Ionising Radiation (Medical Exposure) Regulations 2000. www.legislation.hmso.gov.uk/si/si2000/20001059.htm.

6.   Rasmussen R. Skill, Rule and Knowledge; Signals and Signs and Other Distinctions in Human Performance Models. *IEEE Transactions on Systems, Man and Cybernetics* 1983; SMC-13: 257-266.

7.   Wentink M, Stassen LBS, Alwayn I, *et al*. Rasmussen's model of Human Behaviour in Laparoscopy Training. *Surgical Endoscopy* 2003. In press.

8.   Lingard L, Reznick R, Espin S, Regehr G, DeVito I. Team communications in the operating room; talk patterns, sites of tension and implications for novices. *Acad Med* 2002; 77: 232-237.

9.   Sjoerdsma W. Surgeons at work; time and action analysis of the laparoscopic surgical process. 1998 Delft: PhD Thesis DUT.

10. Bakker NH, Tanase D, Reekers JA, *et al*. Evaluation of vascular and interventional procedures with time action analysis: a pilot study. *J Vasc Intervent Radiol* 2002; 13: 483-488.

Chapter 8

Natural history of thoracic aneurysms and the role of surgery

Aaron M Ranasinghe, MRCS, Research Fellow, Cardiothoracic Surgery

Robert S Bonser, FRCP FRCS FESC, Consultant Cardiothoracic Surgeon

Queen Elizabeth Hospital, University Hospital Birmingham NHS Trust, Birmingham, UK

Introduction

The presence of thoracic aneurysmal disease is associated with a reduced life expectancy. For patients with untreated chronic thoracic aortic aneurysms of either degenerative or dissecting aetiology, the five-year survival is quoted between 13% and 39% [1-3], with the main cause of death being due to rupture. Elective surgery to repair or replace the aneurysm appears to increase long-term survival, but there are no published randomised studies. The timing of surgery for these patients was previously based on clinical judgement without the guidance of relevant scientific data. Advances in surgical technique and end organ protection have reduced the risks associated with operation but they still remain hazardous. When to intervene is a critical question that faces the surgeon. Intervention is based upon an assessment of the risk of rupture. This risk of rupture is related to the site, size, aetiology and expansion rate of the aneurysm.

Aetiology

An aneurysm is defined as a persistent localised dilatation of a blood vessel caused by stretching of the vessel wall, with an at least 50% increase in diameter compared to the normal diameter of the aorta according to the age, sex and body surface area of the patient, and taking into account the location of the aneurysm within the course of the aorta. Dilatation of the vessel wall implies an intrinsic weakness of that wall with an increase in wall tension.

The exact aetiology of aortic aneurysms remains unknown, but is probably multifactorial in the majority, with genetic and environmental components. There is currently a rigorous search underway to identify candidate genes that may predict abdominal aortic aneurysmal disease. It is also likely that thoracic aneurysmal disease has a genetic component. Even when excluding families with known connective tissue disorders, there is a proportion of patients (up to 21%) with a positive family history of aneurysmal disease or a sudden death [4].

The majority of thoracic aneurysms are associated with medial degenerative disease (40%) or chronic dissection (50%) [2]. Degenerative aneurysms are associated with, though not necessarily caused by, atherosclerotic disease [5] and may be multifocal in 12-30% of cases reflecting generalised aortic disease [1,2,6]. They involve all three layers of the aortic wall and are therefore true aneurysms by pathological definition. The majority of degenerative thoracic aneurysms are located in the descending thoracic aorta (89%) [7] compared with dissecting aneurysms which are predominantly located in the ascending aorta and arch (57%) [7].

Post-traumatic aneurysms may occur if an aortic tear and haematoma is contained by the adventitia or pleura. The formation of such false aneurysms at the site of injury may go unnoticed and untreated for several years and diagnosis is usually made on incidental abnormal chest radiograph findings. Nearly 85% of patients with acute traumatic aortic rupture die before reaching hospital. The remaining 15% have a contained rupture and less than 5% of these patients develop a chronic aneurysm.

The connective tissue disease, Marfan's syndrome, relates to a deficiency of the protein fibrillin, which acts as a scaffold for elastin fibres. Thus, aneurysm development occurs at the site of maximum elasticity in the aorta, primarily the aortic root and the first few centimetres of the ascending aorta. Other connective tissue disorders such as Ehlers Danlos [8], tuberous sclerosis [9] and osteogenesis imperfecta [10] also predispose to thoracic aneurysm formation.

Inflammatory disorders such as Bechet's syndrome, Takayasu's and Giant Cell arteritis are all documented in the process of thoracic aneurysm occurrence [11,12].

Bacterial and fungal infections of the aortic wall may either cause aneurysmal change or colonise pre-existing aneurysms. Staphylococcus and salmonella species are the most common organisms involved, being present in 46% and 15% of mycotic aneurysms respectively [13]. Aneurysms involving salmonella species tend to be spontaneous and staphylococcal aneurysms occur predominantly following previous surgical grafting. Syphilitic aneurysms are now rare [14]. They most commonly involved the aortic root, ascending aorta and arch.

The most frequent entities that present to referring centres are those of degenerative aneurysm and chronic dissection [1,15,16].

According to site of the aorta the most common aetiologies found are:-

◆ Root and ascending thoracic aorta - annuloaortic ectasia, Marfan's syndrome and chronic dissection.
◆ Arch and descending thoracic aorta - dissection, atherosclerosis, non-infectious aortitis, medial degeneration and Marfan's syndrome.

It is important to remember that aneurysmal disease of distinct pathologies may co-exist in a single patient, including the development of dissection within a degenerative aneurysm and the development of degenerative abdominal aortic aneurysm disease in patients with a proximal dissection.

Prevalence and incidence of aortic aneurysm disease

Abdominal aortic aneurysm

In abdominal aortic aneurysms, population-based screening and follow-up studies have been possible utilising ultrasonography. The absence of such a readily acceptable and non-invasive investigation has frustrated the documentation of the natural history of thoracic aortic aneurysms. The prevalence of abdominal aortic aneurysms within the population is estimated to be between 1.3 and 8.4% [17]. Their pathological profile is less diverse than that of thoracic aneurysms with the majority of them being degenerative [18]. Their mean expansion rates are between 1.7 and 5.7mm/year [19] and their expansion rates increase exponentially with increasing initial aortic diameter. Thoracic and abdominal aortic aneurysms share common factors that are associated with expansion and rupture, such as initial size, smoking, chronic obstructive pulmonary disease (COPD) and hypertension. Risk of rupture is mainly dependent on aneurysm size and increase in size [17].

Studies of small asymptomatic aneurysms have been carried out [20] and the rupture rate for these small aneurysms is low, considerably less than is associated with the risk of surgery. This supports a policy of routine and careful surveillance in this group of patients and if this data were available for patients with thoracic aneurysms it would facilitate management and allow for the risk benefit analysis of intervention.

Thoracic aortic aneurysm

Prevalence estimates of thoracic aortic aneurysm disease are based largely on postmortem studies. A study of 58,000 postmortems (1958-1985) calculated the prevalence of thoracic aortic aneurysm disease to be 489 per 100,000 postmortems in males and 437 per 100,000 in females [21].

Incidence of thoracic aneurysm disease, i.e. the number of *de novo* cases developing is harder to quantify. The nearest estimate to true incidence is based on a study of patient population derived from validated autopsy, operation and clinical presentation records in a relatively fixed population between 1951 and 1980 [1]. The estimated age- and sex-adjusted incidence of all thoracic aneurysms was 5.9 per 100,000 patient years. Recent follow-up to this study between 1980 and 1994 suggests that the incidence of thoracic aneurysmal disease has increased to 10.4 per 100,000 patient years [16]. A possible explanation for the observation of increasing incidence of thoracic aneurysmal disease may be due to improvements in imaging available to clinicians leading to the detection of smaller aneurysms.

The natural history of thoracic aneurysms

The presumed natural progression of thoracic aneurysm disease is expansion, rupture and death. The larger the aneurysm, the greater is the risk of rupture and death. Over 80% of thoracic aneurysms detected at postmortem have ruptured and follow-up series of large unoperated aneurysms have a dismal prognosis (<20% five-year survival) with the main mode of death being rupture [3,22]. However, not all aneurysms are either large or symptomatic when first detected. Therefore, knowledge of the natural history is fundamentally important when weighing the risks and benefits of prophylactic surgery in an asymptomatic population. Moreover, the very factors that influence expansion rate and risk of rupture also

increase the risk of surgery, eg. age, COPD. Management of these patients is, therefore, a careful balance between weighing the risk of rupture against the complications associated with operative intervention. Studies of the natural history of thoracic aneurysmal disease are confounded by selection bias, unknown true incidence of the disease, failure to standardise non-operative medical therapy and the retrospective nature of the available studies. Selection bias is due to the parallel development of sophisticated imaging and surgical techniques. The majority of studies on expansion rates in thoracic aneurysms exclude patients with rupture and those who have already reached criteria for surgery. Inclusion of aortic dissections without considering site, size or speed of onset of presentation leads to further bias. Inclusion of type A dissections in follow-up studies skews mortality towards a higher rate of early deaths. There are, therefore, no definitive studies available on thoracic aneurysm history.

Aneurysm expansion rates

Factors that may affect aneurysm expansion rate can be divided into patient and aneurysmal factors. The aneurysmal factors can be further subdivided into dimensional and non-dimensional (Table 1).

Maximal cross-sectional diameter is strongly associated with increased rate of expansion. Aneurysmal disease is frequently a multifocal phenomenon within the aorta [1,2,6] and expansion is a three-dimensional process. Overall, median expansion rates for thoracic aneurysms are between 1-4.3mm/year [4,15,23] and expansion rates increase

Table 1. Dimensional and non-dimensional factors associated with aneurysm expansion.

Aneurysm	Patient
Dimensional	Smoking
Absolute cross-sectional diameter	Age
Non-dimensional	Hypertension
Location	COPD
Pathology	ß blockers

Table 2. Exponential formulae describing aortic aneurysm expansion rates.

DaPunt [23]:   expansion rate = 0.0167 (initial aortic diameter) $^{2.1}$

Coady [24]:   final aortic diameter = initial diameter x $e^{0.001395 \times time}$

Hirose [25]:   final aortic diameter = 1.0192 x initial aortic diameter x $e^{0.0032 \times time}$

Shimada [15]:   final aortic diameter = initial diameter x $e^{0.00367 \times time}$

exponentially with incremental increases in aortic diameter. Higher initial aneurysm size is associated with an increased rate of expansion. Aneurysms with a greater than 50mm maximal cross-sectional diameter expand at a far greater rate than those less than 50mm in diameter; 7.9mm/year in comparison to 1.7mm/year respectively [23]. Several formulae are available for calculating expansion rates of thoracic aneurysms, all taken from different populations (Table 2) [15,23-25]. The fundamental part of all these equations is the initial aortic diameter.

Location of the aneurysm not only has important considerations with regard to expansion rate but also relates to the operative risk particularly for paraplegia. There is controversy regarding the effect of site on expansion rate. Some studies have shown that thoracic arch aneurysms expand at a greater rate than those of the ascending aorta which in turn expand quicker than those located within the descending thoracic aorta, irrespective of their initial size [26]. Other studies have shown that aneurysmal segments of the descending aorta expand at a greater rate than more proximal segments [27]. These differences are explained by the relatively small numbers with follow-up data and the heterogeneity of populations. Average expansion rates for the aneurysmal thoracic aorta are quoted at 1mm/year, with rates of 1.9mm/year in the descending aorta and 0.7mm/year in the ascending aorta [4].

Patients with connective tissue disorders such as Marfan's syndrome, in which an alteration in the deposition of elastin within the aortic wall due to the deficiency of the glycoprotein fibrillin occurs, are more likely to develop aneurysms of the elastic arteries [28] and aortic root dilatation is present in up to 80% of these patients by their twenties. These patients also have a greater maximal aortic diameter than age and sex-matched controls without Marfan's [29]. Life expectancy is reduced by a third in this group with 90% of deaths being related to aneurysm rupture [30]. This has important consequences when considering the timing of elective surgery for this group.

There is evidence that chronic type B dissections have a faster expansion rate (3.7mm/year) compared to non-dissecting aneurysms (0.9mm/year) independent of initial size [24]. This however, has not been universally accepted [23,27]. Presence of a patent or closed false lumen after dissection also impacts on the rate of expansion of the aneurysm with the presence of a perfused false lumen conferring a greater expansion rate [31].

Presence of calcification within the aortic wall is believed by some to confer protection against expansion and rupture. Studies have, however, demonstrated that calcification does not prevent expansion [27,32,33]. Presence of thrombus within the aortic wall is also associated with an increase in rate of expansion for ill understood reasons [27,34,35].

Patient factors that have been shown to impact on expansion rate are smoking, age, hypertension, COPD and use of ß blockers. Smoking is consistently noted to have a positive influence on the rate of aneurysm expansion in several studies [23,36,37]. The mechanisms behind this increase in expansion rate are poorly understood, but may be secondary to the influence of smoking on connective tissue properties [38]. Diastolic hypertension is linked to initial aneurysm development and a larger aneurysm diameter at initial diagnosis [23]. However, those patients that have controlled hypertension do not appear to have an increased expansion rate [27] and medical management of hypertension in these patients appears to be of fundamental importance. In the management of chronic type B dissections, prescription and tolerance of ß blocker therapy leads to a reduction in late complication rates [39]. Chronic obstructive pulmonary disease is associated with an increase in the rate of aneurysm expansion. This may be due to connective tissue effects or the inability to prescribe ß blockers within this population.

Rupture

Rupture is the most serious consequence of thoracic aneurysm disease. It is the single most common cause of death in these patients [27] and is almost uniformly fatal [3]. However, there are a small number of patients who survive the initial event and may be referred to specialist centres for treatment [40]. For these patients, operative mortality is high between 10% and 40% [40-43]. It is therefore important to identify patients who are at an increased risk of rupture, so that elective surgery (with a lower mortality and morbidity) can be considered. The factors that influence expansion also influence the risk of rupture.

As aneurysm size increases so does the probability of rupture. This correlates to the law of LaPlace that relates the pressure (P) on a cylinder to its wall thickness (t), wall tension (T) and radius (r) by the equation:-

$$P = (2txT)/r$$

Thus, at a given pressure, any increase in dimension with associated wall thinning leads to an increase in wall tension until rupture.

The risk over time of rupture is 25 times greater in those patients with an aneurysm diameter of ≥60mm when compared to those of 40-49mm. Even aneurysms within the 50-59mm range are associated with 11 times the risk of rupture when compared to those in the 40-49mm range [44]. For every 10mm increase in maximal aortic diameter the risk of rupture increases by a factor of 1.9 [45]. For aneurysms less than 50mm in diameter the yearly rate for risk of rupture is close to zero. This rupture rate rises to 1.7% and 3.6% per year for aneurysms between 50mm and 59mm and those greater than 60mm respectively [44]. Rapid expansion rate is also a risk factor for rupture [46].

More proximally located aneurysms have a higher rate of rupture than those located in the descending thoracic aorta for any given size.

Pathology also has an influence on rupture with dissecting aneurysms more likely to rupture at a smaller median size of 60mm than non-dissecting [3,24,47], although not all authorities agree on this [23]. Aneurysms in patients with Marfan's syndrome rupture at a smaller size than degenerative aneurysms regardless of their position within the thoracic aorta and the majority of premature deaths in patients with Marfan's syndrome are related to aortic rupture. These patients are therefore treated in a more aggressive fashion and early elective repair of aneurysms is frequently carried out in this group at a lower threshold [32].

There is a steady increase in the risk of rupture with age [14]. Smoking increases the risk of rupture by 6.5 times independently of COPD [36] and the presence of COPD increases the risk of rupture by 3.6 times [45,47]. Not only do these factors increase the risk of rupture but they also lead to an increase in operative risk.

Untreated hypertension may also be a risk factor for rupture and it would seem to be appropriate that those patients who are hypertensive should receive appropriate medical therapy to control their hypertension.

Non-specific pain in the presence of aneurysmal disease is also of prognostic significance. In a study of non-operated aneurysms [45], the presence of vague or uncharacteristic pain emerged as an independent risk factor for rupture in patients with non-dissecting aneurysms.

Timing of surgery

Criteria for surgical intervention include rupture, symptoms (such as pain, compression of adjacent organs and aortic incompetence in association with ascending aortic aneurysm), size, expansion rate and dissection. Elective repair of thoracic aneurysmal disease has superior outcomes when compared to emergency surgery for rupture [24]. However, elective operation for thoracic aneurysmal disease is not without risk and a careful assessment of the balance of rupture risk versus operative risk (i.e. mortality and permanent neurological deficit) is necessary. Morbidity associated with operative intervention

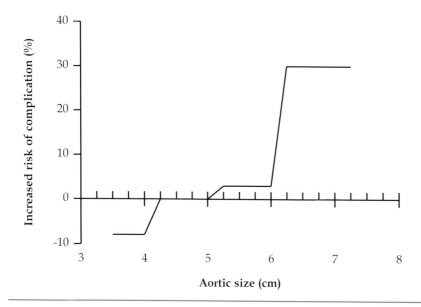

Figure 1. Influence of ascending aortic size on cumulative, lifetime incidence of natural complications of aortic aneurysm [4].

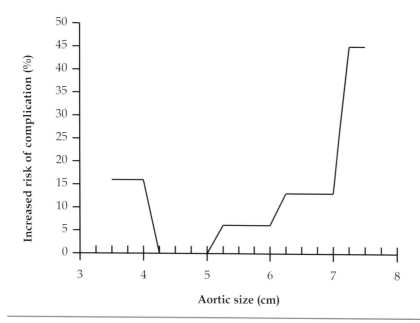

Figure 2. Influence of descending aortic size on cumulative, lifetime incidence of natural complications of aortic aneurysm [4].

Table 3. Equation to estimate the rate of rupture (λ) after CT scan [45].

Ln λ = -21.055 + 0.093 (age) + 0.841 (pain) + 1.282 (COPD) + 0.643 (descending diameter, cm) + 0.405 (abdominal diameter, cm)

Pain and COPD are 1 if present and 0 if absent.
Probability of rupture within 1 year = $1 - e^{-\lambda(365)}$

includes myocardial infarction, stroke, paraplegia, respiratory and renal failure. Even in large centres that perform a large number of these procedures, operative mortality for elective repair can be significant. For ascending aneurysms mortality is quoted between 2.5-12.8% and for the descending thoracic aorta and thoracoabdominal aneurysms, between 8-31% [4,48]. Stroke risk of 8% for ascending and 5% for descending aortic operations are typical of the reported literature, with a further 4.5-8% risk of paraplegia for descending thoracic aortic operations [4,49]. These figures are all increased in patients undergoing emergency surgery for rupture. Therefore, in order to perform thoracic aortic surgery it is essential that the balance of risk of complication from leaving the aneurysm, i.e. risks of rupture or dissection with emergency surgery is appropriately weighed against the risks of elective surgery.

Surgery should be offered at a point when the risk of rupture approaches or exceeds the expected mortality and permanent neurological deficit rate of surgery. Not all patients will reach these criteria and some may die of non-aneurysm-related causes. For some patients the expected mortality from elective surgery may be prohibitively high. The decision to operate is reached by consideration of all the factors that influence rupture. A formula for rupture risk has been calculated based on some of these risk factors that allows for the calculation of the probability of rupture for patients based on age, pain, COPD, and maximal thoracic and abdominal aortic diameter (Table 3) [45]. However, the main factor that determines the need for intervention is the aortic diameter. Recommendations for intervention based on the expected rate of complication (Figures 1 and 2) (Table 4) are 55mm and 65mm for asymptomatic patients in the ascending and descending aorta respectively. These points are arbitrarily lowered in Marfan's patients to 50mm and 60mm because of the

Table 4. Complications based on aortic size [4].

	Aortic size			
Yearly risk	>3.5cm	>4cm	>5cm	>6cm
Rupture	0.0%	0.3%	1.7%	3.6%
Dissection	2.2%	1.5%	2.5%	3.7%
Death	5.9%	4.6%	4.8%	10.8%
Any of the above	7.2%	5.3%	6.5%	14.1%

Figures 1, 2 and Table 4 are reproduced with permission from the Society of Thoracic Surgeons. Elefteriades JA. Natural history of thoracic aortic aneurysms: Indications for surgery, and surgical versus nonsurgical risks. Ann Thorac Surg 2002; 74(5): S1877-S1880.

increased rates of expansion and rupture in this patient population.

Conclusions

Our current understanding of the natural history of thoracic aneurysms is incomplete. The prognosis for patients with large thoracic aneurysms is poor without operative intervention. The risk of aneurysm rupture is dependent upon site, size and co-morbidity, and assessment of these factors allows identification of an appropriate time-point when intervention should be considered. The combined risk of interventional mortality and permanent neurological deficit should be weighed against the risk of rupture. Further studies are required to accurately define best management in smaller asymptomatic aneurysms and should include studies of natural history and interventional outcomes in these patients.

Summary

◆   Natural history of thoracic aneurysmal disease is incomplete.

◆   Prognosis without intervention is poor in large aneurysms.

◆   Factors that affect expansion and rupture are both aneurysm and patient-related.

◆   Aneurysm size is the most important factor in determining expansion rate and risk of rupture.

◆   Factors that affect interventional outcome are dependent on site, extent, pathology and co-morbidity.

◆   Surgical intervention still carries a significant risk of mortality and permanent neurological deficit.

References

1. Bickerstaff LK, Pairolero PC, Hollier LH, *et al*. Thoracic aortic aneurysms: a population-based study. *Surgery* 1982; 92(6): 1103-8.

2. Pressler V, McNamara JJ. Aneurysm of the thoracic aorta. Review of 260 cases. *J Thorac Cardiovasc Surg* 1985; 89(1): 50-54.

3. Perko MJ, Norgaard M, Herzog TM, Olsen PS, Schroeder TV, Pettersson G. Unoperated aortic aneurysm: a survey of 170 patients. *Ann Thorac Surg* 1995; 59(5): 1204-9.

4. Elefteriades JA. Natural history of thoracic aortic aneurysms: Indications for surgery, and surgical versus nonsurgical risks. *Ann Thorac Surg* 2002; 74(5): S1877-S1880.

5. Zarins CK, Glagov S. *Atherosclerotic processes and aneurysms formation*. Appleton, Norwalk, 1994.

6. Crawford ES, Cohen ES. Aortic aneurysm: a multifocal disease. Presidential address. *Arch Surg* 1982; 117(11): 1393-400.

7. Pressler V, McNamara JJ. Thoracic aortic aneurysm: natural history and treatment. *J Thorac Cardiovasc Surg* 1980; 79(4): 489-98.

8. Sheiner NM, Miller N, Lachance C. Arterial complications of Ehlers-Danlos syndrome. *J Cardiovasc Surg* (Torino) 1985; 26(3): 291-6.

9. Shepherd CW, Gomez MR, Lie JT, Crowson CS. Causes of death in patients with tuberous sclerosis. *Mayo Clinic Proceedings* 1991; 66(8): 792-796.

10. Ohteki H, Ohtsubo S, Sakurai J, Koga N, Kohchi K, Itoh T. Aortic regurgitation and aneurysm of Sinus of Valsalva associated with osteogenesis imperfecta. *Thoracic & Cardiovascular Surgeon* 1991; 39(5): 294-295.

11. Sharma S, Rajani M, Shrivastava S, *et al*. Non-specific aorto-arteritis (Takayasu's disease) in children. *Br J Radiol* 1991; 64(764): 690-698.

12. Matsumoto T, Uekusa T, Fukuda Y. Vasculo-Behcet's disease: a pathologic study of eight cases. *Hum Pathol* 1991; 22(1):45-51.

13. Blebea J, Kempczinski RF. Mycotic Aneurysms. In: *Aneurysms - New findings and treatments*. Yao JST, Pearce WH, Eds. Appleton and Lange, 1994.

14. Johansson G, Markstrom U, Swedenborg J. Ruptured thoracic aortic aneurysms: a study of incidence and mortality rates. *J Vasc Surg* 1995; 21(6): 985-988.

15. Shimada I, Rooney SJ, Pagano D, *et al*. Prediction of thoracic aortic aneurysm expansion: validation of formulae describing growth. *Ann Thorac Surg* 1999; 67(6): 1968-1970.

16. Clouse WD, Hallett JW, Jr., Schaff HV, Gayari MM, Ilstrup DM, Melton LJ. Improved prognosis of thoracic aortic aneurysms: a population-based study. *JAMA* 1998; 280(22): 1926-9.

17. Wilmink AB, Quick CR. Epidemiology and potential for prevention of abdominal aortic aneurysm. *Br J Surg* 1998; 85(2): 155-62.

18. Reed D, Reed C, Stemmermann G, Hayashi T. Are aortic aneurysms caused by atherosclerosis? *Circulation* 1992; 85(1): 205-11.

19. Wilson KA, Woodburn KR, Ruckley CV, Fowkes FG. Expansion rates of abdominal aortic aneurysm: current limitations in evaluation. *Eur J Vasc Endovasc Surg* 1997; 13(6): 521-6.

20. Mortality results for randomised controlled trial of early elective surgery or ultrasonographic surveillance for small abdominal aortic aneurysms. The UK Small Aneurysm Trial Participants. *Lancet* 1998; 352(9141): 1649-55.

21. Svensjo S, Bengtsson H, Bergqvist D. Thoracic and thoracoabdominal aortic aneurysm and dissection: an investigation based on autopsy. *Br J Surg* 1996; 83(1): 68-71.

22. Cambria RA, Gloviczki P, Stanson AW, *et al*. Outcome and expansion rate of 57 thoracoabdominal aortic aneurysms managed nonoperatively. *Am J Surg* 1995; 170(2): 213-7.

23. Dapunt OE, Galla JD, Sadeghi AM, *et al*. The natural history of thoracic aortic aneurysms. *J Thorac Cardiovasc Surg* 1994; 107(5): 1323-32.

24. Coady MA, Rizzo JA, Hammond GL, *et al*. What is the appropriate size criterion for resection of thoracic aortic aneurysms? *J Thorac Cardiovasc Surg* 1997; 113(3): 476-91.

25. Hirose Y, Hamada S, Takamiya M. Predicting the growth of aortic aneurysms: a comparison of linear vs exponential models. *Angiology* 1995; 46(5): 413-9.

26. Hirose Y, Hamada S, Takamiya M, Imakita S, Naito H, Nishimura T. Aortic aneurysms: growth rates measured with CT. *Radiology* 1992; 185(1): 249-52.

27. Bonser RS, Pagano D, Lewis ME, *et al.* Clinical and patho-anatomical factors affecting expansion of thoracic aortic aneurysms. *Heart* 2000; 84(3): 277-283.

28. Marsalese DL, Moodie DS, Vacante M, *et al.* Marfan's syndrome: natural history and long-term follow-up of cardiovascular involvement. *J Am Coll Cardiol* 1989; 14(2): 422-8.

29. Hwa J, Richards JG, Huang H, *et al.* The natural history of aortic dilatation in Marfan's syndrome. *Med J Aust* 1993; 158(8): 558-62.

30. Murdoch JL, Walker BA, Halpern BL, Kuzma JW, McKusick VA. Life expectancy and causes of death in the Marfan syndrome. *New Engl J Med* 1972; 286(15): 804-808.

31. Marui A, Mochizuki T, Mitsui N, Koyama T, Kimura F, Horibe M. Toward the best treatment for uncomplicated patients with type B acute aortic dissection: a consideration for sound surgical indication. *Circulation* 1999; 100(19 Suppl): 275-80.

32. Coselli JS, de Figueiredo LF. Natural history of descending and thoracoabdominal aortic aneurysms. *J Card Surg* 1997; 12(2 Suppl): 285-9.

33. Masuda Y, Takanashi K, Takasu J, Morooka N, Inagaki Y. Expansion rate of thoracic aortic aneurysms and influencing factors. *Chest* 1992; 102(2): 461-6.

34. Wolf YG, Thomas WS, Brennan FJ, Goff WG, Sise MJ, Bernstein EF. Computed tomography scanning findings associated with rapid expansion of abdominal aortic aneurysms. *J Vasc Surg* 1994; 20(4): 529-35.

35. Krupski WC, Bass A, Thurston DW, Dilley RB, Bernstein EF. Utility of computed tomography for surveillance of small abdominal aortic aneurysms. Preliminary report. *Arch Surg* 1990; 125(10): 1345-9.

36. Strachan DP. Predictors of death from aortic aneurysm among middle-aged men: the Whitehall study. *Br J Surg* 1991; 78(4): 401-4.

37. MacSweeney ST, Ellis M, Worrell PC, Greenhalgh RM, Powell JT. Smoking and growth rate of small abdominal aortic aneurysms. *Lancet* 1994; 344(8923): 651-2.

38. Cohen JR, Mandell C, Margolis I, Chang J, Wise L. Altered aortic protease and antiprotease activity in patients with ruptured abdominal aortic aneurysms. *Surg Gynecol Obstet* 1987; 164(4): 355-8.

39. Genoni M, Paul M, Jenni R, Graves K, Seifert B, Turina M. Chronic beta-blocker therapy improves outcome and reduces treatment costs in chronic type B aortic dissection. *Eur J Cardiothorac Surg* 2001; 19(5): 606-10.

40. Lewis ME, Ranasinghe AM, Revell MP, Bonser RS. Surgical repair of ruptured thoracic and thoracoabdominal aortic aneurysms. *Br J Surg* 2002; 89(4): 442-5.

41. Mastroroberto P, Chello M. Emergency thoracoabdominal aortic aneurysm repair: clinical outcome. *J Thorac Cardiovasc Surg* 1999; 118(3): 477-81.

42. von Segesser LK, Genoni M, Kunzli A, *et al.* Surgery for ruptured thoracic and thoraco-abdominal aortic aneurysms. *Eur J Cardiothorac Surg* 1996; 10(11): 996-1001.

43. Bradbury AW, Bulstrode NW, Gilling-Smith G, Stansby G, Mansfield AO, Wolfe JH. Repair of ruptured thoracoabdominal aortic aneurysm is worthwhile in selected cases. *Eur J Vasc Endovasc Surg* 1999; 17(2): 160-165.

44. Davies RR, Goldstein LJ, Coady MA, *et al.* Yearly rupture or dissection rates for thoracic aortic aneurysms: simple prediction based on size. *Ann Thorac Surg* 2002; 73(1): 17-27.

45. Juvonen T, Ergin MA, Galla JD, *et al.* Prospective study of the natural history of thoracic aortic aneurysms. [erratum appears in *Ann Thorac Surg* 1997 Aug; 64(2): 594]. *Ann Thorac Surg* 1997; 63(6): 1533-1545.

46. Lobato AC, Puech-Leao P. Predictive factors for rupture of thoracoabdominal aortic aneurysm. *J Vasc Surg* 1998; 27(3): 446-453.

47. Juvonen T, Ergin MA, Galla JD, *et al.* Risk factors for rupture of chronic type B dissections. *J Thorac Cardiovasc Surg* 1999; 117(4): 776-786.

48. The Society of Cardiothoracic Surgeons of Great Britain and Ireland. National Adult Cardiac Surgical Database Report 2000-2001. October 2002 ed. Dendrite Clinical Systems Ltd, 2002.

49. Coselli JS, LeMaire SA, Miller CC3, *et al.* Mortality and paraplegia after thoracoabdominal aortic aneurysm repair: a risk factor analysis. *Ann Thorac Surg* 2000; 69(2): 409-14.

Chapter 9

The development of thoracic stents: current availability and recommendations

Peter R Taylor, MA MChir FRCS, Consultant Vascular Surgeon
Guy's & St. Thomas' Hospital, London, UK

Introduction

The first publication on the endovascular treatment of the infrarenal aorta was from Parodi et al [1]. This detailed mainly animal experiments but also included their initial experience of implanting stent grafts in the infrarenal aorta of five patients. Only a proximal stent was used to secure a polyester tube graft. It quickly became apparent that a distal stent to secure the graft material was essential if the infrarenal aortic aneurysm was to be excluded. Further experience has shown that the best results are obtained when the devices for infrarenal abdominal aortic aneurysms are bifurcated and secured distally in the iliac arteries. At the time of Parodi's report, Volodos et al had published their experience of using stent grafts for arterial disease in the Russian literature [2-4]. The last report, also from 1991, included two patients who had had devices inserted into the thoracic aorta, one five years previously. Therefore, although Parodi and his colleagues have been awarded the accolade for developing and publicising the first stent grafts for treatment of aneurysms of the infrarenal aorta, Volodos and his team must be credited with the first implant for thoracic aortic disease.

Initial experience

The group with the most experience in the West is from Stanford, California, where Dake and his colleagues started to implant thoracic stent grafts from 1992 [5]. They used home-made devices comprising uncrimped woven polyester with Gianturco-Z stents made from stainless steel. They reported their initial experience using these 'first-generation' stent grafts for aneurysms of the descending thoracic aorta in 13 patients. The aetiology of the aneurysms included a mixed bag of degenerative atherosclerotic, anastomotic, post-traumatic and aneurysms related to previous dissections. The mean diameter was 6.1cm, and each device was custom-made for each patient. The device was successfully implanted in all patients, and resulted in thrombosis of the aneurysm in 12 patients. Two devices were used in two patients to gain the required length to adequately exclude the aneurysm. The initial results were encouraging with no deaths, strokes or paraplegia, although the follow-up was short at 11.6 months.

Further publications from the same group using the home-made device confirmed the efficacy of stent grafts in treating diseases of the thoracic aorta [6]. This

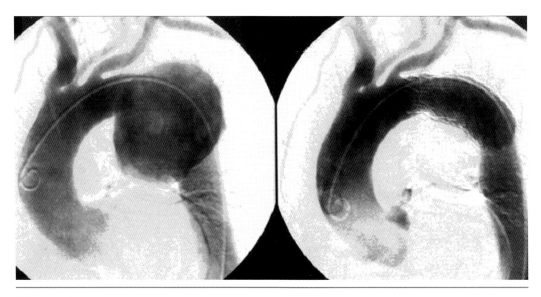

Figure 1. Pre- and post-angiograms showing successful thoracic stent graft placement.

paper followed 103 patients for an average of 22 months. Conventional open surgery was not considered to be an option in 60% of these patients. Complete thrombosis was achieved in 83% and the 30-day mortality was 9%. They also experienced serious complications such as paraplegia in 3% and stroke in 7% of patients. Two patients had myocardial infarctions and 12 suffered respiratory insufficiency. One patient developed a new (more proximal) aortic dissection. The actuarial survival rates were 81% at one year and 73% at two years. Only 53% of patients were free from 'treatment failure' at 3.7 years. The major problems with the home-made device were related to the large size of the delivery sheath, the difficulty of accurate deployment, the lack of column strength which could cause the device to collapse entirely within the aneurysm sac, and an initial endoleak rate of 24%.

The Stanford group also reported their results for acute aortic dissection using a home-made device [7]. The stent grafts were positioned to cover the primary tear in order to reduce the pressure in the false lumen and divert the blood flow into the true lumen exclusively. Four patients had acute type A aortic dissections with the primary entry tear distal to the left subclavian artery origin, and 15 patients presented with acute type B aortic dissections. The dissections compromised branches in 14 of the 19 patients, and multiple, symptomatic branch vessel ischaemia was

present in seven. Technical success was achieved in all 19 patients and complete thrombosis of the thoracic aortic lumen occurred in 15 patients. The finding of complete thrombosis of the false lumen in the thoracic aorta is associated with the best long-term outcome. Revascularisation of branch vessel ischaemia was achieved in 76% of compromised vessels. Partial thrombosis of the false lumen occurred in the remaining four patients during the average 13-month follow-up. These excellent results using home-made devices, compared with open surgery, encouraged commercial companies to develop stent grafts specifically for use in the thoracic aorta (Figure 1).

Commercially available devices

The first two stent grafts which were made by commercial companies, designed specifically for the treatment of thoracic disease, were the 'Excluder', manufactured by W. L. Gore Associates, Inc., and the Talent thoracic device made by Medtronic AVE. The Excluder device was made from a nitinol stent covered with polytetrafluoroethylene. The major advantages of this stent graft was its flexibility, a low profile and the ease and speed with which it could be deployed by pulling a ripcord which opened a sheath holding the device in place. Uniquely, this started the deployment from the middle of the graft, which took less than a second to fully deploy. This prevented the device migrating distally caused by the force of the blood flow, as it was still securely held both proximally and distally to the central axis. The device was pliable and could be successfully positioned in difficult, tortuous aortic arch anatomy. The downside of this device was its lack of radial strength, and the inability to change its position once deployed. Early experience showed that the device could move distally unless the guidewire took the longest course (i.e. the outer diameter of the curve) around the aortic arch. Long-term studies have shown that the metal stent was prone to fracture [8], and the company voluntarily withdrew the device from the commercial market in November 2001. The second generation Gore device, renamed TAG, was made available in Europe in April 2004.

The Talent device consists of polyester secured to a nitinol frame. The thoracic device can be manufactured in diameters of up to 46mm, whereas the Gore Excluder had a maximum diameter of 40mm. The Talent thoracic device has a strong radial force and good column strength. These advantages ensure that it will not move distally on deployment as it is held firmly by the sheath, has good column strength and attains excellent apposition to the native aorta. The Talent device is only available to a maximum of 13cm, which is a disadvantage compared with the Gore Excluder which could reach 20cm in length. The short length of the Talent device is dictated by the friction generated by enclosing the device in a sheath, which causes difficulty in deployment. The device is relatively rigid compared with the Gore Excluder, and will try to straighten along its main axis. This can lead to problems if the thoracic aorta is tortuous. Occasionally, it is necessary to start the deployment of the Talent device in the descending thoracic aorta where the anatomy is relatively straight, before positioning the device more proximally to its definitive position around the arch before fully deploying it. The device sheath may lengthen during deployment in difficult tortuous aortic anatomy. The recommended overlap for the Talent device is half the length of the device, i.e. 5cm. This can mean that multiple devices may have to be used if a long length of aorta is to be covered. Even if adequate overlap is ensured when multiple devices are deployed, they may still become dislocated from each other, leading to a type III

endoleak. The device can be ordered with a bare stent proximally which should ensure a firm fixation. However, this has caused problems, and in one case report, the bare stent ruptured through the aortic arch [9]. Again, long-term studies of the Talent thoracic device have shown that the metal stent can fracture [8]. This can lead to the metal perforating the fabric causing type III endoleaks.

The latest device for the thoracic aorta is the Endofit manufactured by Endomed, which is made from a nitinol stent covered with polytetra-fluoroethylene. This device also has a bare stent proximally and suffers from a lack of column strength so that it can jump back distally after the first two covered stent rings are deployed. Distal migration is particularly encountered in tortuous anatomy when the device needs to be deployed in the distal part of the aortic arch. This migration does not seem to be a problem when the device is deployed in the descending thoracic aorta. The Endofit comes in the form of a cartridge which is loaded into a sheath previously positioned at the deployment site. If the sheath is brought back too far distally, then either the device has to be deployed in this suboptimal position, or the whole assembly has to be withdrawn and another device used. The Endofit device has recently been modified and is now produced without the bare spring. In addition, it is now available on a pre-loaded purpose built sheath.

Cook have developed a stent graft for use in the thoracic aorta. Unlike the other devices, it has barbs to secure it in place and to decrease the chances of migration. The device is similar to the Zenith infrarenal device, being manufactured from stainless steel stents covered with polyester. Anson Medical is also developing thoracic devices and other companies have prototype devices in various stages of development. In particular, Medtronic AVE are developing a successor to the Talent thoracic device.

Mid-term results

Thoracic stent grafts are not immune from the problems found with infrarenal devices. Proximal and distal endoleaks have been reported and can usually be treated by using further devices [8, 10-13]. Excluded aneurysms can decrease in size, but not all do so. An increase in sac size is a cause for concern, and investigations should be performed to identify any endoleak. Type II endoleaks are relatively rare in the thoracic aorta compared with the infrarenal aorta. Proximal and distal migration of the device has been shown in one series [13]. This was associated with dilatation of both the proximal and distal fixation sites. Migration of the graft was associated with kinking of the device, and suggests that column strength may be important in aneurysm exclusion in the mid-term. There is an increasing understanding that endoleaks are device-specific from observations of stent grafts in the infrarenal aorta. It is highly likely that this finding will also apply to thoracic aortic devices.

Problems with thoracic stent grafts

The large size of the current devices and the sheaths required for their use (22-24F) can lead to problems with the access arteries. Rupture of the iliac arteries particularly in women has been reported as has dissection and distal embolisation. All the large series report an incidence of paraplegia and stroke. Instrumentation of the aortic arch may cause loose debris to embolise to the cerebral circulation. Clearly therefore, the smaller and more flexible the device, the lower the likelihood of this occurrence. Intimal damage to the more proximal aorta may convert a type B dissection into a type A with lethal consequences. Deaths have been reported from rupture of the aortic arch during placement of a rigid device, and from massive atheroembolisation causing mesenteric ischaemia.

Future developments

Branched stent grafts are being developed to cope with the aortic arch branches proximally and the visceral and renal arteries distally [14-16]. This may well establish endoluminal treatment for both type A dissections and for thoracoabdominal aneurysms, both of which lie outside the current realm of endovascular repair. Clearly, there is some considerable development required before thoracic devices are perfected. The two main indications for endoluminal treatment at the present time are aneurysms and complicated type B dissection. These two indications have different requirements of stent grafts for successful treatment. Thoracic aneurysms require strong fixation both proximally and distally to the landing zones. Hooks and barbs may be required to prevent proximal and distal migration, which in turn may be related to poor column strength. They may also allow treatment of aneurysms with shorter landing zones than the 2cm currently recommended. Clearly, aneurysms affecting the relatively straight descending thoracic aorta can be treated with a device which is relatively rigid. Those affecting the distal arch require a device which is flexible and which would therefore conform to the tortuous anatomy. Dissections require devices which have a relatively strong fixation proximally, but do not require this distally. Bare stents are to be avoided in dissections, as these may tear the flap so causing further fenestrations between the true and false lumens. Hooks and barbs are also to be avoided in dissections.

One of the most encouraging areas in endoluminal treatment of thoracic aortic pathology is in the treatment of 'mycotic' or infected aneurysms. Reports of successful long-term outcome following stent grafts are increasing in number [17,18]. Theoretically, polytetrafluoroethylene may be more resistant to infection than polyester, but conversely, polyester may bind antibiotics which can be used to flush the device before implantation [18]. Stent grafts have been used to treat false aneurysms related to *Staphylococcus aureus* and salmonella infections. They have also been used to exclude secondary aorto-bronchial fistulas and secondary aorto-oesophageal fistulas following open surgical repair. The low morbidity and mortality associated with endoluminal repair compared with the heroic open surgical alternative may allow stent grafts to attain an important role relatively quickly in this field.

Clearly in time the devices will reduce in size and percutaneous access to the groin vessels will become established. The smaller size will cause less disruption to the access vessels, and a greater degree of flexibility will allow tortuous anatomy to be readily accessed. Devices which are tapered to accommodate differing aortic diameters proximally and distally will be developed. Small diameter stent grafts need to be manufactured to cope with young patients presenting with transection, or aneurysms related to previous coarctation repair [19,20].

Current availability and recommendations

At the time of writing, there is a dearth of decent devices for the thoracic aorta. The Gore Excluder has been withdrawn, and its successor, the TAG, was launched in Europe in April 2004. Cook have just made available the TX-1 one piece device in a range of sizes from 22-42mm in diameter and up to 231mm in length. The extensions are 80mm in length. The Cook TX-2 two piece device (variable length), although CE marked, is not yet available and is awaiting the release of a new sheath and valve.

The other available devices for the treatment of thoracic aneurysms are the Talent and the Endofit thoracic stents. The Talent device is relatively rigid and is suitable for aneurysms of the descending aorta. There are problems in deploying this device around the aortic arch, and its short length means that multiple devices frequently have to be used. The rigidity does not make it useful for tortuous anatomy, and it may cause overlapping devices to dislocate resulting in type III endoleaks. The Endofit thoracic stent graft also has some drawbacks. It lacks column strength, and is therefore liable to migrate distally on deployment, particularly around the aortic arch. The device does not come with its own sheath, so that once the cartridge is loaded into the sheath, further advancement of the device more proximally cannot be undertaken safely. The sheath may damage the intima of the proximal aorta in acute dissections with the theoretical risk of converting a type B dissection into a type A. The bare proximal stent does not seem to be strong enough to anchor the device firmly in position, and again may cause damage to the intima in dissections. The device can be ordered without the bare proximal stent if so desired. Endomed have taken note of these problems and have recently made available their improved device (pre-loaded within a sheath and no proximal bare metal stent). Experience with this modified device is awaited.

Summary

♦ Endoluminal treatment is mainly used for aneurysms of the distal aortic arch and the descending thoracic aorta and for complicated type B dissection.

♦ Aneurysms and dissections probably require different types of endoluminal devices for successful treatment.

♦ Two stent grafts, the Talent and the Endofit, are widely available for the thoracic aorta, but neither is ideal.

♦ The Gore TAG device was launched in Europe in April 2004 and the Cook TX-1 one piece device is also now available.

♦ Branched stent grafts will become available which will allow the treatment of type A dissections and thoracoabdominal aneurysms.

♦ Encouraging results have been reported from endoluminal treatment of infected or 'mycotic' aneurysms.

♦ The development of small, flexible devices should allow the procedure to be performed percutaneously.

♦ Fixation with hooks and barbs may allow aneurysms to be treated with shorter landing zones.

References

1. Parodi JC, Palmaz JC, Barone HD. Transfemoral intraluminal graft implantation for abdominal aortic aneurysms. *Ann Vasc Surg* 1991; 5: 491-9.

2. Volodos NL, Shekhanin VE, Karpovich IP, *et al.* A self-fixing synthetic blood vessel endoprosthesis. *Vestnik Khirurgii Imeni i - i - Grekova* 1986; 137:123-5.

3. Volodos NL, Karpovich IP, Shekhanin VE, *et al.* A case of distant transfemoral endoprosthesis of the thoracic artery using a self-fixing synthetic prosthesis in traumatic aneurysm. *Grudnaia Khirurgiia* 1988; 6: 84-6.

4. Volodos NL, Karpovich IP, Troyan VI, *et al.* Clinical experience of the use of self-fixing synthetic prostheses for remote endoprosthetics of the thoracic and the abdominal aorta and iliac arteries through the femoral artery and as intraoperative endoprosthesis for aorta reconstruction. *Vasa* - Supplementum. 1991; 33: 93-5.

5. Dake MD, Miller DC, Semba CP, *et al.* Transluminal placement of endovascular stent-grafts for the treatment of descending thoracic aortic aneurysms. *N Engl J Med* 1994; 331: 1729-34.

6. Dake MD, Miller DC, Mitchell RS, *et al.* The 'first generation' of endovascular stent-grafts for patients with aneurysms of the descending thoracic aorta. *J Thorac Cardiovasc Surg* 1998; 116: 689-703.

7. Dake MD, Kato N, Mitchell RS, *et al.* Endovascular stent-graft placement for the treatment of acute aortic dissection. *N Engl J Med* 1999; 340: 1546-52.

8. Ellozy SH, Carroccio A, Minor M, *et al.* Challenges of endovascular tube graft repair of thoracic aortic aneurysm: midterm follow-up and lessons learned. *J Vasc Surg* 2003; 38: 676-83.

9. Malina M, Brunkwall J, Ivancev K, *et al.* Late aortic arch perforation by graft-anchoring stent: complication of endovascular thoracic aneurysm exclusion. *J Endovasc Surg* 1998; 5: 274-7.

10. Orend KH, Scharrer-Pamler R, Kapfer X, *et al.* Endovascular treatment in diseases of the descending thoracic aorta: 6-year results of a single center. *J Vasc Surg* 2003; 37: 91-9.

11. Bell RE, Taylor PR, Aukett M, *et al.* Mid-term results for second-generation thoracic stent grafts. *Br J Surg* 2003: 90: 811-817.

12. Criado FJ, Clark NS, Barnatan MF. Stent graft repair in the aortic arch and descending thoracic aorta: a 4-year experience. *J Vasc Surg* 2002; 36: 1121-8.

13. Resch T, Koul B, Dias NV, *et al.* Changes in aneurysm morphology and stent-graft configuration after endovascular repair of aneurysms of the descending thoracic aorta. *J Thorac Cardiovasc Surg* 2001; 122:47-52.

14. Chuter TA, Gordon RL, Reilly LM, *et al.* Multi-branched stent-graft for type III thoracoabdominal aneurysm. *J Vasc Intervent Radiol* 2001; 12: 391-392.

15. Inoue K, Hosokawa H, Iwase T, *et al.* Aortic arch reconstruction by transluminally placed endovascular branched stent graft. *Circulation* 1999; 100 (suppl 19): II 316-321.

16. Chuter TAM, Schneider DB, Reilly LM, *et al.* Modular branched stent graft for endovascular repair of aortic arch aneurysm and dissection. *J Vasc Surg* 2003: 38: 859-863.

17. Bell RE, Taylor PR, Aukett M, *et al.* Results of urgent and emergency thoracic procedures treated by endoluminal repair. *Eur J Vasc Endovasc Surg* 2003; 25; 527-531.

18. Stanley BM, Semmens JB, Lawrence-Brown MMD, *et al.* Endoluminal Repair of Mycotic Thoracic Aneurysms. *J Endovasc Ther* 2003; 10: 511-515.

19. Bell RE, Taylor PR, Aukett M, *et al.* Endoluminal repair of aneurysms associated with coarctation. *Ann Thorac Surg* 2003; 75: 530-533.

20. Taylor PR, Bell RE, Reidy JF. Aortic transection due to blunt trauma: evolving management using endoluminal techniques. *IJCP* 2003; 57: 652.

Chapter 10

The prevention of paraplegia during endovascular thoracic aneurysm repair

Geert Willem H Schurink, MD PhD, Consultant Vascular Surgeon

Michiel H de Haan, MD PhD, Consultant Radiologist

Michael J Jacobs, MD PhD, Consultant Vascular Surgeon & Professor of Surgery

University Hospital Maastricht, Maastricht, the Netherlands

Introduction

Paraplegia is the most devastating complication in the treatment of diseases of the thoracic aorta. Due to several changes in approach and technique, the paraplegia rate in open thoracic and thoraco-abdominal aortic repair has declined in recent years.

Although endovascular repair of the thoracic aorta is an exciting technique, with a lot of potential benefit for the patient, paraplegia remains a problem. Nevertheless, by careful patient selection and by the implementation of techniques learnt from open repair, paraplegia rates after endovascular repair can be kept to a minimum.

Spinal cord vascularisation

The spinal cord circulation is formed by a single anterior and two posterior spinal arteries. The anterior spinal artery supplies up to 75% of the spinal cord, including the dorsal horn grey matter and the corticospinal tracts. The posterior spinal arteries supply the dorsal columns and the head of the posterior horns. The anterior spinal artery originates from both vertebral arteries.

In the middle or lower thoracic region of the spinal cord, the diameter of the anterior spinal artery decreases in most cases. In some cases, the anterior spinal artery has been described as anatomically and functionally discontinuous. The diameter of the anterior spinal artery just proximal to the anastomotic point of the arteria radicularis magna is small, whereas distally it is relatively wide.

The anterior spinal artery can receive blood supply from approximately 25 pairs of segmental arteries that arise from the aorta. In healthy individuals, in the cervical and upper thoracic regions, the anterior spinal artery is supplied by multiple branches of both vertebral and several radicular arteries. Usually one radicular artery provides the mid-thoracic spinal cord, with three to five supplying the anterior spinal artery in the lower thoracic and lumbar area.

The arteria radicularis magna is the major radicular artery supplying the thoracolumbar spinal cord (artery of Adamkiewicz) and usually arises between T8-12. In 10% of the cases it can arise between L1-2, but occasionally this artery can originate from any of the other segments between T5 and L5 (Figure 1).

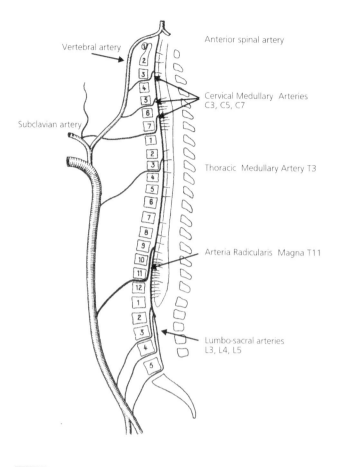

Figure 1. Representation of anterior spinal artery and feeding segmental arteries (from: Strategies to protect the spinal cord during thoraco-abdominal aortic aneurysm repair, SAG Meylaerts, 2000, Thesis, University of Amsterdam.)

During the advancement of chronic aortic disease, a number of collateral pathways can develop when segmental ostia become occluded. These collateral channels can form in a number of ways. Not only do segmental arteries develop connections in the muscles along the vertebral column, but they can also form anastomoses between the anterior and posterior spinal arteries. The third collateral system is dependent on the branches of the internal iliac arteries.

Paraplegia prevention in open surgery

The extent of the diseased aortic segment determines the risk of paraplegia following open surgical repair. The Crawford classification describes type I, II, III and IV thoraco-abdominal aortic aneurysms, according to their anatomical extent. Inevitably, the most extensive type (II) carries the highest risk of paraplegia.

In addition to the extent of the aneurysm, other factors can influence the neurological outcome of open aortic repair. In the surgical treatment of thoracic aortic aneurysms, there is substantial evidence that continued distal aortic perfusion during thoracic aortic cross-clamping can significantly reduce neurological deficits during the perioperative period [1]. With the use of distal aortic perfusion, the paraplegia rate following open repair of thoracic aortic aneurysms varies from 0-6 % [2].

Neurological deficit following thoraco-abdominal aortic aneurysm repair reflects a different disease entity. For example, in type II aneurysms the incidence of paraplegia rises to 30% without adjunctive procedures, but can be reduced to 10%-15% with additional distal aortic perfusion and spinal fluid drainage techniques [3, 4].

The incidence of paraplegia increases significantly after emergency surgery for acute dissections. The main cause for this increased risk is poor aortic wall quality, and difficulty with reattachment of the intercostal arteries during the procedure. This results in spinal cord ischaemia and leads to neurological deficit in 16%-56% [5].

Chronic descending aortic dissection is treated according to the same general guidelines as for descending aortic aneurysms. The results with respect to neurological deficit are comparable.

Disturbance to the anatomy of the intercostal and lumbar arteries in thoracic and thoraco-abdominal aneurysms has a major impact on spinal cord blood supply. In our experience, the mean number of patent segmental arteries along the entire thoracic and abdominal aorta was only three in type I and seven in type II aneurysms. This indicates that, in the absence

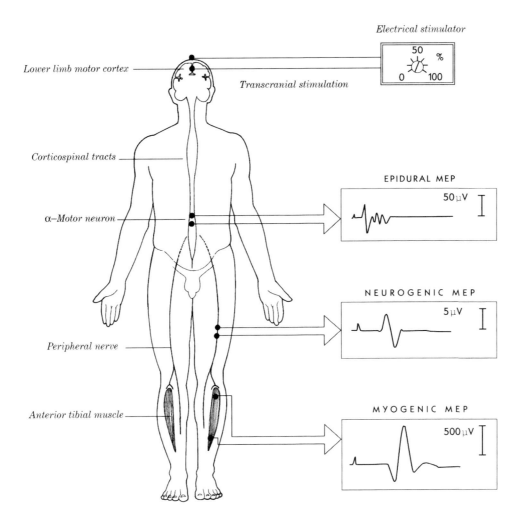

Figure 2. Schematic representation of monitoring motor evoked potentials. *Reproduced with permission from Futura, Blackwell Publishing Ltd. Evoked potential monitoring to assess spinal cord ischemia during TAAA repair. In: Surgical and endovascular treatment of aortic aneurysms. Branchereau A, Jacobs M, Eds.*

of the arteria radicularis magna or other radiculomedullary arteries, collateral circulation is extremely important in feeding the anterior spinal artery [6].

Monitoring spinal cord motor evoked potentials can provide evidence that a substantial part of the spinal collateral blood supply is provided by the iliac and lumbar arteries arising between L3 and L5. These crucial networks are not involved in thoracic aortic aneurysms and during cross-clamping with distal aortic perfusion, they remain a major source of spinal blood supply. This is likely to explain the significantly lower rates of neurological complications noted after descending thoracic aortic repair.

Motor evoked potentials (MEPs) reflect spinal cord motor function and motor tract blood supply (Figure 2) and can be elicited by electrical or magnetical transcranial stimulation (tc-MEPs). Compound muscle action potentials are recorded from the skin over the left and right anterior tibial muscles and from the skin over the left and right thenar muscles. Baseline tc-MEPs are measured every five minutes until the aorta is cross-clamped and every minute during and after cross-clamping. A reduction of tc-MEPs amplitude of the tibial anterior muscle to less than 25% of baseline, during or after the aortic cross-clamp period, is considered an indication of ischaemic spinal cord dysfunction.

If MEPs decrease below 25% during surgery, the mean distal aortic pressure can be raised above 60mmHg in order to regain adequate MEP amplitudes and preserve spinal cord perfusion. If this is not successful, more extensive intercostal or lumbar artery reattachment can be performed. Additional techniques include aortic endarterectomy and selective bypasses to previously occluded intercostal arteries, until MEPs return to normal. Using this protocol, the paraplegic rate in our unit is 2.4% following major thoraco-abdominal aortic surgery [7].

Risk for paraplegia

The endovascular treatment of thoracic aortic pathology is a promising technique. Obvious advantages over the open repair are the absence of a thoracotomy, aortic cross-clamping and distal aortic perfusion techniques. This should result in a more rapid recovery of the patient. Disadvantages include the inability to reattach intercostal arteries into the aortic graft. Thus, coverage of the lower intercostal arteries (Th8-Th12) is a potential risk for disturbing spinal cord blood supply and can lead to paraplegia. However, several publications report on uncomplicated coverage of the Th8-Th12 aortic section [8, 9], although covering an extensive part of the thoracic aorta is mentioned as a risk factor for paraplegia [10-12]. Conversion to open repair is also an event associated with an increased paraplegia rate [10, 11, 13].

As previously mentioned, in patients with a diseased aorta, the spinal cord blood supply frequently depends on a collateral circulation. Theoretically, therefore, occlusion of vertebral, proximal intercostal, lumbar and hypogastric arteries can lead to paraplegia.

In addition, pathology of the infrarenal aorta has been recognised as a potential risk for paraplegia after endovascular treatment of the thoracic aorta.

Both co-existing abdominal aortic aneurysm (AAA) and prior repair of an AAA are associated with an increased risk of paraplegia following endovascular repair of the thoracic aorta [13-15].

Paraplegia has been reported in significant numbers in cases with concomitant endovascular repair of a thoracic aortic aneurysm and open repair of an AAA [13-16]. The largest series is from Stanford University and reports 103 patients treated for descending thoracic aortic aneurysms (TAAs) [15]. Within this group, 19 patients underwent simultaneous open repair of their abdominal aortic aneurysm. The most striking difference between the group with isolated TAA treatment and the group with the concomitant treatment of AAA and TAA was the difference in paraplegia rate. Two of the 19 patients (11%) suffered early paraplegia in contrast to one case of paraplegia in the remaining 84 patients (1%). This last patient had undergone aortic aneurysm repair in the past. Nevertheless, the paraplegia rate in the Stanford experience for concomitant repair of abdominal and descending thoracic aortic aneurysms is 11%. This is considerably higher than the figure of 0-6% reported for open repair of the thoracic aorta, but compares to the 10-15% paraplegia rate of thoraco-abdominal aortic repair, with the use of distal aortic perfusion and cerebrospinal fluid (CSF) drainage.

Prevention of paraplegia during endovascular repair

The first step in the prevention of paraplegia is the selection of the patients at risk. For this subgroup, the threshold for treating the thoracic aortic disease should be higher than for the low-risk group. For those patients deemed unsuitable for endovascular treatment, open repair with reattachment of intercostal arteries should be considered. For the patients who undergo endovascular treatment, several adjunctive measures can be taken.

Cerebrospinal fluid (CSF) drainage is widely used in open thoraco-abdominal aortic aneurysm repair. Although, during endovascular treatment, CSF drainage is mainly used after the paraplegia has occurred, it has been advised during procedures

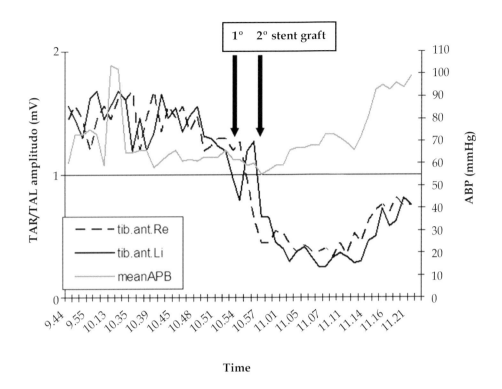

Figure 3. Registration of motor evoked potentials during endovascular treatment of a descending TAA. Amplitudes of right and left anterior tibial muscle (TAR/TAL amplitudo) decrease after stent graft deployment and partially return after elevation of the mean arterial blood pressure (ABP).

involving stenting of an extensive length of the thoracic aorta [12], and for concomitant endovascular thoracic and open abdominal aortic repair [13]. The latter group also undergoes a period of aortic cross-clamping, potentially causing an even more severe initial spinal cord ischaemia, as well as adding an element of reperfusion to the ischaemic insult.

During thoracic endovascular procedures, spinal cord function tests such as the measurement of motor evoked potentials can be performed. Although attempted in 'home-made' devices [17, 18], not one of the commercially available devices is retrievable. Should MEP registration show impaired spinal cord function after stent graft deployment, blood pressure elevation is the first step in trying to restore spinal cord perfusion. Figure 3 illustrates a case of a 72-year-old male with a mid-thoracic aortic aneurysm and a juxtarenal abdominal aortic aneurysm. The juxtarenal aneurysm was treated by an open insertion of a tube

graft. The thoracic aneurysm was treated endovascularly in a second operation. During this procedure, MEP registration of the lower legs showed a significant drop after stent graft deployment (30% of initial amplitude) and returned to 50% after blood pressure elevation. A CSF drainage catheter was left for three days. No clinical signs of paraplegia developed. If blood pressure regulation does not have the desired effect, conversion to open repair, removal of the stent graft and intercostal artery reattachment is the only chance to improve spinal cord perfusion and subsequent function [19].

MEP monitoring during temporary balloon exclusion of the thoracic aneurysm with axillofemoral bypass (as distal aortic perfusion) could be a way to predict the spinal cord function outcome in these patients [20, 21]. This could enable the stent graft placement to be abandoned in the presence of inevitable spinal cord ischaemia.

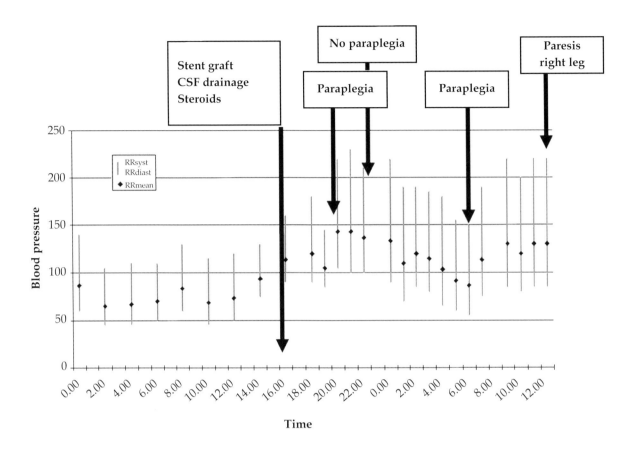

Figure 4. Blood pressure registration after endovascular treatment of a ruptured type B aortic dissection. Paraplegia develops four hours after stent graft treatment and resolves after elevation of blood pressure. A second period of paraplegia occurs after blood pressure decrease, with partial recovery.

Other methods generally used in open thoraco-abdominal aneurysm repair, such as the administration of steroids, could also reduce paraplegia risk in the endovascular repair of descending thoracic aneurysms. Our protocol for distal descending TAAs (Th8-Th12) mirrors our open TAAA protocol, including preoperative installation of CSF drainage and administration of steroids. In addition, spinal cord function control by the measurement of the motor evoked potentials (MEP) is performed.

Salvage post-paraplegia

In most cases, paraplegia after endovascular treatment of the thoracic aorta is not apparent directly after the operation. Only in cases with intra-operative complications and conversion to open repair is early paraplegia described [11, 14, 15]. By far most cases of paraplegia develop in the postoperative period [12-14, 16, 22-24]. This period varies between four hours and ten weeks. Postoperative periods of hypotension have been described as a cause for the delayed paraplegia seen after both open [25] and endovascular repair of the thoracic aorta [16].

Following the development of postoperative paraplegia, conversion to open repair with reattachment of the intercostal arteries is the last available option. As mentioned above, CSF drainage has been described in endovascular TAA cases in an attempt to reverse paraplegia [12,13,23,24,26,27]. Nevertheless, in some cases, elevated CSF pressure up to 45mmHg has been described [24, 26]. This is probably the result of reperfusion of the spinal cord.

Blood pressure management can also alter the outcome following the development of paraplegia. For example, a patient with a low thoracic aortic rupture of an acute type B dissection was treated endovascularly using local anesthesia. The thoracic aorta was covered from the subclavian artery down to the level of Th12. In addition, the patient underwent preoperative CSF drainage and steroid administration. Four hours after successful stent graft placement, the patient developed a dense bilateral lower limb paraplegia. His mean blood pressure was raised to 160mmHg, resulting in complete resolution of his paraplegia. Unfortunately, during the night, a period of relative hypotension again resulted in bilateral paraplegia. On this occasion, blood pressure elevation only resulted in partial resolution (Figure 4).

Summary

◆ The risk of paraplegia after the endovascular treatment of thoracic aortic aneurysms is similar to that seen following open repair using distal aortic perfusion and CSF drainage techniques.

◆ For patients with low risk of spinal cord ischaemia, the reflected paraplegia risk is low (approximately 1%).

◆ For patients with a distorted spinal cord collateral circulation, the paraplegia risk compares to that of open thoraco-abdominal repair (approximately 10%).

◆ Adjunctive measures, like perioperative CSF drainage and blood pressure control can improve outcome.

◆ Postoperative blood pressure control can prevent delayed paraplegia.

◆ The use of motor evoked potentials during stent graft placement can help to evaluate the need for the adjunctive measures and can influence the timing for conversion to open repair with intercostal artery reattachment.

◆ The future may be a combination of spinal cord function monitoring with retrievable stent grafts. However, no commercially available retrievable devices have yet been produced.

References

1. Safi HJ, Subramaniam MH, Miller CC, *et al*. Progress in the management of type I thoracoabdominal and descending thoracic aortic aneurysms. *Ann Vasc Surg* 1999; 13(5): 457-62.

2. Jacobs M, Elenbaas T, Schurink GW, de Mol B, Mochtar B. Complications of descending thoracic aortic surgery. In: *Complications in vascular and endovascular surgery (part I)*. Branchereau A, Jacobs M, Eds. Futura Publishing Company Inc, 2001: 201-9.

3. Schepens MA, Vermeulen FE, Morshuis WJ, *et al*. Impact of left heart bypass on the results of thoracoabdominal aortic aneurysm repair. *Ann Thorac Surg* 1999; 67(6): 1963-7; discussion 1979-80.

4. Coselli JS, Lemaire SA, Koksoy C, Schmittling ZC, Curling PE. Cerebrospinal fluid drainage reduces paraplegia after thoracoabdominal aortic aneurysm repair: results of a randomized clinical trial. *J Vasc Surg* 2002; 35(4): 631-9.

5. Panneton JM, Hollier LH. Dissecting descending thoracic and thoracoabdominal aortic aneurysms: Part II. *Ann Vasc Surg* 1995; 9(6): 596-605.

6. Jacobs MJ, Meylaerts SA, de Haan P, de Mol BA, Kalkman CJ. Strategies to prevent neurologic deficit based on motor-evoked potentials in type I and II thoracoabdominal aortic aneurysm repair. *J Vasc Surg* 1999; 29(1): 48-57; discussion 57-9.

7. Jacobs MJ, Elenbaas TW, Schurink GW, Mess WH, Mochtar B. Assessment of spinal cord integrity during thoraco-abdominal aortic aneurysm repair. *Ann Thorac Surg* 2002; 74(5): S1864-6; discussion S1892-8.

8. Heijmen RH, Deblier IG, Moll FL, *et al*. Endovascular stent-grafting for descending thoracic aortic aneurysms. *Eur J Cardiothorac* Surg 2002; 21(1): 5-9.

9. Lambrechts D, Casselman F, Schroeyers P, De Geest R, D'Haenens P, Degrieck I. Endovascular treatment of the descending thoracic aorta. *Eur J Vasc Endovasc Surg* 2003; 26(4): 437-44.

10. Carroccio A, Marin ML, Ellozy S, Hollier LH. Pathophysiology of paraplegia following endovascular thoracic aortic aneurysm repair. *J Card Surg* 2003;18(4): 359-66.

11. Greenberg R, Resch T, Nyman U, *et al*. Endovascular repair of descending thoracic aortic aneurysms: an early experience with intermediate-term follow-up. *J Vasc Surg* 2000; 3 1(1 Pt 1): 147-56.

12. Tiesenhausen K, Amann W, Koch G, Hausegger KA, Oberwalder P, Rigler B. Cerebrospinal fluid drainage to reverse paraplegia after endovascular thoracic aortic aneurysm repair. *J Endovasc Ther* 2000; 7(2): 132-5.

13. Gravereaux EC, Faries PL, Burks JA, *et al*. Risk of spinal cord ischemia after endograft repair of thoracic aortic aneurysms. *J Vasc Surg* 2001; 34(6): 997-1003.

14. Bell RE, Taylor PR, Aukett M, Sabharwal T, Reidy JF. Mid-term results for second-generation thoracic stent grafts. *Br J Surg* 2003; 90(7): 811-7.

15. Dake MD, Miller DC, Mitchell RS, Semba CP, Moore KA, Sakai T. The 'first generation' of endovascular stent-grafts for patients with aneurysms of the descending thoracic aorta. *J Thorac Cardiovasc Surg* 1998; 116(5): 689-703; discussion 703-4.

16. Kasirajan K, Dolmatch B, Ouriel K, Clair D. Delayed onset of ascending paralysis after thoracic aortic stent graft deployment. *J Vasc Surg* 2000; 31(1 Pt 1): 196-9.

17. Ishimaru S, Kawaguchi S, Koizumi N, Obitsu Y, Ishikawa M. Preliminary report on prediction of spinal cord ischemia in endovascular stent graft repair of thoracic aortic aneurysm by retrievable stent graft. *J Thorac Cardiovasc Surg* 1998; 115(4): 811-8.

18. Watanabe Y, Ishimaru S, Kawaguchi S, *et al*. Successful endografting with simultaneous visceral artery bypass grafting for severely calcified thoracoabdominal aortic aneurysm. *J Vasc Surg* 2002; 35(2): 397-9.

19. Reichart M, Balm R, Meilof JF, de Haan P, Reekers JA, Jacobs MJ. Ischemic transverse myelopathy after endovascular repair of a thoracic aortic aneurysm. *J Endovasc Ther* 2001; 8(3): 321-7.

20. Midorikawa H, Hoshino S, Iwaya F, Igari T, Satou K, Ishikawa K. Prevention of paraplegia in transluminally placed endoluminal prosthetic grafts for descending thoracic aortic aneurysms. *Jpn J Thorac Cardiovasc Surg* 2000; 48(12): 761-8.

21. Bafort C, Astarci P, Goffette P, *et al*. Predicting spinal cord ischemia before endovascular thoracoabdominal aneurysm repair: monitoring somatosensory evoked potentials. *J Endovasc Ther* 2002; 9(3): 289-94.

22. Chuter TA, Gordon RL, Reilly LM, Pak LK, Messina LM. Multi-branched stent-graft for type III thoracoabdominal aortic aneurysm. *J Vasc Intervent Radiol* 2001; 12(3): 391-2.

23. Fleck T, Hutschala D, Weissl M, Wolner E, Grabenwoger M. Cerebrospinal fluid drainage as a useful treatment option to relieve paraplegia after stent-graft implantation for acute aortic dissection type B. *J Thorac Cardiovasc Surg* 2002; 123(5): 1003-5.

24. Hutschala D, Fleck T, Czerny M, *et al*. Endoluminal stent-graft placement in patients with acute aortic dissection type B. *Eur J Cardiothorac Surg* 2002; 21(6): 964-9.

25. Maniar HS, Sundt TM, 3rd, Prasad SM, *et al*. Delayed paraplegia after thoracic and thoracoabdominal aneurysm repair: a continuing risk. *Ann Thorac Surg* 2003; 75(1): 113-9; discussions 119-20.

26. Fuchs RJ, Lee WA, Seubert CN, Gelman S. Transient paraplegia after stent grafting of a descending thoracic aortic aneurysm treated with cerebrospinal fluid drainage. *J Clin Anesth* 2003; 15(1): 59-63.

27. Oberwalder PJ, Tiesenhausen K, Hausegger K, Rigler B. Successful reversal of delayed paraplegia after endovascular stent grafting. *J Thorac Cardiovasc Surg* 2002; 124(6): 1259-60; author reply 1260.

Chapter 11

Stent grafts for dissections: indications and results

Robert Morgan, MRCP FRCR, Consultant Radiologist

St. George's Hospital, London, UK

Introduction

Aortic dissection is a major clinical emergency with an incidence of 20 cases per million population per year [1]. Hypertension as a major precipitating factor is present in 70-90% of cases. There is a male: female preponderance of 3:1, and most dissections occur between the ages of 40 and 70 years of age [2]. The other main causes of aortic dissection are cystic medial necrosis which occurs in Marfan's and Ehler's Danlos syndrome, pregnancy, atherosclerosis and trauma. Dissections may complicate acute aortic ulcers and intramural haematoma and there is speculation that these three pathological entities form a clinical spectrum of disease of the aortic wall. Without treatment, the mortality at 48 hours is 36-72%, and 62-91% of patients die within one week [3].

For years, the main method of treatment of dissections has been the aggressive control of blood pressure, with surgery reserved for dissections involving the ascending aorta and complications arising from the dissection. However, surgical treatment of thoracic aortic dissection is a major undertaking and its use has generally been limited to the relatively small number of patients with favourable cardiorespiratory status who are able to withstand the surgical assault. There are also a variety of minimally invasive interventional techniques available to treat complications of aortic dissection. These include the insertion of metallic stents for branch vessel ischaemia, metallic stenting of the true lumen to counteract true lumen compression and various methods to create a communication or fenestration between the true and the false lumen to equalize the pressure between the two lumens. However, the availability of these radiological techniques varies depending on local personnel and expertise.

The development of stent grafts for placement in the thoracic aorta has led to their use in aortic dissection with encouraging results. Thus, patients can be treated without the need for open thoracic and abdominal surgery with the potential for reduced procedural mortality and morbidity. This enables patients to be treated by endovascular methods who would generally not be considered for conventional surgery because of their comorbidity. Most interventions are performed in patients with acute dissections. Stent grafts may also be indicated in the setting of chronic dissection when there is aneurysm formation. The aim of this chapter is to provide an overview of the current status of stent grafting in patients with aortic dissection.

Pathophysiology

Aortic dissection results from a tear in the intima, which leads to blood entering the media through the tear and splitting the layers of the media. This gives rise to separation of the intima from the adventitial layer which results in an intimal flap, a false lumen and a true lumen. The dissection may be focal or may extend distally or proximally (or both) from the site of the initial intimal tear.

The wall of the false lumen is relatively thin and is at a higher risk of rupture compared with the normal aortic wall. The thin wall of the false lumen is also prone to aneurysmal dilatation over time. Rupture or aneurysmal dilatation of the false lumen occurs in 20-50% of patients managed conservatively within five years of the dissection [2].

Another potential complication of dissection is ischaemia of branch vessels arising from the aorta (eg. coeliac artery, renal artery, iliac artery). This may occur through two processes. Static obstruction occurs when the dissection flap extends into the vessel. This results in the false lumen ending in a blind sac which may obstruct the true lumen and result in organ ischaemia. The other method of branch vessel ischaemia is dynamic obstruction. This occurs when the dissection does not extend into the branch, but the origin of the branch (usually supplied by the true lumen) is compromised by compression of the aortic true lumen by the false lumen [4]. True lumen compression occurs when the pressure in the false lumen is higher than the true lumen and usually occurs when there is no large distal fenestration to relieve the high pressure in the false lumen.

Classification

Previously, aortic dissections were categorised using the DeBakey classification. This classification divides dissections involving the ascending aorta into those involving the entire aorta (type I) and those involving the ascending aorta alone (type II), with dissections restricted to the descending aorta classified as type III dissections. However, the DeBakey classification has largely been superseded by the Stanford classification which divides aortic dissections into those which involve the ascending aorta and proximal aortic arch and are referred to as type A dissections (60-70% of all dissections); and those which involve the aorta distal to the left subclavian artery, which are called type B dissections (30-40% of dissections) [5].

Dissections can also be classified according to their age: acute when less than 14 days, subacute from 14 days to two months, and chronic when older than two months [6].

The major determinant of mortality is whether the dissection involves the ascending aorta and aortic arch. In this situation, there is a major risk of retrograde dissection to the aortic valve which may result in acute aortic valve regurgitation, pericardial effusion leading to tamponade and extension of the dissection into the coronary arteries. For this reason, the standard treatment for type A dissections is surgery which has a mortality of up to 30%. The mortality of conservative management of dissections involving the aorta distal to the aortic arch is around 20%, while the surgical mortality for type B dissections is around 35%. This difference in mortality rates for conservative and surgical therapy between the two types of dissection has resulted in the current standard management strategy of surgery for patients with type A dissections, and conservative management (based on the control of blood pressure), for patients with uncomplicated type B dissections [5].

Until recently, patients with complications associated with type B dissection have also been treated by surgery or by one of the variety of endovascular methods such as fenestration mentioned earlier. However, there is increasing enthusiasm for the use of stent grafts in patients with contained rupture, aneurysm formation, branch vessel ischaemia and continuing pain.

Treatment with stent grafts

Thoracic stent grafts were initially developed for the treatment of aneurysmal disease. In 1999, two papers on the use of stent grafts in aortic dissection appeared in the same issue of the *New England*

Journal of Medicine in 1999[7,8] and stimulated interventionalists to expand the indications for thoracic stent grafting to aortic dissection.

The main rationale in using a stent to treat an aortic dissection is to cover the main entry tear and, as a result, to substantially reduce the pressure in the false lumen. This may have several effects:-

♦ the risk of rupture of the wall of the false lumen may be reduced;
♦ the risk of aneurysm formation may be reduced; and
♦ branch vessel ischaemia caused by dynamic and to a lesser extent, static obstruction by the dissection flap may be relieved.

The use of stent grafts to treat complicated aortic dissection is limited to type B dissections. Some dissections which seem to extend to the proximal aortic arch or even the ascending aorta may in fact have the main entry tear distal to the left subclavian artery and no further tear proximally. These types of dissections may also be treated by stent grafts. There are reports of the use of branched stent grafts in the aortic arch [9]. However, the design and deployment of branched devices is technically challenging and research in this area remains ongoing. For practical purposes, type A dissections are not amenable to treatment with currently available devices.

Current indications for stent grafts in aortic dissection

♦ Contained rupture. This group of patients is at high risk of a further, possibly catastrophic leak and should be treated as soon as possible.
♦ Aneurysm formation. This is usually a late sequela of aortic dissection. Similar to the approach to atherosclerotic aneurysms, the size threshold for treatment is above 5.5cm or 6cm.
♦ The treatment of end-organ ischaemia.
♦ Persistent back pain signifying ongoing dissection.
♦ Inability to control blood pressure in a patient with an acute dissection.

♦ Prophylaxis. This latter indication is controversial. It is possible that placing a stent graft across the main tear at presentation may reduce or prevent complications such as aneurysm formation and rupture in the long-term. There are a number of studies currently in progress looking at this issue.

Stent graft types

There are several makes of stent graft available for use in Europe at the current time:-

♦ Talent stent graft (Medtronic, Santa Rosa, CA, USA). This device comprises thin-wall polyester graft material with an external skeleton of nitinol stents. The device has a bare spring at the upper end and is available in non-tapered and slightly tapered versions. The device is contained in a delivery system which utilises a pull-back method of deployment. The delivery sheath is moderately flexible and is 22-25 French depending on the diameter of the stent graft. The device is available in 22-46mm diameter and 13cm length.
♦ The Thoracic Excluder (W.L. Gore, Flagstaff, AZ, USA) is constructed of PTFE graft material and nitinol stents. The delivery system utilises a drawstring system of release. It is available up to 20cm in length and up to 40mm diameter. The device was withdrawn in 2002 because of reports of several stent fractures and has recently been relaunched with several modifications.
♦ The Cook Thoracic stent graft (William Cook Europe, Bjaeverskov, Denmark) is a relatively new device and is similar to the Zenith abdominal device in that it consists of a series of stainless steel Gianturco stents and polyester graft material. The upper end of the device contains barbs to aid fixation. This latter feature makes the device less suited to the treatment of aortic dissection because of the potential risk of causing a tear of the thin flap by the barbs.
♦ The Endofit stent graft (Endomed, Phoenix, AZ, USA) is a relatively new device which consists of a nitinol stent and ePTFE graft material in a sutureless design. The first generation device has recently been modified and results of the use of this device in clinical practice are awaited.

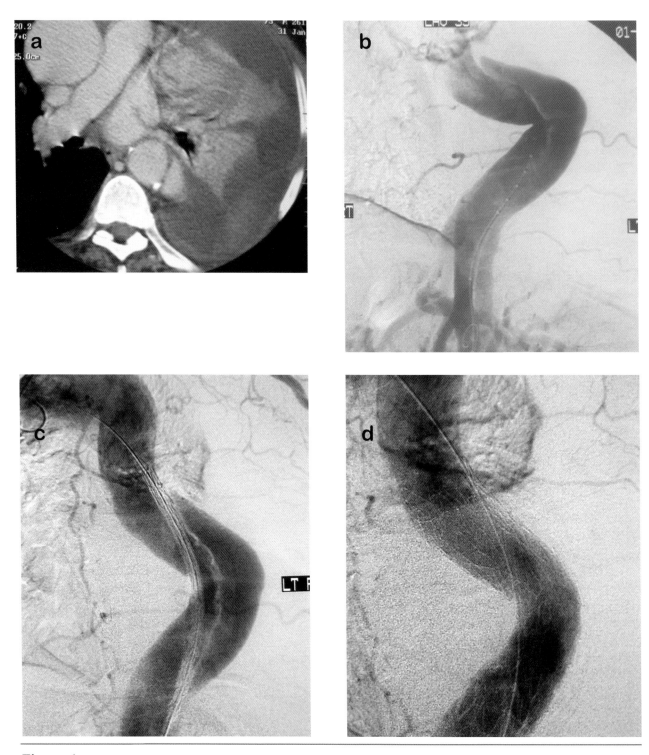

Figure 1. a) A 79-year-old man presented with back pain of four days duration and shortness of breath. The CT scan showed an aortic dissection and a left haemothorax consistent with a contained rupture. b) This thoracic aortogram confirms the presence of a type B aortic dissection with the main entry tear in the mid descending thoracic aorta. c) and d) The entry tear was covered by a single Gore Excluder stent graft. The patient remains well three years later.

Imaging prior to stent grafting

The aims of imaging are to diagnose the presence of aortic dissection, to distinguish between type A and B dissection, to assess for the presence of complications of dissection and finally, to evaluate for the suitability for endovascular therapy. The main imaging methods used to achieve the above are CT and MR. Angiography and transoesophageal echocardiography are also useful but these more invasive tests are generally performed when either CT or MR are unable to provide all of the diagnostic information required. If state of the art machines are available, there is little to choose between the two modalities for imaging of the thoracic aorta. An exhaustive discussion of the imaging of aortic dissection is outside the scope of this chapter. The discussion will be confined to the evaluation for suitability for stenting.

The main entry tear can be easily visualised with thin section CT and MR. It is usually possible to see the main entry tear on the axial images, although reconstructed images in the sagittal oblique plane may often be very helpful. In the majority of cases, there is usually a single main entry tear in the thoracic aorta (Figure 1), although there may be more than one. The main tear is often located just distal to the origin of the left subclavian artery (Figure 2). However, this is by no means invariable and the main tear may be in the mid or distal descending thoracic aorta (Figure 3). There are usually natural fenestrations between the true and false lumen at the levels of the origins of the intercostals vessels, although these are usually small and do not contribute significant flow between the two lumens. Below the diaphragm there are also natural fenestrations at the level of the renal arteries, the coeliac and the superior mesenteric arteries.

In the assessment for suitability for treatment with a stent, there should be a length of normal aorta to function as a landing zone for the ends of the stents above and below the site of the main entry tear. Most operators stipulate a landing zone of 2cm in length and of 'normal' aortic diameter. The widest currently available stent graft is 46mm (Talent device). Therefore, the diameter of the landing zone cannot be wider than this diameter.

The main issue that is encountered regarding landing zone length occurs when the main entry tear is close to the origin of the left subclavian artery. In this situation, the length of the landing zone can be increased by covering the left subclavian artery with the upper end of the stent graft. Previously, interventionalists were reluctant to cover the left subclavian artery because of the theoretical risk of ensuing left arm ischaemia. However, symptomatic arm ischaemia requiring treatment occurs in a negligible proportion of patients. Gorich *et al* investigated the effects of covering the left subclavian artery in 23 patients. None of the patients experienced left arm ischaemia in the immediate post-operative period or during follow-up, intermittent dizziness occurred in one patient and exercise-dependent paraesthesia occurred in another patient [10]. As a result of this, most operators would now adopt a policy of covering the left subclavian artery with no prior subclavian bypass. If patients become symptomatic after stent deployment, carotid-subclavian bypass can then be performed electively. In selected circumstances, the landing zone length can be increased even further by performing left common carotid to right common carotid bypass. The carotid and vertebral arteries should be assessed by duplex ultrasound prior to stent insertion if it is considered necessary to cover the left subclavian artery. This is a precaution to ensure that there is not generalised carotid and vertebral disease with the potential for stroke if the left vertebral artery is covered, and this vessel is the dominant supply to the brain.

Finally, the calibre of the femoral and iliac arteries should be assessed either by duplex ultrasound or as part of the CT or MR protocol. Most stent graft delivery systems require iliac arteries of 8mm diameter or more. If the iliac arteries are smaller than this, the devices can be inserted into the iliac arteries or aorta via a surgical conduit at open surgery.

Device selection

The main decision to be made concerns the diameter of the device to be implanted. In aneurysmal disease, the device is generally oversized by 10-20% relative to the size of the normal calibre aorta. In aortic dissection, this is not thought to be necessary and the diameter of device chosen is that of the diameter of the normal aorta (combined true and false lumen). If

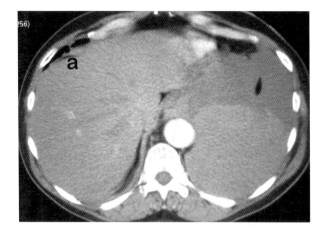

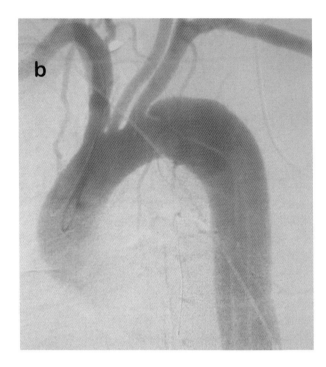

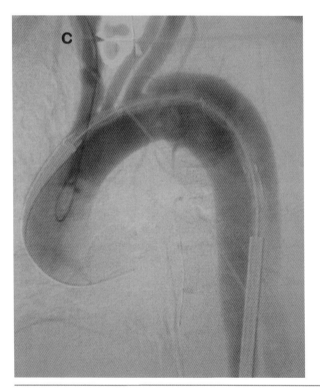

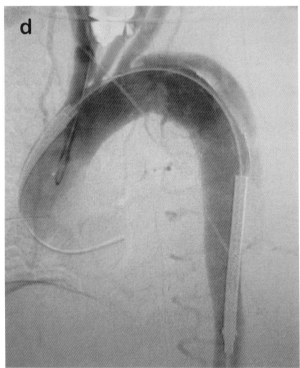

Figure 2. a) This 71-year-old man was admitted with an acute type B aortic dissection and a left haemothorax. b) This angiogram indicates that the main entry tear is located just distal to the left subclavian artery. c) and d) The entry tear was closed with a single Talent stent graft. At one year follow-up, the false lumen in the mid and upper descending thoracic aorta is thrombosed.

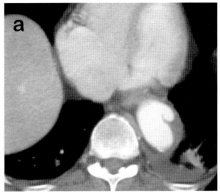

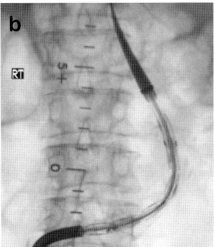

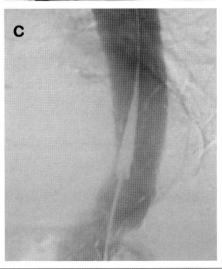

Figure 3. a) In this patient with an acute type B dissection and a contained rupture, the main entry tear was in the distal thoracic aorta. b) The patient also had a small very tortuous aneurysm of the abdominal aorta. This image shows a Talent device being passed through the tortuous aorta to the site of the entry tear. c) This image has been obtained after deployment of the stent graft and closure of the entry tear. The patient is well at one year follow-up.

the aorta is aneurysmal at the site of the main tear, the diameter of the normal calibre aorta, usually at the level of the aortic arch, is used to select the appropriate caliber device. Regarding device length, at least 2cm of device should be placed either side of the tear to be covered.

Technique

We usually place a pigtail catheter in the ascending aorta via the left brachial artery (or the right brachial artery if the intention is to cover the left subclavian artery). Although most stent graft procedures are performed under general anaesthesia, many operators place the devices with the aid of regional or local anaesthesia. The standard technique involves a femoral artery cutdown followed by catheterisation of the femoral artery using either the seldinger technique or a formal arteriotomy. A selective catheter (eg. cobra catheter) and standard or hydrophilic guidewire are manipulated up the abdominal aorta into the ascending aorta and the guidewire is exchanged for a 260cm long extra stiff guidewire (eg. Lunderquist wire, William Cook). It is important that the catheter and wire are passed up the true lumen. Angiography with the catheter in the upper abdominal aorta is the best method to ensure that the true lumen has been cannulated. It may be helpful to view the angiogram in combination with the CT images to confirm catheter placement in the true lumen. The device is advanced over the guidewire to the site of the main entry tear and deployed with the aid of angiography via the brachial catheter. The procedure is deemed technically successful if completion angiography shows correct siting of the deployed stent graft over the site of the main entry tear and no entry of contrast into the false lumen from this location. If there is a further large communication in the thorax, this should also be covered with a stent graft. The false lumen will often continue to fill via communications below the diaphragm at the level of the visceral vessels. This is usual and reduces during follow-up in the majority of cases.

Outcomes of stent grafting

There is as yet relatively limited literature on the outcomes of stent grafts for aortic dissection. Most authors report the results of this technique in patients with complications of acute dissection. There are also little data on the efficacy of stent grafting for patients with chronic dissection. The majority of series in the literature involve under 30 patients, although larger series are now being published [11-13]. However, the reported outcomes of this treatment to date are encouraging. Deployment of stent grafts is possible in virtually every case. Closure of the main entry tear is achieved in 86-100% of patients [7,8,14-17].

In Dake's series, 19 patients were treated with stent grafts (15 true type B, four patients with type A with entry tear in descending thoracic aorta). Technical success was achieved in all patients with a 30-day mortality of 16%. Revascularisation of ischaemic branch vessels occurred in 76% of patients. At a mean follow-up of 13 months, complete thrombosis of the false lumen occurred in 79% of cases [8].

Nienaber treated 12 patients with subacute or chronic dissection with stent grafts with zero mortality and morbidity compared with a surgical cohort who had 33% mortality. At three months follow-up there was complete thrombosis of the false lumen [7].

We have treated 13 dissections with stent grafts at our institution. Ten were acute dissections and three were chronic dissections. The indications for treatment were contained rupture (11 patients) and aneurysm formation (two patients). Successful stent graft insertion and closure of the main entry tear was achieved in all cases. Two patients died within 30 days. One of these sustained an occult type A dissection during the procedure and died two days after stent insertion and the other patient died 29 days after stenting, at home.

Regarding thrombosis of the false lumen after stent insertion, thrombosis usually occurs in the upper thoracic aorta. Distally, there is often residual filling of the false lumen from natural fenestrations below the diaphragm at the level of the visceral vessels.

Complications

Although paraplegia is cited as one of the main complications of stent grafting for thoracic aortic aneurysms, reports of it occurring for aortic dissection are limited to one report [11].

The 30-day mortality of stent grafting is reported in up to 16% [8,11-13,18]. Mortality is usually related to organ ischaemia as a result of branch vessel involvement and associated comorbidity rather than a complication of the stent graft procedure itself. Retrograde aortic dissection as happened in one of our cases, is a recognised, though uncommon complication of stenting [17].

Manipulation of catheters, guidewires and large delivery systems in the aortic arch may provoke emboli into the cerebral circulation and procedural stroke has been reported after thoracic stent grafting [12,19]. Device migration is very rare [20].

Conclusions

There is reasonable evidence, though none of it backed by large randomised trials, that the endovascular treatment with stent grafts for patients with complications of acute and to a lesser extent chronic dissection is an effective and probably safer alternative to surgery. However, there are several issues that need addressing, particularly, uncertainty regarding the durability of the stents themselves, and the lack of an ideal device with regard to delivery system size and ease of deployment around the aortic arch. There is relatively little data on the efficacy of endovascular treatment for aneurysm formation in patients with chronic dissection. Finally, it is not known whether the indications for placement of stent grafts should be limited to the complications of dissection or whether they should be placed prophylactically in all patients to prevent complications at a later date.

Summary

◆ The main indications for stent grafts in patients with aortic dissection are contained rupture, aneurysm formation, the treatment of end organ ischaemia.

◆ Closure of the main entry tear with a stent graft reduces the pressure in the false lumen.

◆ The available data suggests that stent grafting is effective and associated with reduced complications compared with surgery.

References

1. Pate JW, Richardson RJ, Eastridge CE. Acute aortic dissection. *Ann Surg* 1976; 42: 395-404.

2. Chavan A, Lotz J, Oelert F, *et al.* Endoluminal treatment of aortic dissection. *Eur Radiol* 2003; 13: 2521-2534.

3. Anangostopoulos CE, Prabhakar MJS, Kittle CF. Aortic dissections and dissecting aneurysms. *Am J Cardiol* 1972; 30: 263-273.

4. Williams DM, Lee DY, Hamilton BH, *et al.* The dissected aorta: percutaneous treatment of ischemic complications: principles and results. *J Vasc Intervent Radiol* 1997; 8: 605-625

5. Kee ST, Dake MD, Paddon AJ. Endovascular repair of thoracic and dissecting aneurysms and aortic coarctation. In: *Textbook of Endovascular Procedures.* Dyet, Nicholson, Ettles, Wilson, Eds. Churchill Livingston, 2000: pp439-455.

6. Borst HG, Heinemann MK, Stone CD, Eds. *Surgical treatment of aortic dissection.* Churchill Livingstone, New York, USA.

7. Nienabr CA, Rossella F, Lund G, *et al.* Nonsurgical reconstruction of thoracic aortic dissection by stent-graft placement. *New Engl J Med* 1999; 340; 1539-1545.

8. Dake MD, Kato N, Scott Mitchell R, *et al.* Endovascular stent-graft placement for the treatment of acute aortic dissection. *New Engl* J Med 1999; 340: 1546-1552.

9. Innoue K, Hosokawa H, Iwase T, *et al.* Aortic arch reconstruction by transluminally placed endovascular branched stent graft. *Circulation* 1999; 100: 316-321.

10. Gorich J, Asquan Y, Seifarth H, *et al.* Initial experience with intentional stent-graft coverage of the subclavian artery during endovascular aortic repairs. *J Endovasc Ther* 2002; 9 suppl 2:II39-43.

11. Beregi J-P, Haulon S, Otal P, *et al.* Endovascular treatment of acute complications associated with aortic dissection: mid-term results from a multicenter study. *J Endovasc Ther* 2003; 10: 486-493.

12. Kato N, Shimono T, Hirano T, *et al.* Mid-term results of stent-graft repair of acute and chronic aortic dissection with descending tear: the complication specific approach. *J Cardiothorac Surg* 2002; 124: 306-312.

13. Buffolo E, da Fonseca JH, de Souza JA, *et al.* Revolutionary treatment of aneurysms and dissections of descending aorta: the endovascular approach. *Annals of Thoracic surgery* 2002; 74: S1815-1817.

14. Kato N, Shimono T, Hirano T, *et al.* Transluminal placement of endovascular stent-grafts for the treatment of Type A aortic dissection with the entry tear in the descending thoracic aorta. *J Vasc Surg* 2001; 34: 1023-1028.

15. Hausegger KA, Tiesenhausen K, Schedlbauer P, *et al.* Treatment of acute aortic type B dissection with stent-grafts. *Cardiovasc Intervent Radiol* 2001; 24: 306-312.

16. Sailer J, Peloschek P, Rand T, *et al.* Endovascular treatment of aortic type B dissection and penetrating ulcer using commercially available stent-grafts. *AJR* 2001; 177: 1365-1369.

17. Czermak BV, Waldenberger P, Fraedrich G, *et al.* Treatment of Stanford type B dissection with stent-grafts: preliminary results. *Radiology* 2000; 217: 544-550.

18. Orend KH, Scharrer - Pamler R, Kapfer X, *et al.* Endovascular treatment in diseases of the descending thoracic aorta: 6-year results of a single center. *J Vasc Surg* 2003; 37: 91-99.

19. Taylor PR, Gaines PA, McGuiness CL, *et al.* Thoracic aortic stent-grafts - early experience from two centers using commercially available devices. *Eur J Vasc Endovasc Surg* 2001; 22: 70-76.

20. Shim WH, Koo BK, Yoon YS, *et al.* Treatment of thoracic aortic dissection with stent-grafts: midterm results. *J Endovasc Ther* 2002; 9: 817-821.

Chapter 12

Aortic arch branch vessel disease: the role of endovascular surgery

David Kessel MA, MRCP, FRCR, Consultant Vascular Radiologist
St James's University Hospital, Leeds, UK

Introduction

This chapter concerns itself with the clinical manifestations of disease of the proximal great vessels of the aortic arch, their management and how to image them.

In comparison to the lower limb arteries and the carotid bifurcation, the great vessels arising from the aortic arch are relatively spared from atheromatous disease. In a large study, only 17% of patients with extracranial carotid arterial disease had >30% stenosis of either the subclavian or innominate arteries [1]. Tandem lesions involving the ipsilateral common carotid or innominate artery occur in only 1-2% [2]. Ultrasound studies have shown that subclavian and innominate arterial disease is usually slowly progressive [3]. Subclavian artery stenosis and occlusion is asymptomatic in about 75% of patients [4], but otherwise presents with arm ischaemia or vertebrobasilar insufficiency. Common carotid artery disease usually gives rise to cerebral manifestations identical to those caused by internal carotid stenosis, namely anterior circulation transient ischaemic attack, amaurosis fugax and stroke. Innominate artery lesions can present with anterior or posterior cerebral circulatory disturbance or arm ischaemia.

Upper limb vascular insufficiency accounts for only 2-4% of vascular surgical operations and patients have an increased long-term survival compared to patients with lower limb arterial disease [5]. The distribution of disease in the upper limb is also very different and diffuse disease, as seen in the superficial femoral artery, is very unusual. In the arm, atheromatous disease tends to be focal and typically affects the ostium and proximal portions of the innominate and subclavian arteries. The left subclavian artery is affected more commonly than the right but when innominate artery lesions are also considered, both sides are equally affected. Some of the pathologies that affect the arm are rare in the lower limb. Non-ostial disease suggests an alternative aetiology such as fibromuscular hyperplasia (FMH), thoracic outlet syndrome, arterial spasm, Takyasu's disease, post-irradiation fibrosis and giant cell arteritis. Asymmetry of the arm pulses and brachial blood pressure are sure indicators of significant arterial obstruction.

Treatment options in patients with upper limb ischaemia

Angioplasty and stenting are relatively modern forms of treatment and it is worth considering the medical and surgical alternatives.

Conservative therapy

One of the largest reported series [6] retrospectively reviewed outcomes of 274 patients with symptomatic subclavian artery stenoses. Sixty percent were treated conservatively, with the remainder treated by angioplasty. After a median follow-up of 42 months, patients treated with angioplasty had a reduced risk of haemodynamically significant stenosis but the risk of a clinically symptomatic stenosis was the same in both groups. This indicates that patients with arm ischaemia will often improve spontaneously with conservative treatment. The implication from this is that endovascular and surgical therapy should be reserved for those patients with the most severe ischaemic symptoms. Those most likely to benefit will have critical ischaemia, blue digit syndrome and severe vertebrobasilar insufficiency. As always, attempts must be made to modify risk factors for vascular disease in order to minimise stroke and myocardial infarction. In this context it is worth noting that treatment of subclavian steal does not seem to prevent stroke.

The difficulty facing the clinical team is which form of treatment to offer. The most important factors to consider are technical success, procedure-related mortality and morbidity and patency rates. Clearly, conservative therapy has an important role to play in the management of patients with milder symptoms.

Surgery

Contemporary surgical reconstruction of the great vessels to the head, neck and upper limbs can be performed via a transcervical approach or a transthoracic approach. Transthoracic surgery has largely been replaced by extrathoracic approaches and endarterectomy is rarely performed. Transcervical operations such as carotid-subclavian transposition and bypass grafting are best suited to disease affecting a single vessel leaving the remaining vessels as potential 'healthy donors'. When there is disease affecting multiple branches, transthoracic surgery may be advantageous albeit at the cost of an increase in morbidity and mortality.

Cina [7] performed a systematic review of transcervical surgical options of bypass grafting and arterial transposition for subclavian artery disease. Arm claudication was the primary indication in 44%. The review demonstrated an advantage to transposition; in particular, there was a reduction in rates of thrombosis. In his study of 72 patients examined for disease of the subclavian artery, only 27 (38%) had surgery. Cina did not treat patients with arm claudication, indicating the benign nature of this condition.

Berguer [8] reports his experience with the transcervical approach in 182 patients. Straightforward single vessel disease was present in 103 (57%). A more complex group included 79 patients with cardiorespiratory disease and greater than one diseased vessel. Overall, primary patency was in excess of 80% at seven years, 92% of patients were stroke-free and there was 72% survival at five years. Berguer concludes his paper with the statement: 'Use of endovascular techniques in this location can only be justified if their performance matches the results obtained with surgical reconstruction'. His results are impressive but we must look at the morbidity and mortality. This is not minor surgery. There was an average ITU stay of 1.5 days, a hospital stay of 5.6 days and the perioperative morbidity was 26%. There were seven non-fatal perioperative strokes and six myocardial infarctions, all in patients with a preoperative history of cardiac disease. Two patients suffered pulmonary emboli and six developed pleural effusions requiring drainage. Four neck haematomas required evacuation. There were five cases of transient Horner's syndrome, four recurrent laryngeal nerve injuries and one case of reflex sympathetic dystrophy. The overall major stroke and death rate was 4%. This rose to a 9% stroke rate and 1.5% death rate in the complex group.

Endovascular therapy: supra-aortic angioplasty and stenting

Endovascular therapy dates back to Bachman's 1980 case report [9] describing treatment of subclavian steal by balloon angioplasty. Angioplasty and stenting of the subclavian and innominate arteries is an attractive option as they are large high-flow vessels similar to the iliac arteries and similar high patency rates are to be expected. Huttl [10] retrospectively reviewed outcomes of angioplasty of the innominate artery in 89 patients with a variety of presentations (upper limb claudication, transient ischaemic attack, vertebrobasilar insufficiency). In this series, the total stroke (2%) and transient ischaemic attack (6%) rate was 8% and the primary patency was 93% at 16 months. Henry [11] reported 113 patients undergoing percutaneous balloon angioplasty +/- stenting of subclavian occlusive lesions for a variety of indications (vertebrobasilar insufficiency 62%, arm ischaemia 44%). There was a 0.9% major stroke and death rate and an 8-year primary patency rate of 75%. Stenting yielded slightly improved patency rates. These results indicate that endovascular treatments have a reasonable outcome in selected patients but do not demonstrate superiority over the surgical alternative.

Conventional surgery or endovascular surgery?

At first inspection the results of endovascular surgery seem favourable to conventional surgery. However, there are no studies directly comparing surgery and endovascular procedures in the upper limb. In a systematic review of the outcomes of surgery and stenting, Hadjipetrou [12] reviewed 52 surgical series (2496 patients) and seven radiological series (108 patients). Differences in selection criteria, procedure and follow-up make direct comparison impossible. The published results may also be misleading. For example, in one of the surgical series there appeared to be a 4% stroke rate associated with subclavian arterial surgery. Nevertheless, careful analysis showed that all these patients had undergone combined carotid and subclavian surgery. Conversely, in a series on supra-aortic stents there were no

strokes, but the common carotid artery was clamped to prevent embolisation when treating innominate artery lesions. Clearly, his results are not directly applicable to percutaneous stenting. Like most authors Henry [11] found complete subclavian occlusion technically challenging to treat. It can be very difficult to cross the occlusion from either the arm or femoral approach and most authors report only 30-50% success rates. The majority of patients in surgical series have occlusions of the subclavian artery. Inevitably therefore, with formal analysis on an intention to treat basis, surgery will have a higher technical success rate. Both the endovascular and the surgical figures must be viewed with caution.

It is difficult to draw meaningful conclusions from this data, but it seems likely that surgery offers a slightly more durable result than endovascular therapy at the cost of an increased morbidity and mortality (Table 1). Endovascular therapy and surgery are, as always, complementary techniques. When deciding on the best treatment each case should be considered on its own merits and management decisions will be influenced by several factors. Surgery may offer a more durable solution for a young patient, whose livelihood depends on the use of their arm. In addition, in the presence of significant tissue loss, some form of surgery is usually required. Endovascular treatment is appropriate in patients who are poor candidates for surgery, or because of age and co-morbidity will not require such long-term patency. When blue digit syndrome is due to an arterial stenosis, angioplasty will prevent further emboli, although some adjunctive therapy may be needed. Sometimes in the acute situation an endovascular option will reduce the risk to the patient, but is unlikely to prevent subsequent surgery.

Clinical presentations of supra-aortic arterial disease

It is helpful to consider some of the presentations of aortic branch vessel disease. Each of these conditions should be assessed according to its clinical merit. Just like carotid arterial disease and peripheral vascular disease, investigation and treatment should be based on risk of stroke, symptomatology and quality of life considerations.

Table 1. Outcomes of surgery, angioplasty and stenting in upper limb ischaemia.

Outcome	Surgery	Angioplasty	Stenting
Technical success	88-100%	40**-100%	88-100%
Mortality	0-3% extrathoracic	0%	0%
	6-19% transthoracic		
Stroke	3%	0-1%	0%
Other complications*	6% extrathoracic	<5%	0-14%
	19% transthoracic		
Patency 2-5 years	83%	54-97%	-
Recurrence	10-18%	-	0-13%

* Other complications include:-

   • Surgical - damage to the phrenic and recurrent laryngeal nerves, lymphocoele, graft infection, pleural effusion and wound haematoma and infection.
   • Radiological - distal embolisation, puncture site and other vessel.

** Lower technical success rates in the presence of complete occlusion.

The therapeutic options for supra-aortic disease include medical therapy, endovascular options and surgery. Steps should always be taken to modify the risk factors for arterial disease.

Upper limb ischaemia

Chronic upper limb ischaemia is often relatively asymptomatic and treatment should be reserved for those with significant disability. Many patients will improve spontaneously as collaterals develop. Atheromatous disease responds well to angioplasty and stenting. When the ischaemia is due to fibromuscular hyperplasia, there is usually a good response to angioplasty alone. Other unusual conditions have less certain outcomes. Takayasu's arteritis is rarely seen in Europe, but a few small series have suggested that angioplasty and stenting can successfully relieve symptoms. Caution should be exercised as there is a propensity for these patients to develop aneurysms even without the trauma of angioplasty. Patients with arterial trauma can also be managed by endovascular means.

Blue digit syndrome

Blue digit syndrome is common and should be considered as a form of critical limb ischaemia. It represents digital ischaemia due to an acute embolic event usually from a proximal arterial source (Figure 1). The patient should be investigated urgently and the aortic arch, the proximal innominate and the subclavian arteries must be assessed for plaque and stenosis. Echocardiography is performed to exclude a cardiac source. This is particularly important in the context of a recent large myocardial infarction, as a high proportion of patients will develop intracardiac thrombus. Treatment is aimed at preventing recurrent thromboembolism and therapy for the distal ischaemia. The patient is usually anticoagulated following a full thrombophilia screen.

Where there is a proximal arterial stenosis, angioplasty alone has been shown to be effective in preventing recurrent emboli [13]. This is not surprising as remodelling will result in a smooth lumen. Neointimal hyperplasia may cause restenosis but does not usually result in further embolisation. If there is plaque ulceration or evidence of thrombus, then primary stenting should be considered (Figure 2). Adjunctive treatment with vasodilators, such as

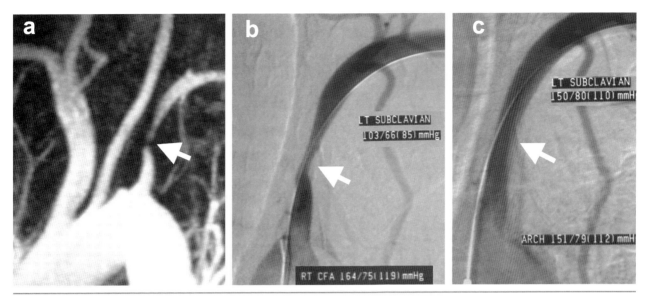

Figure 1. Uncomplicated left subclavian artery stenosis (white arrows) in a patient with blue digit syndrome. a) Contrast-enhanced magnetic resonance angiogram. b) Intra-arterial digital subtraction angiogram. c) Intra-arterial digital subtraction angiogram post-angioplasty.

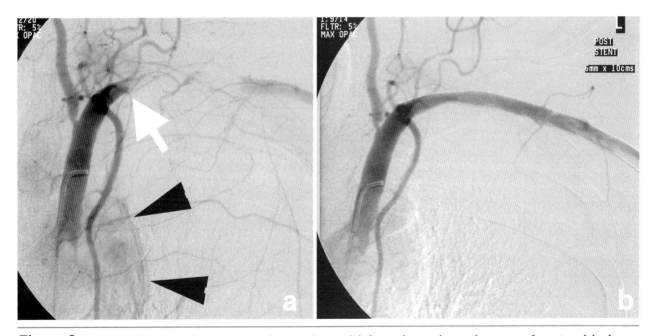

Figure 2. Occluded left subclavian artery in a patient with bronchogenic carcinoma and acute critical arm ischaemia. a) Selective angiogram. Note thrombus in the proximal occlusion (white arrow) and enhancing mediastinal lymph nodes (black arrows). b) Post primary stenting, there is minor residual stenosis; further dilatation was not performed due to pain.

iloprost, transthoracic endoscopic cervical sympathectomy and digital amputation may be required depending on the severity of the distal ischaemia and the potential for reversibility.

Steal syndrome

Steal syndromes resulting in vertebrobasilar and coronary insufficiency are caused by retrograde flow in the vertebral and internal mammary arteries distal to a stenosis or occlusion. Patients with steal syndromes will almost always show reduced blood pressure in the symptomatic limb. A 10% drop in systolic pressure may be sufficient to cause flow reversal. Subclavian steal is a benign condition and many of these patients are asymptomatic. Neurological symptoms or posterior fossa cerebrovascular accident are rare [14]. The subclavian steal syndrome of dizziness, vertigo or visual disturbance during arm exercise usually occurs when there is a significant tandem lesion in another of the cerebral arteries. Most 'dizzy spells' have nothing to do with subclavian steal syndrome. Be guided by expert neurological assessment. If there is doubt as to whether vascular insufficiency is the cause, this must be discussed with the patient prior to treatment. Coronary steal is a similar phenomenon that occurs in patients with an internal mammary artery bypass graft distal to a subclavian stenosis.

Vertebrobasilar insufficiency

Vertebrobasilar insufficiency may also occur when there is a stenosis within the vertebral arteries themselves. Patients need to be formally assessed by a neurologist before proceeding to intervention. Once again, vertebral artery disease tends to be focal and ostial. Unlike the internal carotid artery, vertebrobasilar symptoms tend to be flow-related rather than embolic, hence they would appear to be a suitable target for endovascular intervention. Vertebral artery angioplasty was first described in 1981 [15] long before carotid artery angioplasty. There is only anecdotal evidence from small series for its use. In patients with a strongly suggestive history, angioplasty is recommended in the first instance. This can be readily performed using low profile catheters and balloons (Figure 3). Follow-up with serial ultrasound is helpful but the origin of the vertebral artery can be difficult to demonstrate. Stents are best reserved for symptomatic restenosis and low profile systems allow deployment through a 4 French sheath. There is a relatively low risk of distal embolisation and no evidence to suggest a benefit of cerebral protection devices.

Arterial complications of the thoracic outlet syndrome

Arterial complications of the thoracic outlet syndrome are not rare and result from compression between the clavicle and abnormal ribs or fibrous bands. This typically occurs during arm abduction and repeated trauma leads to subclavian artery aneurysm, thrombosis, distal embolisation and Raynaud's syndrome. Patients with suspected TOS should have plain radiographs of the thoracic inlet looking for abnormal ribs, and a Doppler ultrasound to study the effect of postural manoeuvres on the subclavian vessels. Angiography is required if the ultrasound is abnormal. In particular, one should look for abnormality of the subclavian artery at the site of vascular compression, between the clavicle and first rib. The most valuable signs are aneurysm dilatation or irregularity with the arm in the neutral position. Arm abduction and the Roos manoeuvre (elbow and shoulder flexed 90°, arm dorsiflexed) may show vascular compression or occlusion. False positive arterial compression is present in about 1/3 of normal subjects when the arm is excessively abducted and dorsiflexed. Minor smooth compression during postural manoeuvres is very common in normal subjects and is unlikely to be significant.

The treatment of vascular TOS is surgical and involves resection of either the first rib or a cervical rib and/or division of abnormal fibrous and muscular bands. Although it is tempting to treat TOS-related stenoses and aneurysms by endovascular means, this is best avoided. TOS often affects young patients and a durable solution is required. Stents and stent grafts are likely to fail due to repeated mechanical stress [16] (Figure 4). Only consider stenting in elderly patients who are unfit for surgery. If there is residual stenoses in the artery following surgery, simple angioplasty may

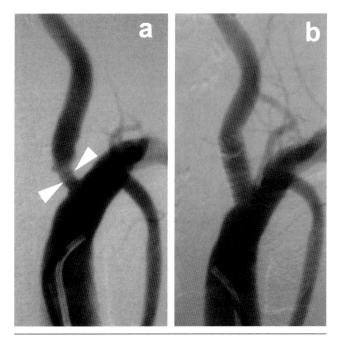

Figure 3. A patient with severe vertebrobasilar ischaemia. a) Recurrent left vertebral artery stenosis (white arrowheads) one year after angioplasty. b) Following stenting; complete symptomatic relief.

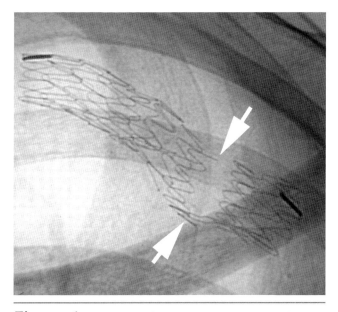

Figure 4. Stent graft used to treat subclavian aneurysm in thoracic outlet syndrome. Arrows show fracture at the point of compression between the first rib and clavicle. The stent graft subsequently thrombosed and open surgical repair was performed.

suffice. Stenting should be reserved for restenosis, and only considered in cases in which vascular compression is no longer demonstrable.

Endovascular therapy: technical considerations

There are special considerations relevant to endovascular therapy in the upper limb and extra equipment is often necessary. It would be negligent not to discuss the risk of stroke with the patient. This probably lies between those associated with carotid angiography and angioplasty, i.e. 1-5%.

Decide whether the optimal approach is from the brachial or femoral artery. It is possible to traverse most stenoses from the femoral approach, but occlusions and tortuous vessels will be much more difficult and sometimes the additional catheter support gained from the arm approach is invaluable. The disadvantage of the brachial approach is that an ischaemic limb may not tolerate even a 6 French sheath. If brachial access is necessary for larger sheaths (eg. stent graft), a surgical cutdown may be preferable to the percutaneous approach. Consider 'bodyflossing' by traversing the lesion from the brachial approach using 4 or 5 French catheters. The next step is to snare the guidewire and bring it out through a femoral sheath of suitable size for the angioplasty balloons and stents. A 'through and through' guidewire greatly increases catheter stability during angioplasty and stenting. It should be remembered that a minimum shaft length of 80cm is required for catheters, angioplasty balloons and stents. Exchange length guidewires up to 260cm may be required.

Balloon inflation time should be kept to a minimum in the innominate artery, or in other situations when cerebral perfusion is likely to be reduced. The indications for stenting are to treat occlusions, cover thrombus and ulcerated plaque, and when angioplasty is technically suboptimal. Pre-dilatation of the lesion with a low profile balloon can be helpful in high-grade stenoses. Stents should be positioned to cover the entire lesion; using a long sheath or guide catheter is invaluable for accurate positioning. Balloon mounted stents are ideal for short proximal lesions but more flexible self-expanding stents are equally acceptable and invaluable when dealing with tortuous vessels.

There is no evidence to support the use of use of cerebral protection devices during routine supra-aortic angioplasty and stenting. Interestingly, flow reversal in the vertebral artery may not be immediate [17], and might confer some protection against posterior circulation embolisation.

When not to treat?

A good example is a calcified lesion involving the origin of both the right subclavian artery and common carotid artery (Figure 5). It is essential to keep the patient's best interests in mind. There are some lesions, ill-suited to endovascular therapy, which should be left alone or have conventional surgery.

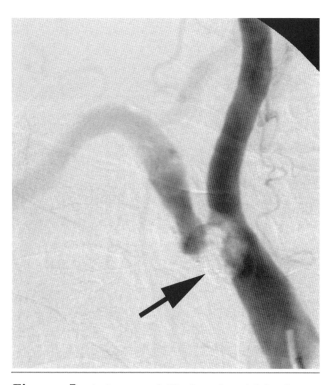

Figure 5. A large calcified polypoidal plaque involving the distal innominate artery and both the right common carotid and subclavian artery origins. The patient had cerebrovascular and arm symptoms and was considered unsuitable for endovascular surgery so underwent open repair.

Imaging supra-aortic arterial disease

The key to successful management of supra-aortic disease is good quality pre-intervention imaging to show the aortic arch, the origins of the great vessels and, where necessary, the distal circulation in the upper limb and brain. Until recently, this was dependent on intra-arterial digital subtraction angiography (IADSA). This procedure is not without risk with a mortality of 0.1% and disabling stroke rate of about 1%. Clearly, a non-invasive alternative is desirable.

Ultrasound

Ultrasound is excellent for the cervical carotid artery and the extrathoracic subclavian artery, but views of the proximal vessels are limited and dependent on the patient's body habitus and the skill of the operator. Ultrasound cannot reliably diagnose or exclude proximal disease of the great vessels.

Contrast-enhanced magnetic resonance angiography (CE-MRA)

CE-MRA and Computed Tomography Angiography (CTA) have added to the diagnostic armamentarium. Wutke et al [18] studied 30 patients with carotid artery disease using both CE-MRA and IADSA. When stenoses were graded in increments of 10%, there was agreement in 25 out of 60 arterial segments. MRA graded stenoses as tighter than IADSA in 34 segments and lower in one segment. This is not altogether surprising as CE-MRA has inferior spatial resolution to IADSA. Typical MRA has a pixel size of about 1.2 x 0.8mm compared to 0.3 x 0.3mm for IADSA. When the stenoses were graded in accordance with NASCET criteria, using a 4 point scale (0-49%, 50-69%, 70-99% and occlusion), there was very good agreement. Unfortunately, in this and other studies, CE-MRA performed poorly at aortic arch level and in the proximal common carotid arterial segments. Image quality made diagnosis uncertain in 15% and uninterpretable in 4%. This appears largely attributable to respiratory motion artifacts and was not observed in patients who were able to breath hold for 30 seconds during data acquisition.

A concern is that magnetic resonance angiography tends to overestimate the degree of stenosis. This artifact is well recognised with time of flight MRA. Turbulent flow leads to signal loss resulting in an apparent increase in the severity of the stenosis and sometimes causing a pseudo-occlusion. Contrast-enhanced MRA is much less prone to the effects of turbulent flow. Randoux [19] found a degree of overestimation of stenosis especially at the ostia of the vertebral arteries but overall correlation with IADSA was high. There is emerging evidence that MRA and rotational angiography demonstrate more high-grade stenoses than conventional two view angiography due to the greater number of angiographic projections [20]. In Wutke's [18] study three of the IADSA studies were found to have underestimated the degree of stenosis due to the angiographic projections not demonstrating the stenosis in true profile. It is possible that when there is a discrepancy in the degree of stenosis, IADSA may actually be an underestimate rather than CE-MRA overestimating it. In this respect the ability to view CT and MRA reconstructions in multiple orientations may offset the inferior spatial resolution.

Conclusions

Upper limb ischaemia is uncommon even in specialist centres and there is unlikely to be a trial to show whether endovascular therapy or surgery is the best treatment. Use CE-MRA in the initial assessment and reserve angiography for patients in whom it is necessary to visualise the distal vessels in the hand. Weigh up the pros and cons of surgery and minimally invasive therapy and discuss them with the patient. Angioplasty and stenting should be considered for the treatment of stenotic disease and will not normally preclude subsequent surgical intervention. Consider approaching the lesion from the arm or using a combined approach. Do not hesitate to use a surgical cutdown. Ultimately, we should not be surprised if the results of endovascular treatment prove not to be as durable as surgery but the advantages of a minimally invasive approach may outweigh this in many clinical scenarios.

Summary

♦   Contrast-enhanced MRA is rapidly becoming the first choice imaging modality for planning endovascular or surgical therapy of the supra-aortic vessels.

♦   There is no direct comparison of surgery and endovascular therapy for supra-aortic intervention.

♦   Surgery probably has better long-term patency at the cost of higher morbidity.

♦   Stenotic disease is usually straightforward to treat by angioplasty or stenting.

♦   Complete occlusion is technically much harder to treat by endovascular means and is more likely to recur.

♦   There are potential advantages for the patient if they can have a minimally invasive procedure but these must be weighed against questions concerning long-term patency.

♦   There is no evidence regarding the use of cerebral protection devices.

References

1. Fields WS, Lemak NA. Joint study of extra-cranial arterial occlusion: VII subclavian steal - a review of 168 cases. *JAMA* 1972; 222: 1139-43.

2. Arko FR, Buckely CJ, Lee SD Manning LG, *et al.* Combined carotid endarterectomy with transluminal angioplasty and primary stenting of the supra-aortic vessels. *J Cardiovasc Surg* 2000; 41: 737-42.

3. Ackerman H, Diener HC, Seboldt H, *et al.* Ultrasonographic follow-up of subclavian stenosis and occlusion: natural history and surgical treatment. *Stroke* 1988; 19: 431-435.

4. Walker PM, Paley D, Harris KA, Thompson A, Johnson KW. What determines the symptoms associated with subclavian artery occlusive disease? *J Vasc Surg* 1985; 2: 154-7.

5. Criqui MH, Langer RD, Fronek AF, *et al.* Mortality over a period of 10 years in patients with peripheral arterial disease. *N Engl J Med* 1992; 326: 381-6.

6. Schillinger M, Haumer M, Schillinger S, *et al.* Outcome of conservative versus interventional treatment of subclavian artery stenosis. *J Endovasc Ther* 2002 Apr; 9(2):139-46.

7. Cina CS, Safar HA, Lagana A, *et al.* Subclavian carotid transposition and bypass grafting: consecutive cohort study and systematic review. *J Vasc Surg* 2002; 35: 422-9.

8. Berguer R, Morasch MD, Kline RA, *et al.* Cervical reconstruction of the supra-aortic trunks: a 16 year experience. *J Vasc Surg* 1999; 29: 239-48.

9. Bachman DM, Kim RM. Transluminal dilatation for subclavian steal syndrome. *AJR* 1980; 135: 995-6.

10. Huttl K, Nemes B, Simonffy A, *et al.* Angioplasty of the innominate artery in 89 patients: experience over 19 years. *Cardiovasc Intervent Radiol* 2002; 25: 109-14.

11. Henry M, Amor M, Henry I, *et al.* Percutaneous transluminal angioplasty of the subclavian arteries. *J Endovasc Surg* 1999; 6: 33-41.

12. Hadjipetrou P, Cox S, Piemonte T, *et al.* Percutaneous revascularization of atherosclerotic obstruction of aortic arch vessels. *J Am Coll Cardiol* 1999; 33: 1238-1245.

13. Swarbrick MJ, Lopez AJ, Gaines PA, *et al.* The endovascular management of blue finger syndrome. *Eur J Vasc Endovasc Surg* 1999; 17: 106-110.

14. Hennerici M, Klemm C, Rautenberg W. The subclavian steal phenomenon a common vascular disorder with rare neurologic deficits. *Neurology* 1988; 38: 669-73.

15. Motarjeme A, Gordon GI. Percutaneous transluminal angioplasty of the brachiocephalic vessels: guidelines for therapy. *Int Angiol* 1993; 12: 260-269.

16. Phipp L, Scott J, Kessel D, *et al.* Subclavian endovascular stents and stent grafts: cause for concern? *J Endovasc Surg* 1999; 6: 223-6.

17. Ringelstein EB, Zeumer H. Delayed reversal of vertebral artery blood flow following percutaneous transluminal angioplasty for subclavian steal syndrome. *Neuroradiology* 1984; 26: 189-98.

18. Wutke R, Lang W, Fellner C, *et al.* High resolution, contrast enhanced magnetic resonance angiography with elliptical centric k-space ordering of supra-aortic arteries compared with selective X-ray angiography. *Stroke* 2002; 23: 1522-9.

19. Randoux B, Marro B, Sourour N, *et al.* Exploration of the origin of supra-aortic arterial trunk: can MR angiography with gadolinium injection replace digital angiography? *J Neuroradiol* 2001; 28: 176-82.

20. Elgersma OE, Wust AF, Buijs PC, *et al.* Multidirectional depiction of internal carotid arterial three dimensional time of flight MR angiography versus rotational conventional digital subtraction angiography. *Radiology* 2000; 216: 511-516.

Chapter 13

The evolution of carotid angioplasty and stenting: where are we now?

Sumaira Macdonald, MRCP FRCR,

Consultant Vascular Radiologist & Honorary Clinical Senior Lecturer

Northern Vascular Centre, Freeman Hospital, Newcastle-upon-Tyne, UK

First reports of carotid angioplasty

Following earlier innovations in peripheral and coronary percutaneous transluminal angioplasty, the technique was trialed in the carotid territory in an animal model in 1977. A new catheter system, comprising a dilatation catheter with a second lumen for simultaneous carotid artery perfusion was shown to be effective in dilating 31 experimental carotid artery stenoses in dogs [1]. Human carotid angioplasty was first reported in 1980, albeit as a combined surgical and endovascular procedure. In this report, proximal common carotid angioplasty was performed via carotid cut-down with concomitant bifurcation endarterectomy [2].

Early reported series and techniques of carotid angioplasty

In the early 1980s the first case reports and small series of carotid angioplasty were reported. The authors of these suggested that fibrodysplastic carotid artery lesions were better suited to angioplasty than to surgery, as they often extended to the skull base and were thus less accessible [3]. Pioneering work by both interventional and neuroradiologists

continued throughout this decade. Series reporting angioplasty of carotid atherosclerotic lesions [4-9], post-endarterectomy restenotic lesions [10-12] and of fibromuscular dysplastic lesions [13-16] were published. In 1990, the feasibility of carotid angioplasty was highlighted by an independent neurologist with the caveat 'its general application to patients with thromboembolic carotid-territory stroke will depend on the risk-benefit ratio compared to carotid endarterectomy or to conventional medical treatment' [17]. During this era of carotid angioplasty, the concept and first reports of procedural cerebral protection arose. Theron and Kachel presented distal balloon occlusion devices based on coaxial systems [18, 19, 20]. Throughout this time, angioplasty in the extracranial carotid territory was performed using guidewires, vascular sheaths and balloons adapted from peripheral use.

Post-angioplasty angiographic assessment of the treated segment necessitated bilateral femoral access. A 7 French sheath was placed in one femoral artery to deliver the balloon catheter. A second catheter placed via a 5 French sheath provided the means for check angiography whilst maintaining guidewire access across the lesion at all times. A steerable extendible 0.035" guidewire was used to cross the lesion under road-mapping performed via a catheter from the 7 French sheath. The catheter was exchanged for a 5mm or 6mm diameter balloon on a standard shaft (which at this time was 7 French). The balloon was sized according to calibrated angiographic measurements. Balloon inflation was performed at high pressure (typically 8 atmospheres) for 15 seconds. Following angioplasty, the balloon was removed and with the wire still across the lesion, check angiography was performed via a catheter from the contralateral 5 French sheath.

The move towards carotid stenting

The endovascular versus surgical treatment in patients with carotid stenosis in the Carotid and Vertebral Artery Transluminal Angioplasty Study (CAVATAS) [21] recruited between March 1992 and July 1997. During this time-frame, the concept of carotid stenting evolved as a natural progression from secondary or 'bail-out' stenting required for significant recoil or a dissection flap with flow limitation following angioplasty through to primary stenting. The procedural details documented during CAVATAS provide a unique insight into endovascular carotid intervention at that time.

Stenting within CAVATAS was permitted from 1994 onwards, whenever it was deemed necessary, either for primary placement or for rescue. Stents were used in a total of 26% of cases within CAVATAS, but the use of stenting clearly increased towards the end of the trial. By the end of recruitment, primary stenting had become accepted as best practice.

The sceptic would dismiss the introduction of carotid stents on the basis of lack of evidence:-

'when you have a new hammer, everything looks like a nail'.

George Bernard Shaw

Certainly, the evidence-base supporting their introduction was limited. Some of the drive for stenting came from interventional cardiology, where there was some evidence that stents reduced the incidence of restenosis compared to angioplasty in the coronary arteries [22, 23]. Subsequent reports supported their use in subacute ischaemic heart disease (especially stable and unstable angina) in order

to reduce the requirement for repeat angioplasty [24], but no positive benefit with respect to major adverse coronary events or death was demonstrated [25]. Proponents of carotid stenting suggested that primary stenting was safer than angioplasty or secondary stenting because plaque rupture, arterial dissection and acute carotid occlusion were less likely to arise [26, 27]. Outside of animal models [28] and limited series [29], these beliefs would seem to be largely based on anecdotal evidence, but it was clear that stenting at least provided a more definitive lumen and therefore, had the potential to reduce the impact of subsequent restenosis caused by neointimal hyperplasia [30]. It would be some time before there was evidence, based on *ex-vivo* human carotid bifurcation samples [31, 32] and on procedural transcranial Doppler during clinical evaluations that carotid stenting is a substantially emboligenic stage of the interventional procedure [33, 34].

The first stents placed were balloon-mounted, articulated Palmaz-Schatz which were quickly superseded by the 7 French rolling membrane Wallstent (Schneider Bülach, Switzerland). Subsequent evidence demonstrated that the stent deformation rate in the extracranial carotid artery could approach 17% for balloon-mounted models [35] although the deformation rate in larger series was later shown to be closer to 2.5% [36]. Much later work showed slightly better patency rates with balloon-mounted compared to self-expanding stents in the carotid arteries [37]. It was acknowledged, however, that balloon-mounted stents would be unlikely to replace self-expanding devices because of their vulnerability to compression [37].

Early in the stenting era, a single guiding catheter (commonly 9 French) was used to maintain secure access to the common carotid artery downstream of the target lesion and allow stent delivery, abrogating the need for a second femoral access point. Pre-dilatation of the lesion using a 4mm or 5mm balloon to prevent 'dottering' the lesion with the relatively high-profile stent delivery system (7 French) became routine.

Shortly after primary stenting became accepted practice, technical advances meant that the system was downsized to be firstly 0.018" guidewire compatible, and subsequently, 0.014" compatible. Coronary-type sub-4 French balloons were used to

Table 1. Dedicated carotid stents which may be used within the ICSS trial.

Stent	Crossing profile	Material	Configuration	OTW/Rx
Carotid Wallstent (Boston Scientific)	5.6F for 8mm 5.9F for 10mm	Elgiloy (chromium/cobalt/nickel alloy)	Straight	OTW (0.018") or Rx (0.014")
Precise (Cordis*)	5.5F for 7mm 6F for 8mm-10mm	Nitinol (nickel/titanium/alloy)	Straight	Rx
Acculink (Guidant**)	4.4F	Nitinol	Straight or tapered	Rx

Key:

*   Cordis Endovascular, a Johnson & Johnson Company, Miami, Florida, USA.

**   Guidant Corporation, Indianapolis, USA

pre-dilate the lesion, commonly to 3mm, with an initial up-sizing to an 0.035" system for stent delivery and post-dilatation. Arrow sheaths (Arrow International Inc., Reading, PA, USA) with their superior flexibility and haemostatic valve were developed and were used in a number of centres in place of guiding catheters.

With the advent of dedicated carotid stents, such as the Carotid Wallstent (Boston Scientific Corporation, Natick, MA, USA), with a crossing profile of 5.6 French for the 8mm stent and 5.9 French for the 10mm stent, these were then used in a substantial number of procedures, initially as the over-the-wire iteration (OTW) and more recently, as the 'Monorail' or rapid exchange device. The rapid exchange platform affords the primary operator absolute control of all placement and exchange manoeuvres. In addition, by avoiding the need for dealing with longer wires, the procedural time may be reduced without compromising control. Arguably this limits the risks caused by patient movement due to discomfort resulting from prolonged immobility on a hard angiographic table, and minimises the risks of thromboembolic 'seeding' from the external surfaces of sheaths, stents, guidewires and protection devices.

From around 2000 onwards, all stages of the procedure gradually became 0.014" compatible. The use of closure devices became routine, namely Angio-

seal (St Jude Medical, Bawcourt, Unit 8, Fletchworth Gate, Coventry, CVS 6SP, Great Britain) and Perclose (Abbott Laboratories Company, Saginaw Dr, Redwood City, CA, USA).

Although as relatively recently as 2001, the consensus was that the optimal stent for use in carotid stenting was not defined [38], a number of dedicated carotid stents have since been developed. Those acceptable for use in the International Carotid Stenting Study (ICSS) are given (Table 1).

The X.Act (Abbott Vascular, Maidenhead, UK) and the Exponent Rx (Medtronic Vascular, Santa Rosa, CA, USA) carotid stents are CE marked but have yet to be subjected to the peer-review mandatory before acceptance for use within ICSS.

Each step-wise technical advance is likely to have had beneficial effects on the adverse event rate. The use of dedicated carotid stents compared to designs adapted from coronary or peripheral designs is an independent factor in the reduction of the atheroembolic neurological event rate. An analysis of patients treated by primary stenting without cerebral protection, reveals a reduction in the combined death and any neurological event rate (including transient ischaemic attack) from 22.2% to 10.2% (X^2 test p=0.05) when adapted stents for the carotid are compared with dedicated carotid stents. The major disabling stroke/all death rate was reduced from 5.9% to 0% (Fisher's Exact test p=0.18) [39].

Pharmacological support

During the advent of carotid angioplasty, periprocedural heparin was routinely given, as was commonplace during peripheral angioplasty, although there was no clear consensus either in the UK [40] or elsewhere on the optimal dose. There was variable use of periprocedural antiplatelets most commonly limited to the use of aspirin as the sole agent. Initially, intravenous heparin was administered for 24 hours post-procedure. The importance of the administration of an anticholinergic prior to endovascular manipulation of the carotid bulb, in order to prevent sinus bradyarrythmias, was emphasized in the early 1990s [41].

As early as 1996, major centres were advocating a dual antiplatelet periprocedural regime namely aspirin and ticlopidine [42]. Ticlopidine was replaced by clopidogrel once the adverse bone marrow suppressive effects of the former were appreciated and dipyridamole was used in aspirin-intolerant patients. Aspirin is a cyclo-oxygenase inhibitor (prostaglandin synthase) and its antiplatelet effect is due to platelet thromboxane sythesis inhibition. Clopidogrel inhibits platelet adenosine diphosphonate (ADP) receptors thus preventing fibrinogen binding. Dual antiplatelet therapy that inhibits more than one pathway of platelet activation is biologically rational and sufficient antiplatelet effect is achieved if clopidogrel is added to aspirin as a loading dose of 300mg six hours before or 75mg daily for one week pre-procedure, to continue for 28 days following stent placement. Previous studies have demonstrated that by 30 minutes following a 375mg loading dose of clopidogrel, there is a 55% platelet inhibition, and that maximal inhibition occurs by five hours. There is some support for this antiplatelet regime from the coronary trials. Those undergoing percutaneous coronary intervention derive early and sustained benefit from treatment with aspirin and clopidogrel following loading with clopidogrel, (the Percutaneous Coronary Intervention in the Clopidogrel in Unstable Angina to Prevent Recurrent Events [PCI-CURE] and the Clopidogrel for Reduction of Events During Observation [CREDO] trials) [43, 44].

The effect of pharmacological regimes on the embolic risk of a carotid stenosis cannot be overemphasised. S-Nitrosoglutathione has been shown to significantly reduce microembolic signals (MES) on Transcranial Doppler (TCD) post-carotid angioplasty compared with placebo in a randomised trial [45].

Intravenous acetylsalicylic acid rapidly reduces MES on TCD in patients with recent stroke of carotid bifurcation origin. A significant drop in MES on the side of the symptomatic carotid stenosis was demonstrated within 30 minutes of a bolus injection of acetylsalicylic acid [46].

With respect to glycoprotein IIb/IIIa inhibitors (abciximab; ReoPro, Eli Lilly & Co, Indianapolis, USA), the promise shown in reducing ischaemic events during coronary interventions has not been borne out in the carotid territory. In fact, a recent retrospective review urged caution against the use of ReoPro during carotid stenting, suggesting that patients receiving this drug were more likely to suffer more numerous and consequential sequelae [47].

From the mid-1990s to date, increasing numbers of carotid stents were placed by interventional cardiologists in Europe and the US, although this has not been the case so far in the United Kingdom. Their involvement has had a positive influence on the accrual of evidence because of the trial-orientation and infrastructure of the specialty.

Evolution of protection devices

Since the earliest reports of the use of protection devices, there has been a pervasive move towards their use as it was perceived that they would enhance the safety profile of the procedure. Interventionists worked closely with the industry to modify and improve each of the three philosophies in mechanical cerebral protection and many of the currently available devices have evolved through many iterations and currently enjoy greatly improved structure and function. In 2001, the consensus amongst opinion leaders in carotid angioplasty and stenting was that protection devices should be used when available [38]. For an in-depth discussion of the use of protection devices during endovascular carotid intervention, the reader is referred to chapter 15.

Evidence - where are we now?

Current recommendations for carotid stenting

Recommendations with respect to carotid stenting have been based on the outcomes from the earliest randomised trials. Two such trials were prematurely stopped [33, 48] and the three completed trials were ongoing [21, 49, 50] when a number of the recommendations were made. To put the 'stopped' trials into concept, it must be appreciated that during the era that endarterectomy was scrutinized, there were at least two trials with negative outcomes [51, 52].

There has been substantial evolutionary change in the technique of percutaneous carotid intervention during the time-frame of the reported randomised trials and consequently, the endovascular limb of the CAVATAS trial is now hardly recognisable compared with current endovascular practice.

The recommendations from various advisory bodies are presented in chronological order.

The American Heart Association Science Advisory Council's statements with respect to carotid stenting and angioplasty dating from 1998 [53] are as follows:-

Despite several large studies...there is still debate about its relative efficacy and applicability compared with surgery, primarily because long-term patency after PTA (angioplasty) is limited by restenosis....

The final statement of this document was:-

The techniques of carotid angioplasty and carotid stenting are available, as are a limited degree of experience and a high level of interest. The existence of a technique, however, does not justify or mandate its use. We must remember a basic tenet of medicine: primum non nocere - first do no harm. At this point, with few exceptions, use of carotid stenting should be limited to well-designed, well-controlled randomised studies with careful, dispassionate oversight.

This recommendation is dated because it was based largely on the results of carotid angioplasty

results and it can no longer be stated that there is limited experience; there is a substantial body of experience albeit within limited centres.

A Cochrane systematic review on percutaneous transluminal angioplasty and stenting for carotid artery stenosis reported in 2000 [54]:-

There is no evidence as yet to assess the relative effects of carotid percutaneous transluminal angioplasty in people with carotid stenosis.

CAVATAS [21], the Lexington trial [49] and SAPPHIRE [50] were yet to report at the time of this review's conclusion.

In 2001, in a document on the current status of carotid bifurcation angioplasty and stenting based on a consensus of opinion leaders [38], it was concluded:-

Carotid bifurcation angioplasty and stenting should not undergo widespread practice, which should await results of randomised trials. Carotid bifurcation angioplasty and stenting is currently appropriate treatment for patients at high risk in experienced centres. Carotid bifurcation angioplasty is not generally appropriate for patients at low risk.

There were divergent opinions regarding the proportions of patients acceptable for stenting, ranging from 5% to 100% with a mean of 44%.

In 2002, an Intercollegiate Working Party for Stroke (Royal College of Physicians, London, United Kingdom) produced guidelines on secondary stroke prevention as part of the National Clinical Guidelines for Stroke [55]. It was stated that:-

Carotid angioplasty or stenting is an alternative to surgery but should only be carried out in centres with a proven low complication rate.

This was a grade A recommendation and reflects an early subtle change in emphasis. There was no stipulation that carotid stenting must be limited to trials or to patients deemed to be at high surgical risk.

The most recent documented recommendations date from 2003, from the European Stroke Initiative Recommendations for Stroke Management - Update

2003 [56]. With respect to asymptomatic disease it was stated:-

Carotid angioplasty, with or without stenting, is not routinely recommended for patients with asymptomatic carotid stenosis. It may be considered in the context of randomised clinical trials.

With respect to symptomatic disease, it was concluded that:-

The use of carotid angioplasty and stenting should be limited to well-designed, well-conducted, randomised trials.

The specific recommendations were:-

◆ Carotid percutaneous transluminal angioplasty may be performed for patients with contraindications to endarterectomy or with stenosis at surgically inaccessible sites (level IV).
◆ Carotid percutaneous transluminal angioplasty and stenting may be indicated for patients with restenosis after initial endarterectomy or stenosis following radiation (level IV).
◆ Patients should receive a combination of clopidogrel and aspirin immediately before, during and at least one month after stenting (level IV).

Level I evidence supporting the safety of carotid angioplasty/stenting

Just over 20 years on from the initial case report, the first completed randomised trial comparing carotid angioplasty (with or without stenting) to CEA reported immediate and intermediate-term outcomes. The relative speed with which this new procedure went from first report to first randomised trial reflects a number of things: firstly, it had to compete with a reasonably well-evaluated gold standard; secondly, the efforts of the interventionists involved; and lastly, the prevailing milieu of evidence-based practice.

The completed randomised trials include CAVATAS [21], the Lexington trial set in a community hospital [49] and the SAPPHIRE trial (Stenting and Angioplasty with Protection in Patients at High Risk for Endarterectomy) [50]. CAVATAS and the Lexington trial reported fully in 2001. The 12-month results of SAPPHIRE were presented in March 2003 [50].

CAVATAS was a multicentre clinical trial that randomised 504 patients with symptomatic carotid artery stenosis which the investigators 'believed needed treatment' between endovascular and surgical treatments. In the endovascular limb, stents were used in 26% of cases. The rates of major outcome events within 30 days of first treatment did not differ significantly between endovascular and surgical treatment (6.4% versus 5.9%, respectively for disabling stroke or death; 10% versus 9.9% for any stroke lasting more than seven days, or death). Cranial neuropathy was reported after endarterectomy (8.7%), but not after endovascular treatment (p<0.0001). Major groin or neck haematoma occurred less often after endovascular treatment than after surgery (1.2% versus 6.7%, p<0.0015). It was concluded that carotid surgery and angioplasty were equivalent in safety and efficacy, but that angioplasty had advantages with respect to nerve injury and cardiac complications [57]. Detractors of this study point out that the confidence intervals were wide and that the surgical event rate was higher than expected. The authors of the trial conceded that a clinically important difference in favour of either treatment could not be ruled out. With respect to the surgical event rate, it was concluded that the surgeons and anesthesiologists involved in CAVATAS were likely to have had similar skills and used similar techniques to those in NASCET; indeed, many CAVATAS centres had collaborated in ECST and NASCET. The rate of non-stroke related adverse events in CAVATAS and NASCET were very similar. The high morbidity rate in both limbs of the trial was attributed to the inclusion of patients at higher than average risk from treatment; case mix is known to be an important factor in surgical risk [58]. The great strength of CAVATAS, apart from its randomised design, was the independent neurological review common to NASCET and ECST but often lacking in many self-audited, single-centre experiences. The addition of a neurologist to the authorship of a paper evaluating outcomes following endarterectomy has been shown to significantly increase the reported neurological event rate [59].

One hundred and four patients with symptomatic carotid artery stenosis >70% (NASCET criteria) were randomised to carotid stenting versus endarterectomy within the Lexington trial. There was one death (from myocardial infarction) following endarterectomy and one transient ischaemic attack (following stenting). In the surgical limb, four surgical patients suffered peripheral neurological injury and one had a neck haematoma requiring surgical intervention. Primary stenting was performed after routine predilatation, without cerebral protection but with a dual antiplatelet regime. The conclusions were that carotid stenting was equivalent to endarterectomy in reducing carotid stenosis without increased risk for major complications of death/stroke. Stenting was also considered to have potential benefits with respect to shortened hospitalisation and convalescence, if a reduction in costs could be achieved.

SAPPHIRE enrolled patients from 29 US centres. Patients were enrolled if they had at least one feature that would make them a high surgical risk (age >80 years, the presence of congestive heart failure, severe COPD, previous endarterectomy with restenosis, previous radiation therapy or radical neck surgery, or lesions proximal or distal to the bulb/proximal internal carotid artery). Asymptomatic patients with >80% stenosis on ultrasound or symptomatic patients with >50% stenosis were included. A total of 307 patients were randomised, 156 to carotid stenting, 151 to endarterectomy. The trial was stopped prematurely because of slowing enrollment, with increasing resistance on the part of both physicians and patients to randomisation. The primary outcome was the composite end-point of myocardial infarction, any stroke and death. There was a significant overall reduction in the stenting limb, 5.8% versus 12.6% in the surgical limb (p=0.05), with reductions in adverse events that did not reach statistical significance for a subset analysis for symptomatic and asymptomatic populations. There was no significant difference in the rates of major bleeding or transient ischaemic attack, but a significant reduction in cranial nerve injury in the stented limb (p<0.01).

A systematic review published in 2000 and evaluating articles published between 1990 and 1999, concluded that the risk of stroke was significantly greater with angioplasty than with endarterectomy (7.1% versus 4%) [60]. This review

was not prepared for the Cochrane Collaboration and was not based on level I evidence. The studies included were non-randomised, heterogeneous, sometimes single-centre and often self-audited. The reviewers did not assess the quality of the included studies, dual independent review was lacking and there was no discussion of consistency, just a pooling and/or averaging of results. The patient populations treated by angioplasty and by endarterectomy were different. Endovascular treatments were also heterogeneous.

In a Cochrane review evaluating only level I evidence, stopped, unreported and unpublished trials would all necessarily contribute to the final body of evidence and the uncompleted trials must thus be considered.

The Wallstent trial [61] aimed to compare carotid stenting and endarterectomy in patients with high-grade symptomatic carotid disease, but was stopped after only 219 patients out of the proposed 700 were recruited. The event rate in the stenting group was unacceptably high with an ipsilateral stroke, procedure-related death or vascular death rate at one year of 12.1% versus 3.6% for endarterectomy (p=0.02). Primary stenting was performed without predilatation or cerebral protection and the Wallstent was not a dedicated carotid device. The Leicester trial [33] which randomised patients with high-grade disease between surgery and stenting, was expected to recruit 300 patients but was stopped after only 17 had been treated because of an unacceptable complication rate in the stenting limb. Ten endarterectomies were performed without complication, but five of the seven patients undergoing stenting suffered a stroke. The structure of this study deserves comment because the outcomes were disparate compared with those of many other centres during the same period. No prior imaging of the origin of the major vessels was undertaken to exclude disease that would ordinarily constitute a contraindication to an endovascular approach. Only a single antiplatelet agent was employed prior to carotid stenting, whereas major units were already recommending combining aspirin with clopidogrel or ticlopidine [42]. The interventionist had limited experience of stenting within the carotid territory, whereas the surgeons involved had considerable expertise. Pre-dilatation was not routine and it is observed from the data that of five of the cases in whom there was failed initial passage of the stent, four suffered a stroke. A non-dedicated Wallstent was used. It is clearly not possible to pass a 7 French device (2.3mm) through a 70% stenosis (best residual channel of 1.8mm) without some uncontrolled plaque disruption. Cerebral protection was not used.

Currently, a number of trials and registries are ongoing and ought to yield reliable data. The Carotid Revascularization Endarterectomy Versus Stenting Trial (CREST), the International Carotid Stenting Study (ICSS or CAVATAS-II), Stent-protected Percutaneous Angioplasty of the Carotid Versus Endarterectomy (SPACE) and the Endarterectomy Versus Angioplasty in patients with severe symptomatic carotid stenosis (EVA-3S) study are all multicentre randomised trials comparing carotid stenting and endarterectomy for symptomatic patients.

CARESS (Carotid Revascularization with Endarterectomy or Stenting Systems) is an observational study designed to include those patients excluded from CREST and include some asymptomatic patients. This is a multicentre prospective non-randomised clinical trial designed as an equivalent cohort study with concurrent controls and independent review and it has recently reported [62]. It evaluated outcomes from surgical or endovascular intervention in a broad risk population of patients with symptomatic and asymptomatic carotid stenosis. There was no significant difference in the 30-day combined all-cause mortality and stroke rate by Kaplan-Meier estimate between endarterectomy (2%) and stenting (2%). There was no significant difference in the secondary endpoint of combined 30-day all-cause mortality, stroke, and myocardial infarction rate between endarterectomy (3%) and stenting (2%).

SECURITY (Registry Study to Evaluate the NeuroShield™ Bare Wire Cerebral Protection System and X-Act™ Stent in Patients at High Risk for Carotid Endarterectomy) and ARCHER (ACCULINK™ for revascularization of carotids in High-Risk Patients) are registries evaluating protected carotid stenting in surgically high-risk patients.

Large-series experience has gradually accrued within high-throughput centres and the reported outcomes are favourable but do highlight the influence of both learning curve and the technological advances on the event rate. Many show a reduction in adverse event rate in more recently treated patients. A survey reporting outcomes of 12,392 carotid stent procedures worldwide (11,243 patients) demonstrated a combined all stroke/procedure-related death of 4.75% [63]. This was largely self-audited and thus some caution must be exercised in the interpretation of this study. What is evident from the current available literature is that event rates from stenting may be comfortably below those recommended by the American Heart Association for endarterectomy [64].

Efficacy at preventing future stroke: level I evidence

At present there are limited data on long-term outcomes following carotid stenting arising from randomised trials. Essentially, these data comprise the results of CAVATAS and the Lexington trial. There have been some concerns on the restenosis rate following carotid angioplasty/stenting. However, some important factors should be appreciated. Firstly, the majority of patients treated within the endovascular limb of CAVATAS underwent angioplasty alone. Angioplasty may provide a less definitive lumen initially compared to stenting and may result in greater immediate recoil. This must be differentiated from 'true' restenosis as caused by neointimal hyperplasia or atheromatous disease-progression. Secondly, there may be very different true restenosis rates following primary stenting compared to angioplasty, due to the difference in mechanism of vascular wall injury.

At 1-year after treatment in CAVATAS, severe (70-99%) ipsilateral carotid stenosis was more usual after endovascular treatment than surgery (14% versus 4%), p<0.001. However, results from the survival analysis showed that both surgery and endovascular treatment were equally effective at preventing stroke. At three years' follow-up, the rate of death or disabling stroke (any territory) including treatment-related events was 14.3% in the endovascular group and 14.2% in the surgery patients. Survival analyses were done by Cox's proportional hazards regression, with adjustment for sex, age and trial centre. For any disabling stroke or death, the hazards ratio (endovascular treatment/surgery) was 1.03 (95% CI

Table 2. Intermediate and longer-term outcomes from carotid angioplasty/stenting trials, registries and larger series.

Trial/ Series	Int.	Duration of follow-up	Endpoint	Rate of outcome event	Restenosis	Independent review	Asymptomatic patients included
CAVATAS [21]	PTA/ Stent	3 years	Death/disabling stroke any territory	14.3%	(70-99%) 14%	Yes	No
	CEA			14.2%	(70-99%) 4%		
SAPPHIRE [50]	Protected stenting	1 year	MI/any stroke/death	11.9%	-	Yes	Yes
	CEA			19.9%			
Wholey registry [61]	Stent	3 years	All stroke/stroke related death	1.7%	(>50%) 2.4%	No	Yes
Roubin et al [73]	Stent	3 years	Fatal and non-fatal stroke*	11% (symptomatic) 14% (asymptomatic)	-	Yes	Yes
McKevitt (Gaines) et al [39]	PTA/Stent	1 year	All-stroke *post-procedure* Ipsilateral stroke *post-procedure*	2.8% 0.8%	(>50%) 17.7% (>70%) 6.7% (100%) 2.9% (70-100%) 15.5%	Yes	No
Ahmadi et al [74]	Stent	1 year	All-stroke *post-procedure* Ipsilateral stroke *post-procedure*	0.7% 0.3%	(>70%) 3%	Yes	Yes
Gray et al [75]	Stent	2 years	Ipsilateral stroke (including procedural) Ipsilateral stroke Ipsilateral stroke (major)	3.9% 1.3% 0%	(>50%) 4.8%	Yes	Yes
Cremonesi et al [76]	PTA/Stent	3 years (6-36 months)	All-stroke Stroke mortality	6.7% 0%	(>50%) 5.04%	Yes	Yes
Bequemin et al [77]	Stent	3 years	Minor persistent stroke Major ipsilateral stroke	2.6% 1.8%	(>50%) 7.5%	Yes	Yes
	CEA		Minor persistent stroke Major ipsilateral stroke	1.4% 0.5%	1.4%		

Key:

MI = myocardial infarction

PTA = percutaneous transluminal angioplasty

CEA = carotid endarterectomy

INT = intervention

* Fatal and non-fatal stroke were chosen by Roubin et al as the most appropriate outcome measure rather than stroke and all-cause mortality. This choice was made as selection criteria in trials of CEA often precluded life-threatening illnesses: cancer, lung disease and coronary ischaemia, whereas these factors did not exclude patients from carotid stenting. Survival analysis in terms of all-cause mortality for carotid stenting may therefore reflect levels of co-morbidity rather than efficacy of technique.

0.64-1.64, p=0.09). Secondary analyses were done for two other survival outcomes. For ipsilateral stroke lasting more than seven days the hazards ratio was 1.04 (95% CI 0.63-1.70, p=0.9). For disabling or fatal ipsilateral stroke, with other causes of treatment-related death excluded, the hazard ratio was 1.22 (95% CI 0.63-2.36, p=0.4).

Provisional analysis of further follow-up data within CAVATAS suggests that the benefit of carotid angioplasty or stenting persists for up to eight years following treatment.

Patients treated within the Lexington trial [49] have reported follow-up for 24 months to date. There were no strokes in either treatment limb within this period of follow-up and no evidence of asymptomatic focal cerebral ischaemia on magnetic resonance imaging (MRI). The 24-month patency of the reconstructed artery was reported as 'satisfactory' as determined by carotid ultrasound.

Twelve-month results have now been presented for the SAPPHIRE trial [50]. In this population, deemed to be at high surgical risk, the 12-month major adverse event rate was 11.9% in patients randomised to stent plus embolic protection device compared with 19.9% in patients randomised to endarterectomy.

There is a growing body of level II evidence providing data on the efficacy of stenting at preventing ipsilateral stroke in the intermediate term. There are some sizeable single-centre series with independent review to between three and five years. Intermediate and longer-term outcomes from carotid stenting trials, registries and larger series are given in Table 2.

Restenosis

Currently, the limiting factor in the wider application of carotid stenting is the perceived problem of restenosis. The pragmatic approach to restenosis is the consideration of clinical relevance. Arguably, neointimal hyperplasia is not generally accepted to be an emboligenic surface and the rationale for treatment in the carotid artery is for embolic risk and not, in the majority, for hypoperfusion issues. Furthermore, care must be taken in the evaluation of carotid restenosis in a stented vessel. A study on the haemodynamic effects of internal carotid artery stenting using color-coded duplex sonography demonstrated a number of important findings most notably relating to changes in the ICA to CCA velocity ratio which may be misinterpreted as restenosis on the basis of increased velocities [65].

Following stenting, restenosis would appear to be infrequently symptomatic [66, 67]. This mirrors the lack of correlation between late stroke and recurrent stenosis within the asymptomatic carotid atherosclerosis study (ACAS) [68]. Initial hyperglycaemia in the stented diabetic population is a predictor of more pronounced neointimal hyperplasia [69]. Increasing age, female sex, multiple stents and post-procedural percent stenosis may be associated with an increased incidence of restenosis [70]. There are also some data to suggest that patients who develop restenosis after endarterectomy are also more likely to restenose post-stenting [71]. However, it would appear that symptomatic restenoses are likely to be amenable to further endovascular intervention.

A recent study evaluated healing of the stented carotid artery on duplex [72]. Three phases of carotid stent incorporation were defined: an early unstable period soon after stent placement with an echolucent (thrombotic) layer which is seen to become negligible by 30 days; a moderately unstable phase with ingrowing neointima (1-12 months); and lastly, a stable phase from the second year on. These data may indicate the need for different intensities of therapy and surveillance intervals.

Conclusions

The evolutionary change of each element of the endovascular technique as applicable to the carotid territory has been both profound and precipitous. The emerging data on the efficacy of carotid stenting with respect to survival free of ipsilateral stroke is encouraging. The restenosis rate does not necessarily parallel the recurrence of symptoms.

Summary

◆ There has been a profound and precipitous evolutionary change in the technique of percutaneous carotid intervention.

◆ This evoution has been driven by both the industry and by the involved interventionists in order to enhance the technique's safety profile.

◆ There are level I data to support the safety of carotid stenting.

◆ The emerging data on survival free of ipsilateral stroke are encouraging.

◆ Mechanisms of tissue healing following carotid stenting are being evaluated and understanding of these may further direct optimal post-procedural therapeutic regimes.

◆ Restenosis is asymptomatic in the majority.

References

1. Mathias K. A new catheter system for percutaneous transluminal angioplasty (PTA) of carotid artery stenoses. *Fortschr Med* 1977; 95: 1007-1011.

2. Kerber CW, Cromwell LD, Leohden OL. Catheter dilatation of proximal stenosis during distal bifurcation endarterectomy. *AJNR* 1980; 1: 348-349.

3. Mathias K, Bockenheimer S, von Reutern G, Heiss HW, Ostheim-Dzerowycz W. Catheter dilatation of arteries supplying the brain. *Radiologe* 1983; 23: 208-214.

4. Bockenheimer SA, Mathias K. Percutaneous transluminal angioplasty in arteriosclerotic internal carotid artery stenosis. *AJNR* 1983; 4: 791-792.

5. Wigli U, Gratz O. Transluminal angioplasty of stenotic carotid arteries: case reports and protocol. *AJNR* 1983; 4: 793-795.

6. Frietag G, Frietag J, Koch RD, Wagemann W. Percutaneous angioplasty of carotid artery stenoses. *Neuroradiology* 1986; 28: 126-127.

7. Kachel R, Ritter H, Grossman K, Glaser FH. Results of percutaneous transluminal dilatation of cerebral vascular stenoses. *ROFO Fortschr Geb Roentgenstr Nuklearmed* 1986; 144: 338-342.

8. Vitek J. Percutaneous transluminal angioplasty of the carotid artery. *AJNR* 1986; 7: 1103-1104.

9. Kachel R, Endert G, Basche S, Grossman K, Glaser FH. Percutaneous transluminal angioplasty (dilatation) of carotid, vertebral and innominate artery stenoses. *Cardiovasc Intervent Radiol* 1987; 10: 142-146.

10. Tievsky AL, Druy EM, Mardiat JG. Transluminal angioplasty in postsurgical stenosis of the extracranial carotid artery. *AJNR* 1983; 4: 800-802.

11. Numaguchi Y, Puyau FA, Provenza LJ, Ricahrdson DE. Percutaneous transluminal angioplasty of the carotid artery. Its application to post surgical stenosis. *Neuroradiology* 1984; 26: 527-530.

12. Courtheoux P, Theron J, Tournade A, Maiza D, Henriet JP, Braun JP. Percutaneous endoluminal angioplasty of post endarterectomy carotid stenoses. *Neuroradiology* 1987; 29: 186-189.

13. Hasso AN, Bird CR, Zinke DE, Thompson JR. Fibromuscular dysplasia of the internal carotid artery: percutaneous transluminal angioplasty. *AJR* 1981; 136: 955-960.

14. Garrido E, Montoya J. Transluminal dilatation of internal carotid artery in fibromuscular dysplasia: a preliminary study. *Surg Neurol* 1981; 16: 469-471.

15. Belan A, Vesela M, Vanek I, Weiss K, Peregrin J. Percutaneous transluminal angioplasty of fibromuscular dysplasia of the internal carotid artery. *Cardiovasc Intervent Radiol* 1982; 5: 79-81.

16. Dublin AB, Baltaxe HA, Cobb CA 3rd. Percutaneous transluminal carotid angioplasty in fibromuscular dysplasia. Case Report. *J Neurosurg* 1983; 59: 162-165.

17. Brown MM, Butler P, Gibbs J, Swash M, Waterston J. Feasibility of percutaenous transluminal angioplasty for carotid artery stenosis. *J Neurol Neurosurg Psychiatry* 1990; 53: 238-243.

18. Theron J, Raymond J, Casasco A, Courtheoux F. Percutaneous amgioplasty of atherosclerotic and postsurgical stenosis of the carotid arteries. *AJNR* 1987; 8: 495-500.

19. Theron J, Courtheoux P, Alachkar F, Bouvard G, Maiza D. New triple coaxial catheter system for carotid angioplasty with cerebral protection. *AJNR* 1990; 11: 869-874.

20. Kachel R. Results of Balloon Angioplasty in the Carotid Arteries. *J Endovasc Surg* 1996; 3: 22-30.

21. CAVATAS investigators. Endovascular versus surgical treatment in patients with carotid stenosis in the Carotid and Vertebral Artery Transluminal Angioplasty study (CAVATAS): a randomized trial. *Lancet* 2001; 357: 1729-1737.

22. Serruys PW, De Jaegere P, Kiemeneij F, *et al.* A comparison of balloon-expandable stent implantation with balloon angioplasty in patients with coronary artery disease: Benestent study group. *N Engl J Med* 1994; 331: 489-495.

23. Stent restenosis study investigators. A randomized comparison of coronary-stent placement and balloon angioplasty in the treatment of coronary artery disease. *N Engl J Med* 1994; 331: 496-501.

24. Meads C, Cummins C, Jolly K, Stevens A, Burls A, Hyde C. Executive Summary: coronary artery stents in the treatment of ischaemic heart disease: a rapid and systematic review. *Health Technology Assessment* 2000; Vol 4: No 23.

25. Brophy JM, Belisle P, Joseph L. Evidence for use of coronary stents. A hierarchical Bayesian meta-analysis. *Ann Intern Med* 2003; 138: 777-786.

26. Diethrich EB, Ndiaye M, Reid DB. Stenting in the carotid artery: initial experience in 110 patients. *J Endovasc Surg* 1996; 3: 42-62.

27. Yadav J, Roubin GS, Iyer S, Vitek J, King P, Jordan WD, Fisher WS. Elective stenting of the extracranial carotid arteries. *Circulation* 1997; 95: 376-381.

28. Krupski WC, Bass A, Kelly AB, Hanson SR, Harker LA. Reduction in thrombus formation by placement of endovascular stents at endarterectomy sites in baboon carotid arteries. *Circulation* 1991; 84: 1749-1757.

29. Bergeron P, Chambran P, Benichou H, Alessandri C. Recurrent carotid disease: will stents be an alternative to surgery? *J Endovasc Surg* 1996; 3: 76-79.

30. Gaines PA. Carotid Angioplasty. *Vasc Med* 1996; 1: 121-124.

31. Rapp JH, Pan XM, Sharp FR, et al. Atheroemboli to the brain: Size threshold causing acute neuronal cell death. *J Vasc Surg* 2000; 32: 68-76

32. Coggia M, Goeau-Brissonniere O, Duvall JL, Leschi JP, Letort M, Nagel MD. Embolic risk of the different stages of carotid bifurcation balloon angioplasty: an experimental study. *J Vasc Surg* 2000; 31: 550-557.

33. Naylor AR, Bolia A, Abbott RJ, et al. Randomized study of carotid angioplasty and stenting versus carotid endarterectomy: a stopped trial. *J Vasc Surg* 1998; 28: 326-334.

34. Parodi JC, La Mura R, Ferreira M, et al. Initial evaluation of carotid angioplasty and stenting with three different cerebral protection devices. *J Vasc Surg* 2000;32:1127-1136.

35. Mathur A, Dorros G, Iyer SS, Vitek JJ, Yadav SS, Roubin GS. Palmaz stent compression in patients following carotid artery stenting. *Cathet Cardiovasc Diagn* 1997; 41: 137-140.

36. Wholey MH, Wholey M, Mathias K, et al. Global experience in cervical carotid artery stent placement. *Catheter Cardiovasc Interv* 2000; 50: 160-167.

37. Wholey MH, Wholey MH, Tan WA, Eles G, Jarmolowski C, Cho S. A comparison of balloon-mounted and self-expanding stents in the carotid arteries: immediate and long-term results of more than 500 patients. *J Endovasc Ther* 2003; 10: 171-181.

38. Veith FJ, Amor M, Ohki T, et al. Current status of carotid bifurcation angioplasty and stenting based on a consensus of opinion leaders. *J Vasc Surg* 2001; 33 (2 Suppl): S111-6 Review.

39. McKevitt FM, Macdonald S, Venables G, Cleveland TJ, Gaines PA. Complications following carotid angioplasty and carotid stenting in patients with symptomatic carotid artery disease. *Cerebrovasc Dis* 2004; 17: 28-34.

40. Zaman SM, de Vroos Meiring P, Gandhi MR, Gaines PA. The pharmoacokinetics and UK usage of heparin in vascular intervention. *Clinical Radiology* 1996; 51: 113-116.

41. Gaines PA. Carotid angioplasty and sinus arrythmia. *Clinical Radiology* 1993; 48: 431-433.

42. Yadav JS, Roubin GS, King P, Iyer S, Vitek J. Angioplasty and stenting for restenosis after carotid endarterectomy. *Stroke* 1996; 27: 2075-2079.

43. Mehta SR, Yusuf S, Peters RJ, et al. Effects of pretreatment with clopidogrel and aspirin followed by long-term therapy in patients undergoing percutaneous coronary intervention: the PCI-CURE study. *Lancet* 2001; 358: 527-533.

44. Steinhubl SR, Berger PB, Mann JT III, et al for the CREDO Investigators. Early and sustained dual oral antiplatelet therapy following percutaneous coronary intervention: a randomized controlled trial. *JAMA* 2002; 288: 2411-2420.

45. Kaposzta Z, Clifton A, Molloy J, Martin JF, Markus HS. S-nitrosoglutathione reduces asymptomatic embolization after carotid angioplasty. *Circulation* 2002; 106: 3057-3062.

46. Goertler M, Baeumer M, Kross R, et al. Rapid decline of cerebral microemboli of arterial origin after intravenous acetylsalicylic acid. *Stroke* 1999; 30: 66-69.

47. Wholey HM, Wholey MH, Eles G, et al. Evaluation of glycoprotein IIb/IIIa inhibitors in carotid angioplasty and stenting. *J Endovasc Ther* 2003; 10: 33-41.

48. Alberts MJ. Results of a Multicenter Prospective Randomized Trial of Carotid Artery Senting vs. Carotid Endarterectomy. *Stroke* 2001; 32: 325.

49. Brooks WH, McClure RR, Jones MR, Coleman TL, Breathitt L. Carotid Angioplasty and Stenting Versus Carotid Endarterectomy: Randomized Trial in a Cummunity Hospital. *J Am Coll Cardiol* 2001; 38: 1589-1595.

50. Yadav J. SAPPHIRE 12-month results. Presented at Transcatheter Cardiovascular Therapeutics (TCT) Chicago, March 2003.

51. Fields WS, Maslenikov V, Meyer JS, et al. Joint study of extracranial arterial occlusion. V. Progress report of prognosis following surgery or nonsurgical treatment for transient cerebral ischemic attacks and cervical carotid artery lesions. *JAMA* 1970; 211: 1993-2003.

52. Shaw DA, Venables GS, Cartildge NEF, et al. Carotid endarterectomy in patients with transient cerebral ischemia. *J Neurol Sci* 1984; 64: 45-53.

53. Bettmann MA, Katzen BT, Whisnant J, et al. Carotid stenting and angioplasty: a statement for healthcare professionals from the Councils on Cardiovascular Radiology, Stroke, Cardio-Thoracic and Vascular Surgery, Epidemiology, and Prevention, and Clinical Cardiology, American Heart Association. *Circulation* 1998; 97: 121-123.

54. Crawley F, Brown MM. Percutaneous transluminal angioplasty and stenting for carotid artery stenosis. *Cochrane Database Syst Rev* 2000; (2): CD000515

55. Intercollegiate Working Party for Stroke. National Clinical Guidelines for Stroke. Section 11.3: Secondary prevention-update. February 2002. Copyright to Royal College of Physicians, London.

56. The European Stroke Initiative Executive Committee and EUSI Writing Committee. European Stroke Initiative Recommendations for Stroke Management-Update 2003. *Cerebrovasc Dis* 2003; 16: 311-337.

57. Brown MM. Results of the carotid and vertebral artery transluminal angioplasty study. *Br J Surg* 1999; 86: 710-711.

58. Sundt TM, Sandok BA, Whisnant JP. Carotid endarterectomy: complications and preoperative assessment of risk. *Mayo Clin Proc* 1975; 50: 301-306.

59. Rothwell P, Warlow C. Is self-audit reliable? *Lancet* 1995; 346: 1623.

60. Golledge J, Mitchell A, Greenhalgh RM. Systematic comparison of the early outcome of angioplasty and endarterectomy for symptomatic carotid artery disease. *Stroke* 2000; 31: 1439-1443.

61. Alberts MJ. Results of a Multicenter Prospective Randomized Trial of Carotid Artery Senting vs. Carotid Endarterectomy. *Stroke* 2001; 32: 325.

62. Carotid Revascularisation Using Endarterectomy or Stenting Systems (CARESS): Phase 1 Clinical Trial. *J Endovasc Ther* 2003; 10: 1021-1030.

63. Wholey MH, Al-Mubarak N, Wholey MH. Updated review of the global carotid artery stent registry. *Catheter Cardiovasc Interv* 2003; 60: 259-266.

64. Moore WS, Barnett HJM, Beebe HG, *et al.* Guidelines for carotid endarterectomy. A Multidisciplinary Consensus Statement from the *Ad Hoc* Committee, American Heart Association. *Stroke* 1995; 26: 188-201.

65. Lu CJ, Kao HL, Sun Y, *et al.* The hemodynamic effects of internal carotid artery stenting: a study with color-coded duplex sonography. *Cerebrovasc Dis* 2003;15:264-269.

66. Christiaans MH, Ernst JM, Suttorp MJ, *et al.* Antonius CAROTID Endarterectomy, Angioplasty and Stenting Study Group. *Eur J Vasc Endovasc Surg* 2003; 26: 141-144.

67. Lal BK, Hobson RW 2nd, Goldstein J, *et al.* In-stent recurrent stenosis after carotid artery stenting: life table analysis and clinical experience. *J Vasc Surg* 2003; 38: 1162-1169.

68. Moore WS, Kempczinski RF, Nelson JJ, Toole JF. Recurrent carotid stenosis: results of the asymptomatic carotid atherosclerosis study. *Stroke* 1998; 29: 2018-2025.

69. Willfort-Ehringer A, Ahmadi R, Gessl A, *et al.* Neointinal proliferation with carotid stents is more pronounced in diabetic patients with initial poor glycaemic state. *Diabetologia* 2004 Feb 18 (Epub ahead of print).

70. Khan MA, Liu MW, Chio FL, Roubin GS, Iyer SS, Vitek JJ. Predictors of restenosis after successful carotid artery stenting. *Am J Cardiol* 2003; 92: 895-897.

71. Setacci C, Pula G, Baldi I, *et al.* Determinants of in-stent restenosis after carotid angioplasty: a case-control study. *J Endovasc Ther* 2003; 10: 1031-1038.

72. Willfort-Ehringer A, Ahmadi R, Gschwandtner ME, *et al.* Healing of carotid stents: a prospective duplex ultrasound study. *J Endovasc Ther* 2003 Jun; 10(3): 636-42.

73. Roubin G, Gishel N, Iyer SS, *et al.* Immediate and late clinical outcomes of carotid artery stenting in patients with symptomatic and asymptomatic carotid artery stenosis. A 5-year prospective analysis. *Circulation* 2001; 103: 532.

74. Ahmadi R, Willfort A, Lang W, *et al.* Carotid Artery Stenting: Effect of Learning Curve and Intermediate-Term Morphological Outcome. *J Endovasc Ther* 2001; 8: 539-546.

75. Gray WA, White HJ, Barrett DM, Chandran G, Turner R, Reisman M. Carotid Stenting and Endarterectomy. A Clinical and Cost Comparison of Revascularisation Strategies. *Stroke* 2003; 33: 1063.

76. Cremonesi A, Castriota F, Manetti R, Balestra G, Liso A. Endovascular treatment of carotid atherosclerotic disease:early and late outcome in a non-selected population. *Ital Heart J* 2000; 1: 801-809.

77. Becquemin JP, Ben El Kadi H, Desgranges P, Kobeiter H. Carotid stenting versus carotid surgery: a prospective cohort study. *J Endovasc Ther* 2003; 10: 687-694.

Chapter 14

Carotid endarterectomy or stenting: an overview of the randomised trials

A Ross Naylor, MD FRCS, Professor of Vascular Surgery

Leicester Royal Infirmary, Leicester, UK

Peter A Gaines, FRCP FRCR, Consultant Vascular Radiologist

The Sheffield Vascular Institute, The Northern General Hospital, Sheffield, UK

Introduction

Four multicentre randomised trials have provided level I (grade A) evidence that carotid endarterectomy (CEA) confers significant benefit over 'best medical therapy' in the management of selected patients with symptomatic [1,2] and asymptomatic [3,4] carotid artery disease. Over the last decade, however, the role of CEA as the 'gold standard treatment' has been challenged by the emergence of carotid artery stenting (CAS).

Carotid stenting offers a number of potential advantages over CEA including:-

◆ shorter hospital stay;
◆ avoidance of a wound and its associated complications (pain, infection, numbness, haematoma, patch infection;
◆ avoidance of cranial nerve injury; and
◆ reduced cardiovascular complications (myocardial infarction etc).

However, the principal reason for intervening in the first place is the prevention of long-term stroke. As a consequence, the main concerns regarding CAS relate to whether it is:-

◆ associated with an increased risk of procedural stroke; and
◆ durable in the long-term.

The literature abounds with claim and counterclaim about the relative benefits, longevity and cost-effectiveness of CEA versus CAS. However, the only way to definitively evaluate the two treatments is through randomised trials. This chapter reviews the available data from the seven studies published to date and highlights the key messages and limitations from each study.

The Leicester Trial [5]

Methodology

This study planned to randomise 300 patients with carotid territory symptoms and an ipsilateral carotid stenosis >70% to CEA or CAS with primary stenting. Endpoints were the 30-day risk of death/stroke, cumulative stroke at three years, restenosis rates and impairment of cognitive function. Patients were randomised without preliminary diagnostic angiography. Specific exclusion criteria included asymptomatic patients, patients with crescendo TIAs or stroke in evolution and those unwilling to give informed consent. Stents were employed in all patients (Wallstent, Schneider, Minneapolis, USA), preceded by predilatation where necessary.

Results

The Data Monitoring Committee (DMC) suspended the trial after 23 patients had been randomised, by which time 17 had received their allocated treatment. Ten patients randomised to CEA underwent an uncomplicated procedure (five performed by a supervised trainee). However, 5/7 patients randomised to CAS suffered a procedural stroke (p=0.0034). Four occurred during the procedure, while one patient was readmitted on day eight with a non-disabling stroke. Overall, 3/5 strokes were disabling at 30 days. Following review of the outcomes, the DMC, Ethics Committee and the Investigators were unable to develop sufficient clinical equipoise to resume the trial in an amended format. The main problem was in agreeing what CAS risks should be quoted to future patients in the trial. Accordingly, the study was abandoned.

Comment

This was the first randomised trial to be published. However, while it remains too small to influence clinical practice, it did serve to reinforce the potential problem of treating 'all comers' in a non-selected population. In 1996, no cerebral protection devices had been developed.

CAVATAS [6]

Methodology

The Carotid and Vertebral Artery Transluminal Angioplasty Study (CAVATAS) randomised 504 patients with carotid territory symptoms and an ipsilateral stenosis >50%, although the majority had a stenosis >70%. To qualify for inclusion in the trial, a patient had to have a lesion that was suitable for both CEA and CAS. No record was kept of the number of excluded patients in each centre. Specific exclusion

criteria included patients considered unsuitable for surgery (usually due to severe co-morbidity), patients considered unsuitable for CAS because of hostile anatomy (usually vessel tortuosity), those with suspected thrombus overlying the plaque, patients with a severe intracranial stenosis and those unwilling to give informed consent. The trial started recruiting in 1992, before the routine use of dual antiplatelet therapy, primary stenting, or the development of cerebral protection devices (CPDs) and dedicated stent systems. Accordingly, as technology evolved during the 5-year period of patient recruitment, so too did the endovascular technique. Stents were employed after 1994 and included the Wallstent (Schneider, USA), Streker (Medi-Tech, USA) and Palmaz (Johnson and Johnson, USA). Overall, 26% of patients randomised to CAS were stented primarily. Many of these were, however, placed as a 'bail-out' following a poor angioplasty result rather than as a primary stenting procedure.

Results

The risk of death/any stroke at 30 days for 251 patients randomised to CAS was 10.0%, as compared with 9.9% in the 253 patients randomised to CEA (p=ns). Comparable data for death/disabling stroke were 6.4% and 5.9% respectively (p=ns). Cranial nerve injury was documented in 8.7% of CEA patients and surgical patients were significantly more likely to have their hospital discharge delayed because of wound haematoma (6.7% versus 1.3%, p<0.0015). At one year, patients randomised to CAS were more likely to have a recurrent 70-99% stenosis (14% versus 6.7%, p<0.011), but this did not translate into any difference in the cumulative stroke risk at three years. Including the 30-day risk, cumulative freedom from death or disabling stroke at three years was 86% for both CEA and CAS patients (p=ns). No comparable data were provided regarding the three-year risk of death/any stroke.

Comment

This is the largest, published study to date with each treatment modality showing equivalence in terms of prevention of stroke/death out to three years.

Although restenosis rates were significantly higher following CAS, there was no evidence that this translated into a higher risk of late stroke. However, concerns were voiced regarding the higher than anticipated 30-day risks of death/stroke in both treatment groups. The 10% risk of death/stroke was higher than that observed in ECST (7.5%) and NASCET (5.8%), but there was an overlap in confidence intervals. The trial investigators highlighted a number of reasons for the higher procedural risk following CEA and CAS in this trial. These included:-

◆ CAVATAS patients comprised a much higher risk population than was recruited into ECST and NASCET;
◆ many patients were not stented primarily;
◆ cerebral protection devices were not then available; and
◆ interventionists participating in CAVATAS had not received a standardised training in angioplasty.

If, however, 10% was a true reflection of practice, the overall benefit in terms of stroke prevention is significantly reduced. Based on ECST data in symptomatic patients with 70-99% stenoses, units performing CEA or CAS with a 30-day death/stroke rate of 6% will prevent 72 ipsilateral strokes per 1000 interventions and 14 procedures have to be performed to prevent one stroke [7]. If, however, the initial risk was 10%, only 32 ipsilateral strokes would be prevented per 1000 interventions and 32 procedures would have to be performed to prevent one ipsilateral stroke.

CAVATAS was, thereafter, the catalyst for a number of other randomised trials, not least its much larger successor (the International Carotid Stenting Study [ICSS]), which is now recruiting in the UK and Europe.

The WALLSTENT Study [8]

Methods

This study has only been reported in abstract form, having been abandoned by the commercial sponsors after recruiting 219 patients. It is, however, the third largest randomised trial of its kind. All patients were symptomatic and had to have ipsilateral 60-99% carotid stenoses. Patients randomised to CAS (n=107) underwent primary stenting with the Wallstent endoprosthesis (Schneider, Minn, USA). No CPDs were available for use at that time. Power calculations had suggested that 700 patients would be required to complete the study, but the trial was abandoned because of the excess procedural risk in CAS patients.

Results

The 30-day risk of death/any stroke was 12.1% following CAS as compared with 4.5% for CEA (p=0.049). In addition, CAS patients encountered a 7% incidence of bradycardia during the procedure and a 4% incidence of groin haematoma. The 1-year risk of death/ipsilateral stroke (including the procedural risk) was 12.1% for CAS patients and 3.6% for CEA patients (p=0.022). Comparable 1-year data for death/any stroke was not published in the abstract and there was no data regarding rates of restenosis.

Comment

The abstract detailing the above results was published in the journal, *Stroke,* in 2001. It is very disappointing that the methodology and results of this relatively large trial have never subsequently been published in a peer-reviewed journal.

The Lexington Symptomatic Study [9]

Methods

This randomised trial was undertaken in a community hospital and randomised 104 patients with carotid territory symptoms and an ipsilateral >70% stenosis to either CAS with primary stenting (n=53) or CEA (n=51). The stent used in this study was the Wallstent endoprosthesis (Boston Scientific, USA) and no CPDs were employed in any patient. The study was apparently powered to demonstrate equivalence between the two treatment modalities and patients were followed-up for two years.

Results

Following CAS, there was one transient ischaemic attack and one leg amputation. Following CEA, there was one non-stroke death and four cranial nerve palsies. By two years, no patient in either treatment arm had suffered a stroke.

Comment

This trial was underpowered from the start and is virtually unique in that no patient (irrespective of treatment) suffered a stroke at any time within two years of undergoing his or her allocated intervention.

The EVA-3S Trial [10]

Methods

EVA-3S was a multicentre, randomised trial undertaken in France and supported with national research organisation funding. All patients had to have reported recent carotid territory symptoms and had to have an ipsilateral carotid stenosis >70%. In this study, the track records of the interventionists were assessed before they could randomise in the trial. Interventionists had to have performed either:-

◆ 12 CAS with stenting; or
◆ five CAS cases with stenting plus 30 cases of angioplasty to supra-aortic vessels. Less experienced interventionists were, however, mentored until sufficiently skilled.

CAS was performed with primary stenting. Cerebral protection devices were used at the discretion of the operator. However, in order to use one of these devices, the interventionist was required to use a CPD that had been approved by the technical committee of EVA-3S, and he/she also had to demonstrate experience in using this CPD in at least two patients outwith the trial.

Results

This trial was also unique in that the Data Monitoring Committee recommended suspension of the study following an interim analysis of outcomes in the CAS patients. Their principal concern was that the procedural risk appeared to be higher in patients undergoing unprotected CAS (without using a CPD). No data were provided in patients randomised to CEA. However, the trial reported outcomes in all 80 patients who had been randomised to CAS within EVA-3S. CAS could not be performed in 7.5% of randomised patients because of technical difficulties and all of these patients thereafter underwent CEA. Accordingly, CAS was only performed in 73 randomised patients, of whom, 58 (80%) involved the use of a CPD.

Overall, the 30-day risk of death/any stroke was 13.6% in patients randomised to CAS. However, if one includes the patient who suffered a stroke during a failed CAS, the risk of death/stroke within 30 days was 15%. The main reason for declaring these results prematurely was because the investigators and the DMC felt that the adverse outcomes were primarily due to the non-use of a CPD. In their analysis, the risk of death/stroke following unprotected CAS was 4/15 (26.7%). This compared with 6/58 (10.3%) in patients undergoing CAS using a CPD. Based on these results, the DMC recommended stopping unprotected CAS.

Comment

This is an extraordinary state of affairs. The DMC propose to restart the trial with the recommendation that CAS be performed using CPDs. This is despite the fact that:-

◆ the study was never powered to make this distinction;
◆ the observed differences were not statistically significant; and
◆ the lower limits of the confidence intervals were compatible with an absence of difference.

Accordingly, while one has sympathy with the dilemma faced by the investigators and the DMC, they have now probably rendered continuation of the trial in its amended format all but impossible. They have now revealed the entire outcome data for the CAS limb of the trial (15% death/stroke) and it is almost certain that this figure is higher than was anticipated when the power calculations were made. Accordingly, this clinical alert will inevitably alter the equanimity of the randomising physicians (and surgeons) who are otherwise considering whether they should continue to participate in the study or not.

The SAPPHIRE study [11]

Methodology

This was a randomised trial of CEA versus protected CAS in patients considered 'high-risk' for CEA. 723 patients with a symptomatic stenosis >50% or an asymptomatic stenosis >80% were considered for randomisation. However, two thirds of the study cohort was asymptomatic. Following case review, 416 patients were excluded from the study, 409 patients were treated by CAS and seven by CEA. The remaining 307 patients were randomised within the study. Patients randomised to CAS (n=156) underwent primary stenting (Cordis Precise Nitinol self-expanding stent) in combination with the Angioguard or Angioguard XP Embolus Capture guidewire. The remaining 151 patients were randomised to CEA. Specified endpoints included death/any stroke and (for the first time) death/any stroke/any myocardial infarction (MI).

Results

This trial has not been published in a peer-reviewed journal, but has been the subject of numerous abstracts and media attention. The 'headline' data showed that patients randomised to CAS + CPD were significantly less likely to suffer a death/stroke or MI within 30 days (5.8% versus 12.6%, p=0.047). In addition, the clinically driven restenosis rate was higher in the surgical limb of the trial. The term 'clinically driven' is presumed to mean those that required re-intervention but the precise definition remains elusive. The only other comparable data to be published relate to outcomes in the asymptomatic patients, who otherwise dominated the trial cohort. In this subgroup, the death/stroke rate at 30 days for patients randomised to CAS was 5.8% as compared with 6.1% for CEA (p=ns). No long-term follow-up data have been published.

Comment

This is one of the most provocative of the randomised trials to have been published. This is because surgeons have been rather indignant at the inclusion of 'myocardial infarction' as part of the primary end-point. However, if there is equivalence for the 30 days risk of death/stroke in patients undergoing CEA or CAS, then the fact that the risk of MI can be reduced is surely beneficial to the patient. However, aside from this potential benefit, there are worrying aspects to this study. First is the haphazard cohort of patients (symptomatic, asymptomatic, recurrent stenosis after CEA) and the absence of any standardised definition as to what comprises 'high-risk'. Second is the observation that 60% of patients were not thereafter randomised within the trial. Third, and of most clinical importance, is the very high complication rate observed in asymptomatic patients. It is now generally accepted that if the procedural risk exceeds 4% in asymptomatic individuals, no benefit (in terms of long-term stroke prevention) will be observed [12]. Accordingly, if the SAPPHIRE data is a true reflection on practice, then extrapolation of the results from ACAS show that 45 asymptomatic patients would have to undergo CAS or CEA to prevent one stroke and performing 1000 interventions would prevent only 22 strokes!

The Lexington Asymptomatic Trial [13]

Methodology

This second trial from the community hospital in Lexington randomised 85 patients with an asymptomatic carotid stenosis >80% to unprotected CAS (n=43) with primary stenting (Wallstent, Boston Scientific, USA and Dynalink, Guidant USA) or CEA (n=42). Unusually for this type of study, a neurologist and a clinic co-ordinator performed all neurological examinations. All patients were followed-up for four years.

Results

As with the earlier 'symptomatic' trial, no patient in this study suffered a stroke, either within 30 days of treatment or during the ensuing four years of follow-up. Hypotension and/or bradycardia complicated five

CAS procedures, whilst atrial fibrillation complicated one CEA. Cranial nerve injuries complicated three CEAs. Finally, no patient in this study developed significant restenosis within 48 months of treatment as evaluated by Duplex ultrasound.

Comments

The power calculations must have been very interesting to come out with a predicted cohort of 85 patients to prove equivalence between CAS and CEA. Once again, this study has reported truly remarkable data, especially when you consider that no CPD device was employed!

Conclusions

Seven randomised trials have published their results in peer-reviewed journals (n=5) or as abstracts (n=2). Two trials were abandoned because of poor results in the CAS arm [5,8] and another has been suspended pending a change in practice to recommend the use of CPDs in the future [10], again because of poor results in the CAS limb. Paradoxically, two studies from the same centre have reported zero procedural and long-term neurological complications following CAS and CEA for symptomatic and asymptomatic patients, despite not using a CPD. Publication of the SAPPHIRE study has aroused a lot of debate, much of which will be resolved one way or the other following publication of the full study. There remain, however, significant concerns regarding selection of the patient cohort as a whole and the high complication rate observed in asymptomatic individuals for both CAS and CEA. The only large scale, completed study is CAVATAS. Despite its high procedural risk, it has suggested that the long-term results of CAS are comparable to CEA, i.e. concerns about the durability of CEA may have been overestimated. Inevitably, the key objective for the future is reducing the procedural risk to the minimum. To date, four of the seven trials have reported death/any stroke rates following CAS which are $\geq 10\%$. Colleagues are encouraged to support the ICSS (otherwise known as CAVATAS II) to help determine which is the optimal intervention in our patients.

Summary

◆ Seven randomised trials have reported their results.

◆ Two trials were abandoned and one was suspended (poor results in the CAS arm).

◆ The SAPPHIRE study raised concerns regarding patient selection and the high complication rate (CAS and CEA) in asymptomatic patients.

◆ The CAVATAS study suggests equivalent results for CEA and CAS.

References

1. European Carotid Surgery Trialists Collaborative Group. MRC European Carotid Surgery Trial: interim results for symptomatic patients with severe (70-99%) or with mild (0-29%) carotid stenosis. *Lancet* 1991; 337: 1235-1241.

2. North American Symptomatic Carotid Endarterectomy Trial Collaborators. Beneficial effect of carotid endarterectomy in symptomatic patients with high grade stenosis. *N Engl J Med* 1991; 325: 445-453.

3. Asymptomatic Carotid Surgery Trial Collaborators. The MRC Asymptomatic Carotid Surgery Trial (ACST): carotid endarterectomy prevents disabling and fatal carotid territory strokes. *Lancet* (In press).

4. Executive Committee for the Asymptomatic Carotid Atherosclerosis Study. Endarterectomy for asymptomatic carotid artery stenosis. *JAMA* 1995; 273: 1421-1428.

5. Naylor AR, Bolia A, Abbott RJ, *et al*. Randomized study of carotid angioplasty and stenting versus carotid endarterectomy: a stopped trial. *J Vasc Surg* 1998; 28(2): 326-34.

6. CAVATAS Investigators. Endovascular versus surgical treatment in patients with carotid stenosis in the Carotid and Vertebral Artery Transluminal Angioplasty Study (CAVATAS): a randomised trial. *Lancet* 2001; 357: 1729-37.

7. Naylor AR, Rothwell PM, Bell PRF. Overview of the principal results and secondary analyses from the European and the North American randomised trials of carotid endarterectomy. *Eur J Vasc Endovasc Surg* 2003; 26: 115-129.

8. Alberts MJ. WALLSTENT. Results of a multicenter prospective randomized trial of carotid artery stenting versus carotid endarterectomy (abstract). *Stroke* 2001; 32: 325.

9. Brooks WH, McClure RR, Jones MR, Coleman TL, Breathitt L. Carotid Angioplasty and Stenting versus Carotid Endarterectomy: Randomized Trial in a Community Hospital. *J Am Coll Cardiol* 2001; 38: 1589-95.

10. EVA-3S Investigators. Carotid angioplasty and stenting with and without cerebral protection: Clinical alert from the endarterectomy versus angioplasty in patients with symptomatic severe carotid stenosis. *Stroke* 2004; 35: e18-e20.

11. Ouriel K, Yadav J, Wholey M, Katzen B, Fayad P. The SAPPHIRE randomised trial of carotid stenting versus endarterectomy: a subgroup analysis. Proceedings of the Annual Meeting of the Society for Vascular Surgery and the American Association of Vascular Surgeons. Chicago, 8th-11th June 2003.

12. Barnett HJM, Eliasziw M, Meldrum HE, Taylor DW. Do the facts and figures warrant a tenfold increase in the performance of carotid endarterectomy in asymptomatic patients? *Neurology* 1996; 466: 603-608.

13. Brooks WH, McClure RR, Jones MR, Coleman TL, Breathitt L. Carotid angioplasty and stenting versus carotid endarterectomy for treatment of asymptomatic carotid stenosis: a randomised trial in a community hospital. *Neurosurgery* 2004; 54: 318-324.

Chapter 15

The use of protection devices for carotid angioplasty

Viktor Berczi, MD PhD, Endovascular Fellow

Peter A Gaines, FRCP FRCR, Consultant Vascular Radiologist

Trevor Cleveland, FRCS FRCR, Consultant Vascular Radiologist

The Sheffield Vascular Institute, The Northern General Hospital, Sheffield, UK

Introduction

The currently available published level I evidence supports the concept that carotid artery stenting is an effective alternative to carotid endarterectomy in patients with symptomatic high-grade carotid stenosis [1,2]. Reasons for treating the carotid bifurcation are generally different than those for which other vascular structures undergo angioplasty (PTA). Disease at the carotid bifurcation usually comes to light because the plaque causes thrombus to form in its proximity (eg. because of plaque rupture or blood stasis) and this may then embolise to the brain, with resulting symptoms. Such patients have unstable plaque, or haemodynamics, which make them at risk of distal embolisation. In more than 90% of treatment episodes, emboli are detected by transcranial Doppler. Even so, defined cerebral ischaemia shown by magnetic resonance diffusion-weighted imaging occurs in 15-29% of cases on the ipsilateral side. However, many of them were clinically non-relevant [3-5]. These changes have also been found following carotid endarterectomy in 34% of cases [6].

Strategies to avoid cerebral embolism

Strategies to avoid neurologic events as a consequence to embolism should include the following.

- Stabilization of the plaque (aspirin, ticlopidine, clopidogrel, statins).
- Prevention of plaque dislodgement (careful and minimal manipulation, low profile devices, appropriate selection of patients and lesions, primary stent placement).
- Prevention of debris reaching the brain (cerebral protection devices).

The remainder of this chapter deals with the latter possibility.

Cerebral protection devices

Two approaches to distal cerebral protection have been developed: balloon occlusion systems and filter or basket systems [7-13,28,30] (Table 1).

Table 1. Methods of distal cerebral protection.

A. Occlusive balloons

Distal flow arrest	**Theron Catheter System** - 2.3F microcatheter with distal elasotomeric balloon; aspiration through the guide catheter.
	PercuSurge Guidewire (Medtronic) - elastomeric balloon mounted on 0.014" hypotube attached to floppy-tipped angioplasty wire; 5F Export multiple sidehole aspiration catheter to remove debris.
Proximal flow arrest (flow-reversal)	**Kachel Catheter** - occludes CCA allowing reverse flow down the ICA into the ECA and via aspiration into the guide catheter.
	Parodi Anti-Emboli System (ArteriA) - occludes CCA and ECA, blood is shunted through the guide catheter from the ICA into the femoral vein.
	MOMA (Invatec) - flow arrest.

B. Non-occlusive (filters and baskets)

	EmboShield (Abbot)
	Angioguard (Cordis)
	FilterWire EZ (Boston Scientific)
	TRAP (Microvena)
	Accunet (Guidant)
	Spider (EV3)

Occlusive balloons: distal flow arrest (Figure 1)

This concept was first proposed by Theron [8]. He suggested that by occluding flow in the ICA the embolic particles could be prevented from reaching the brain. This was based on the assumptions that particles which were diverted away from the ICA into the external carotid territory, did not reach the brain; that any particles trapped in the column of blood between the carotid bifurcation and the occlusion balloon could be effectively captured and removed and that patients could tolerate the occlusion of their ICA for the time required to perform their carotid stent. Regarding the former, it has been known for many years that there are connections between the external and internal carotid artery systems, and so embolic particles liberated into the external system may still reach the internal carotid artery and subsequently the brain. Theron's original prototype, and the subsequent commercial version (PercuSurge™, Medtronic) included the placement of a large bore catheter into the ICA following successful stent placement. This catheter allowed suction aspiration to be performed to remove these embolic particles. Nevertheless, subsequent Transcranial Doppler studies have shown that this process is not completely successful [9].

Patient tolerance of these devices depends upon the degree of the remaining disease in the carotid and vertebral arteries, and the completeness of the Circle of Willis. Prediction of who will, and who will not be intolerant is difficult, but series show that intolerance is in the region of 0.5% [10]. However, if selective four vessel angiography is not performed prior to selecting this device, the intolerance rate may be higher [11].

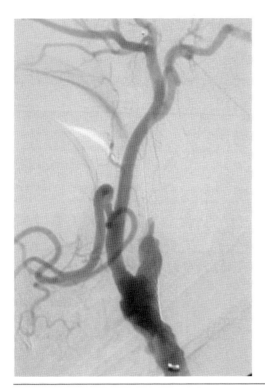

Figure 1. Distal flow arrest occlusive balloon in the internal carotid artery (PercuSurge, Medtronic). The internal carotid artery is not visualised on the angiogram due to the occlusive balloon.

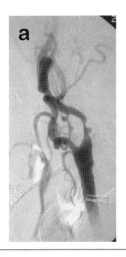 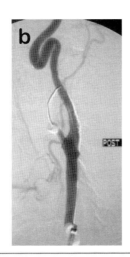

Figure 2. a) Lateral view angiogram shows 80% stenosis with an ulcerated plaque at the origin of the internal carotid artery. Due to the kink on distal ICA (shown better on b), a proximal flow arrest system (Parodi device), rather than a filter, has been used. b) Shows occlusion balloons in the ECA and CCA; the flow in the ICA and CCA is retrograde.

Occlusive balloons: proximal flow arrest (flow-reversal) (Figure 2)

This was first proposed by Kachel [12], and subsequently popularised by Parodi [13]. In the latter version, a guide catheter with a balloon occludes the CCA proximal to the intended site of treatment and another balloon is used to occlude the ECA. The lumen of the guide catheter is connected via a filtered shunt to the femoral vein. This creates a pressure gradient from the ICA to the femoral vein and effectively reverses flow in the ICA. Experimental data from this system indicates that, so long as the shunt is functional, all particulate matter can be retrieved and none reach the brain [14]. However, the systems available require large access catheters (in the region of 10 French) and can be difficult to use, particularly for physicians new to the device. In addition, when the reversed flow is activated, a proportion of patients will have flow-related symptoms.

Non-occlusive devices: filter systems (Figure 3)

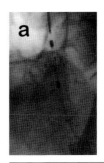 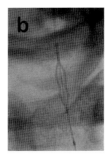 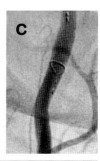

Figure 3. Non-occlusive filter systems placed in the internal carotid artery. a) Angioguard (Cordis). b) EmboShield (Abbot). c) FilterWire EZ (Boston Scientific).

The concept utilised in these systems is to try to place a filter in the ICA above the carotid stenosis. Once this filter is in place blood flow to the brain is preserved, but any particles larger than the size of the holes in the filter will be captured and prevented from causing a stoke. Once the stenting procedure has been completed, the channel at the carotid bifurcation will be considerably improved, and the filter can be collapsed, retaining any debris within it, and removed.

This concept raises a number of issues, which have been addressed in varying degrees by the different devices available.

The profile of the filter delivery system

Clearly until the filter has been introduced and deployed, the carotid stenting procedure remains without specific cerebral protection. The filter in its delivery form has to be passed across the stenosis prior to deployment. The smaller the profile of the system at this stage, the less likely it would be to cause dislodgement of atheroma or other plaque material.

The ability of the system to be steered across the stenosis

Not only is the profile of the delivery system important, but so too is the controllability of the system. The more precise the manoeuvrability of the wire tip, and the more controlled the traversal of the lesion, the less likely are emboli to be generated.

The size of the filter when deployed

The internal carotid artery is usually between 4 and 6mm in diameter. The filters available are designed to expand to fit these diameters. If the filter is too small it will not achieve its goal. Similarly, with most devices, if it is oversized, then there is a tendency for the covering to fold in at the edges, again allowing some blood to remain unfiltered. It is therefore imperative for the internal carotid artery diameter to be accurately measured, and for an appropriate sized filter to be selected.

The ability of the filter to function maximally in a tortuous ICA

Not only is it important for a filter delivery system to be sufficiently flexible to pass along tortuous vessels, but it must also function close to bends.

The size of the pores

It is not known what size of particle is critical to the production of neurological symptoms in the human brain. There are some data on the tolerance of experimental animal model brains to emboli of differing sizes, but how this relates to the human is not known (see below). It would therefore seem sensible to design a filter with the smallest pore size possible. However, this logic does not take into account that platelets and fibrinogen may be activated by the 'foreign' material of the filter, with the resultant deposition onto the filter and blockage of the pores. The holes in the present filter systems (in the range of 80-140 microns) are, therefore, a balance between the need to allow blood to flow freely through the filter and the need to try to capture all of the clinically important particles.

The length of the filter

Whilst the systems for delivering the filters are flexible, the ICA may present too much tortuosity to allow these to be placed well above the index lesion. As a result, there may be restricted space for filter placement. In such circumstances, a filter which is short in length is advantageous. It is necessary to place the filter a sufficient distance above the lesion to allow for stenting.

ICA spasm

The ICA, like the renal artery, is prone to spasm when manipulated. If a filter is placed in the ICA, this may in itself stimulate a degree of spasm. However, if the filter is moved within the ICA once deployed, then this risk of spasm is increased. As a result, antispasmodic agents (such as glycerol trinitrate) should be readily available, and the amount of filter movement minimised.

Retrieval of the filter

Once the CAS procedure has been completed, with stent deployment and post-dilatation, the filter needs to be retrieved causing further potential problems. By this stage, the stenosis should have been treated and instead of a channel less than 2mm in diameter, there should now be a 4-6mm channel. The limits on the size of the retrieval devices are, therefore, less stringent. There is, however, still a need for the retrieval system to pass through the deployed stent. Some stents have a smoother internal channel than others, particularly those that have been used to treat calcified lesions. In addition, the lowest stent struts may not necessarily be well applied to the common carotid artery wall. In such circumstances the retrieval 'cup' may snag on the caudal end of the stent. This has generally been addressed by either the retrieval system having a central stylet, or else it is slightly curved to allow for the cup to be steered away from the artery wall.

Maintaining the debris within the filter during retrieval

After the procedure is complete the filter may contain a variable amount of particulate matter. This must be retained within the filter during withdrawal, otherwise the effectiveness of the system will be compromised. Also the retrieval system must be such that the filter cannot be damaged by the stent struts during the withdrawal process.

Protected carotid stenting - experimental results

In both animal and ex-vivo human models, there are a number of stages in the carotid stenting process during which there is a particular risk of embolic events. Using recently removed carotid endarterectomy specimens, Ohki et al [15] demonstrated that during unprotected CAS procedures particulate emboli are generated during the processes of wire traversal across the stenosis, predilatation, stent placement and subsequent post-dilatation; this was confirmed by Coggia et al [16].

In his experimental model, Ohki was able to test the efficacy of a filter device in the prevention of embolic events during CAS [17]. He obtained atherosclerotic plaques, embedded them in polytetrafluoroethylene, and performed CAS under x-ray screening control.

He found that the mean number of particles released during initial filter passage was 3.1, with a maximum size of 500 microns. Most particles, however, were released at the time of stent placement and the filter was able to capture 88% of them. The material collected appeared to be a mixture of thrombotic material, foam cells and cholesterol clefts [18].

Using a dog model, Ohki et al [14] investigated the efficacy of a proximal balloon occlusion and a reversed flow device. They introduced artificial radio-opaque particles into the common carotid arteries of the animals, and provided that reverse flow could be achieved, by the formation of a shunt to the low-pressure venous system, then all of these particles could be prevented from reaching the brain.

Rapp et al [19] studied the size threshold for causing acute neuronal cell death. They examined the fragments released during ex-vivo carotid angioplasty and separated the smaller and most numerous particles and injected them into rats to determine the tolerance of the brain. The particles were separated into <200 micron particles and 200-500 microns. They found that at one and three days the group receiving particles <200 microns had no neuronal damage, but the group receiving larger emboli had scattered damage. At seven days both groups had a scattered pattern of ischaemic neurones. If saline were administered, no such neuronal damage was observed. They concluded that whilst the brain seems to be surprisingly tolerant to micro-embolisation in the short-term, even small plaque fragments may cause neuronal ischaemia at later time points.

In a recent study [20], the importance of emboli not trapped by carotid angioplasty filtration devices (fragments <100 micron released with ex-vivo angioplasty injected into rat carotid artery) were examined. Brain ischaemia and infarction were assessed by MRI scans (7-T small-bore magnet) and by immunohistologic staining for HSP70 and NueN in these experiments. All five animals injected with 100-200-micron calcified fragments had infarctions; one was lethal. Fragments from calcified plaques cause greater levels of infarction than fragments from fibrous plaques, although ischaemia is common with both fragment types [20]. These results should be extrapolated to humans with caution.

From an experimental viewpoint, it would appear that an attempt should be made to prevent all microemboli from reaching the brain. The Ohki model, described above, indicated that a filter system could be expected to be in the region of 88% effective at removing particles [17], but this does not include particles which pass through the filter by virtue of their small size. On the other hand the experimental model would indicate that the reversed flow system completely retrieved the particles introduced, but only as long as reversed flow could be guaranteed. It has been shown by Al-Mubarak et al, that if distal balloon occlusion is utilised, despite the balloon inflation, particles are able to reach the middle cerebral artery through collateral circulation [21]. In addition, when the balloon is deflated, a number of embolic particles are seen to reach the brain, presumably because the aspiration from the ICA proximal to the occlusion balloon was not 100% effective [9].

Using a human plaque model, Muller-Hulsbeck et al [22] investigated the efficacy of four filtration devices (Angioguard [Cordis], FilterWire EX [Boston Scientific], TRAP [Microvena] and NeuroShield [Mednova]). They found that none of the devices were completely able to prevent embolisation into the ICA. Comparing the designs, the NeuroShield and the FilterWire EX captured the highest percentage of the particles.

Protected carotid stenting - clinical results

It is still not known whether these theoretical and animal considerations translate into a reduction of cerebrovascular events during and after CAS in humans. Table 2 summarises the reported case series of protected CAS (n=1960).

Twenty-six neurological complications occurred at the time of CAS out of 1826 treatments (for 134 cases this information was not available), and persisted longer than 24 hours (i.e. excluding TIAs and intolerance to ICA occlusion or reversed ICA flow). This represents a peri-procedural neurological event rate of 1.4%. Comparable rates of 30-day stroke and death rates are not possible to determine. It is also not possible to reliably identify the proportion of symptomatic and asymptomatic patients.

Several studies have compared neurological complication rates with and without cerebral protection. Castriota [28] reported periprocedural embolic rates of 3.2% (4/125) in the unprotected and 0.7% (1/150) in the protected groups. In addition, one patient in each group suffered a subarachnoid haemorrhage.

Similarly, our group demonstrated that the procedural all-stroke/death rates in the unprotected versus protected groups were 5.3% (4/75) and 2.7% (2/75; p=0.681), while the disabling stroke/death rates were 4% (3/75) and 1.3% (1/75; p=0.620). At 30 days, the all-stroke/death rates were 10.7% (8/75) in the unprotected group and 4.0% (3/75) in the protected group (p=0.117) and the death/major-disability-from-stroke rates were 6.7% (5/75) and 2.7% (2/75), (p=0.442) [30]. Non-significant p numbers probably reflect the low number of cases.

In the most recent publication, the Safety Committee for the EVA-3S trial recommended stopping unprotected CAS, because the 30-day rate of strokes was 3.9 times higher than that of CAS with cerebral protection (4/15 versus 5/58) [40].

Recently, in order to evaluate the efficacy of cerebral protection devices in preventing thromboembolic complications during CAS, a systematic review of studies reporting on the incidence of minor stroke, major stroke, or death within 30 days after CAS was conducted [41]. In 2357 patients a total of 2537 CAS procedures were performed without protection devices, and in 839 patients 896 CAS procedures were performed with protection devices. Both groups were similar with respect to age, sex distribution, cerebrovascular risk factors, and indications for CAS. The conclusion was that protection systems probably reduce the incidence of complications [41].

The development of protective devices has been a major step in the attempt to reduce the number and effect of embolic events during carotid stenting, although it has increased the complexity and the cost of the intervention. In addition, there is a learning curve for the use of protection devices with Roubin et al reporting a 30-day minor stroke rate which decreased from 7.1% during the first year to 3.1% in the fifth [42].

Table 2. Periprocedural and 30-day neurological events related to protected carotid artery stenting.

Name	Year	No of lesions	Neurological events During CAS	30-day	Protection type	Failure to protect
Theron [8]	1996	136	0	-	ICA balloon	Retrospective
Albuquerque [24]	2000	17	0	-	ICA balloon	1/17 (6%)
Parodi [13]	2000	25	0	-	ICA balloon Filter Reverse flow	0
Jaeger [25]	2001	20	0	-	ICA balloon	0
Jaeger [23]	2001	20	0	-	Filter	4 (20%)
Reimers [26]	2001	88	1 (1.2%)	0	Filter	5/88 (6%)
Henry [27]	2002	184	3 (1.6%)	2 (1.1%)	ICA balloon	0.5%
Castriota [28]	2002	150	1 (0.7%)	1 (0.7%)	ICA balloon Filter Reverse flow	Retrospective
Whitlow [29]	2002	75	0	0	ICA Balloon	-
Macdonald [30]	2002	75	1 (1.3%)	2 (2.6%)	Filter	Retrospective
Ohki [31]	2002	31	0	1 (3%)	ICA balloon Filter Reverse flow	1/31 (3%)
Al-Mubarak [32]	2002	164	2 (1.2%)	4 (2%)	Filter	5 (3%)
Grube [33]	2003	36	2 (5.7%)	0	Filter	0
Mudra [34]	2003	100	4 (4%)	5 (5%)	ICA balloon Filter	1/100 (1%)
Piske [35]	2003	47	1(2.1%)	-	ICA balloon	0
Castellan [36]	2003	29	1(3%)	-	Filter	0
Cremonesi [11]	2003	442	9(2%)	5(1.1%)	ICA balloon Filter Reverse flow	Retrospective
Terada [5]	2003	87	1(1.1%)	-	ICA balloon	0
Rath [37]	2003	30	-	2(6.9%)	Filter	1/30 (3.3%)
Bosiers [38]	2003	100	0	1(1%)	Filter	7/100(7%)
Cernetti [39]	2003	104	-	3(2.9%)	-	2/104(1.9%)

By identifying MRI changes in the brains of patients undergoing CAS under protection with the Angioguard system, Jaegar et al have shown that filter devices do not always prevent emboli [28]. Also, it was recently shown that 23% of the patients (n=10) undergoing neuroprotected carotid stenting had silent new ischaemic foci (n=1-3, maximum area 43 mm^2) on post-interventional DWMRI. One patient had sustained a major stroke; for this patient 12 ischaemic foci (maximum area 84.5 mm^2) were exclusively located in the contralateral hemisphere [43].

Lately, our group came out with some surprising results from a randomised study. The mean number of total events (466±160 SD versus 165±100) and the numbers of particulate emboli (300±105 SD versus 92±40) (but not the gaseous emboli) were higher in the protected than in the unprotected group [44]. In a different study we showed that there were no differences in global cognitive function outcomes between protected and unprotected carotid stenting [45].

There are a number of reports of intolerance of the ICA occlusion or reversed flow techniques, but the precise rate of such problems is impossible to determine, as case selection criteria and reporting clarity are variable. There are, unfortunately, no data at present to shed light upon whether protection devices in general are not only effective, but also cost-effective.

Prediction of highly embolic lesions

In order to define a subgroup of patients who do not require cerebral protection, we should be able to predict which type of lesions will release most emboli. We do not have sufficient data in this regard and some of the existing data are contradictory. When debris is collected using temporary balloon occlusion, Henry showed that hypoechoic plaques released the greater number of particles, whereas hyperechoic plaque produced the larger debris [27]. However, in an ex-vivo model, Ohki and colleagues demonstrated that echolucent plaque released a higher number of particles than echogenic plaque [15]. Henry could not find an association with the degree of stenosis yet Ohki could.

Correlation of ultrasonic carotid plaque morphology with the degree of carotid stenosis (n=2460) showed that the higher the degree of stenosis, the more likely it is to be associated with heterogeneous plaques. Heterogeneous plaques were associated with an increased incidence of symptoms than that for homogeneous plaques for all grades of stenoses [46]. Patients with 60% to 69% carotid artery stenosis with heterogeneous plaque had a higher incidence rate of late stroke, TIA, and progression to >70% stenosis than patients with homogeneous plaque [47]. Ultrasonic plaque heterogeneity may serve as one of the tools to predict highly embolic lesions.

If the behaviour of vulnerable atherosclerotic plaques is believed to be closely related to plaque composition, then there is a need for an effective in-vivo technique for examining plaque constituent properties. Multisequence MRI can accurately characterise the in-vivo state of the fibrous cap. This finding supports the use of these noninvasive techniques to prospectively identify vulnerable plaques [48]. In a recent study, Fourier Transform Infrared Spectroscopy using Attenuated Total Reflectance (FTIR-ATR) was used to assess and analyse the biochemical properties of human atherosclerotic plaques. FTIR spectra clearly revealed prominent spectral features corresponding to plaque constituents of interest (lipids, lipid esters, fibrous tissues, calcification). Spectral data examined on a qualitative basis correlated well with both gross tissue anatomy and histologic features [49].

Many studies have linked carotid plaque surface irregularities with stroke risk, but this relationship has been obscured by the limited ability of available imaging modalities to resolve plaque surface morphology. To address this issue, a prospective study correlating the presenting neurologic symptoms of patients with high-resolution Magnetic Resonance Imaging (MRI; 200 microns) was performed on 100 patients. Surface irregularities were revealed by means of submillimeter resolution of the carotid plaques with MRI to be common, but only the presence of major irregularities correlated with the patient having a TIA or stroke. Lumen shape and plaque location did not appear to predict stroke risk, but may affect imaging accuracy in determining the degree of stenosis. These data further define the relationship of plaque irregularity and cerebrovascular symptoms caused by atheroemboli [50].

Summary

◆ Carotid artery stenting is associated with neuroembolic complications.

◆ Cerebral protection systems are capable of collecting atheromatous debris during the stenting procedure.

◆ The number of neuroembolic complications is reduced when using a cerebral protection system.

◆ We cannot yet define a sub-group of patients who do not require cerebral protection.

◆ With the current array of devices available there are no technical reasons why a cerebral protection system cannot be used in most patients; it should be considered in all patients being treated with a carotid artery stent.

References

1. Endovascular versus surgical treatment in patients with carotid stenosis in the Carotid and Vertebral Artery Transluminal Angioplasty Study (CAVATAS): a randomised trial. *Lancet* 2001; 357: 1729-1737.

2. Brooks WH, McClure RR, Jones MR, *et al*. Carotid Angioplasty and stenting versus carotid endarterectomy a randomised trial in a community hospital. *J Am Coll Cardiol* 2001; 38: 1589-1595.

3. Jaeger HJ, Mathias KD, Hauth E, *et al*. Cerebral ischemia detected with diffusion-weighted MR imaging after stent implantation in the carotid artery. *Am J Neuroradiol* 2002; 23: 200-7.

4. Jordan WD Jr, Voellinger DC, Doblar DD, *et al*. Microemboli detected by transcranial Doppler monitoring in patients during carotid angioplasty versus carotid endarterectomy. *Cardiovasc Surg* 1999; 7: 33-8.

5. Terada T, Tsuura M, Matsumoto H, *et al*. Results of endovascular treatment of internal carotid artery stenoses with a newly developed balloon protection catheter. *Neurosurgery* 2003; 53: 617-23.

6. Muller M, Reiche W, Langenscheidt P, *et al*. Ischemia after carotid endarterectomy: comparison between transcranial Doppler sonography and diffusion-weighted MR imaging. *Am J Neuroradiol* 2000; 21: 47-54.

7. Wilentz JR, Amor M. Carotid bifurcation stenting, short-term results: protected vs. unprotected techniques. In: *Carotid artery angioplasty and stenting. A multidisciplinary approach.* Amor M, Bergeron P, Mathias K, Raithel D, Eds. Edizioni Minerva Medica, Torino, 2002: pp235-245.

8. Theron JG, Payelle GG, Coskun O, *et al*. Carotid artery stenosis: treatment with protected balloon angioplasty and stent placement. *Radiology* 1996; 201: 627-636.

9. Al-Mubarak N, Roubin GS, Vitek JJ, *et al*. Microembolization during carotid stenting with the distal-balloon antiemboli system. *Int Angiol* 2002; 21: 344-8.

10. Henry M, Amor M, Henry I, *et al*. Carotid stenting with cerebral protection: first clinical experience using the PercuSurg GuardWire™ system. *J Endovasc Surg* 1999; 6: 321-331.

11. Cremonesi A, Manetti R, Setacci F, *et al*. Protected carotid stenting: clinical advantages and complications of embolic protection devices in 442 consecutive patients. *Stroke* 2003; 34: 1936-41.

12. Kachel R. Results of Balloon Angioplasty in the Carotid Arteries. *J Endovasc Surg* 1996; 3: 22-30.

13. Parodi JC, La Mura R, Ferreira LM, *et al*. Initial evaluation of carotid angioplasty and stenting with three difference cerebral protection devices. *J Vasc Surg* 2000; 32: 1127-36.

14. Ohki T, Parodi J, Veith FJ, *et al*. Efficacy of a proximal occlusion catheter with reversal of flow in the prevention of embolic events during carotid artery stenting: an experimental analysis. *J Vasc Surg* 2001; 33: 504-9.

15. Ohki T, Marin ML, Lyon RT, *et al*. Human ex-vivo carotid artery bifurcation stenting: correlation of lesion characteristics with embolic potential. *J Vasc Surg* 1998; 27: 463-471.

16. Coggia M, Goeau-Brissonniere O, Duval JL, *et al*. Embolic risk of the different stages of carotid bifurcation balloon angioplasty: an experimental study. *J Vasc Surg* 2000; 31: 550-7.

17. Ohki T, Roubin GS, Veith FJ, *et al*. Efficacy of a filter device in the prevention of embolic events during carotid angioplasty and stenting: an ex-vivo analysis. *J Vasc Surg* 1999; 30: 1034-44.

18. Angelini A, Reimers B, Della Barbera M, *et al*. Cerebral protection during carotid artery stenting: collection and histopathologic analysis of embolised debris. *Stroke* 2002; 33: 456-61.

19. Rapp JH, Pan XM, Sharp FR, *et al*. Atherombi to the brain: size threshold for causing acute neuronal cell death. *J Vasc Surg* 2000; 32: 68-76.

20. Rapp JH, Pan XM, Yu B, *et al*. Cerebral ischemia and infarction from atheroemboli <100 micron in size. *Stroke* 2003; 34: 1976-80.

21. Al-Mubarak N, Vitek JJ, Iyer S, *et al*. Embolisation via collateral circulation during carotid stenting with the distal balloon protection system. *J Endovasc Ther* 2001; 8: 354-7.

22. Müller-Hülsbeck S, Jahnke T, Liess C, *et al*. In Vitro Comparison of Four Cerebral Protection Filters for Preventing Human Plaque Embolization during Carotid Interventions. *J Endovasc Ther* 2002; 9: 793-802.

23. Jaeger H, Mathias K, Drescher R, et al. Clinical results of cerebral protection with a filter device during stent implantation of the carotid artery. Cardiovasc Intervent Radiol 2001; 24: 249-56.

24. Albuquerque FC, Teitelbaum GP, Lavine SD, et al. Balloon-protected carotid angioplasty. Neurosurgery 2000; 46: 918-21.

25. Jaeger HJ, Mathias KD, Drescher R, et al. Cerebral protection with balloon occlusion during carotid artery stent implantation - first experiences. (German). ROFO-Fortschritte auf dem Gebiet der Rontgenstrahlen und der Bildgebenden V 2001; 173: 139-46.

26. Reimers B, Corvaja N, Moshiri S, et al. Cerebral protection with filter devices during carotid artery stenting. [Comment]. Circ 2001; 104: 12-5.

27. Henry M, Henry I, Klonaris C, et al. Benefits of cerebral protection during carotid stenting with the PecurSurge GuardWire system: midterm results. J Endovasc Ther 2002; 9: 1-13.

28. Castriota F, Cremonesi A, Manetti R, et al. Impact of Cerebral Protection Devices on Early Outcome of Carotid Stenting. J Endovasc Ther 2002; 9: 786-792.

29. Whitlow PL, Lylyk P, Londero H, et al. Carotid artery stenting protected with an emboli containment system. Stroke 2002; 33: 1308-14.

30. Macdonald S, McKevitt F, Venables GS, et al. Neurological outcomes after carotid stenting protected with the NeuroShield filter compared to unprotected stenting. J Endovasc Ther 2002; 9: 777-85.

31. Ohki T, Veith FJ, Grenell S, et al. Initial experience with cerebral protection devices to prevent embolisation during carotid artery stenting. J Vasc Surg 2002; 36; 1175-85.

32. Al-Mubarak N, Colombo A, Gaines PA, et al. Multicenter evaluation of carotid artery stenting with a filter protection system. J Am Coll Card 2002; 39: 841-6.

33. Grube E, Colombo A, Hauptmann E, et al. Initial multicenter experience with a novel distal protection filter during carotid artery stent implantation. Catheter Cardiovasc Interv 2003; 58: 139-46.

34. Mudra H, Ziegler M, Haufe MC, et al. Percutaneous carotid angioplasty with stent implantation and protection device against embolism - a prospective study of 100 consecutive cases. [German]. Deutsche Medizinische Wochenschrift 2003; 128: 790-6.

35. Piske RL, Ferreira MS, Capos CM, et al. The cerebral protection technique in angioplasty plus stenting of carotid: an effective procedure against cerebral embolism. [Portugese]. Arquivos de neuro-Psiquiatria 2003; 61: 296-302.

36. Castellan L, Causin F, Danieli D, et al. Carotid stenting with filter protection. Correlation of ACT values with angiographic and histopathologic findings. J Neuroradiology 2003; 30: 103-8.

37. Rath PC, Lakshmi G, Agarwala M, et al. Carotid artery stenting with filter protection. Indian Heart J 2003; 55: 241-4.

38. Bosiers M, Peeters P, Verbist J, et al. Belgian experience with FilterWire EX in the prevention of embolic events during carotid stenting. J Endovasc Ther 2003; 10: 695-701.

39. Cernetti C, Reimers B, Picciolo A, et al. Carotid artery stenting with cerebral protection in 100 consecutive patients: immediate and two-year follow-up results. Ital Heart J 2003; 4: 695-700.

40. Mas JL, Chatellier G, Beyssen B; EVA-3S Investigators. Carotid angioplasty and stenting with and without cerebral protection: clinical alert from the Endarterectomy Versus Angioplasty in Patients With Symptomatic Severe Carotid Stenosis (EVA-3S) trial. Stroke 2004; 35: 18-20.

41. Kastrup A, Groschel K, Krapf H, et al. Early outcome of carotid angioplasty and stenting with and without cerebral protection devices: a systematic review of the literature. Stroke 2003; 34: 813-9.

42. Roubin GS, New G, Iyer SS, et al. Immediate and late clinical outcomes of carotid artery stenting in patients with symptomatic and asymptomatic carotid artery stenosis: a 5-year prospective analysis. Circ 2001; 103: 532-537.

43. Schluter M, Tubler T, Steffens JC, et al. Focal ischemia of the brain after neuroprotected carotid artery stenting. J Am Coll Cardiol 2003; 42: 1007-1013.

44. Macdonald S, Cleveland TJ, Evans D, et al. A comparison of the high-intensity signal rate using transcranial Doppler during unprotected and protected carotid stenting (NeuroShield filter) within a randomised controlled trial. CIRSE Annual Meeting, 2003, Abstracts, pp130.

45. Macdonald S, Cleveland TJ, Graham J, et al. Comparison of outcomes of unprotected and protected carotid stenting (NeuroShield filter) within a randomised trial using a neuropsychometric test battery. CIRSE Annual Meeting, 2003, Abstracts, pp165.

46. AbuRahma AF, Wulu JT Jr, Crotty B. Carotid plaque ultrasonic heterogeneity and severity of stenosis. Stroke 2002; 33: 1772-5.

47. Aburahma AF, Thiele SP, Wulu JT Jr. Prospective controlled study of the natural history of asymptomatic 60% to 69% carotid stenosis according to ultrasonic plaque morphology. J Vasc Surg 2002; 36: 437-42.

48. Mitsumori LM, Hatsukami TS, Ferguson MS, et al. In vivo accuracy of multisequence MR imaging for identifying unstable fibrous caps in advanced human carotid plaques. J Magn Reson Imaging 2003; 17: 410-20.

49. Li C, Ebenstein D, Xu C, et al. Biochemical characterization of atherosclerotic plaque constituents using FTIR spectroscopy and histology. J Biomed Mater Res 2003; 64A: 197-206.

50. Troyer A, Saloner D, Pan XM, et al. Assessment of Carotid Stenosis by Comparison with Endarterectomy Plaque Trial Investigators. Major carotid plaque surface irregularities correlate with neurologic symptoms. J Vasc Surg 2002; 35: 741-747.

Chapter 16

The diagnosis and endovascular treatment of carotid and vertebral artery dissections

Christine M Flis, MRCP FRCR, Specialist Registrar
Kings College Hospital, London, UK

H Rolf Jäger, MD FRCR, Reader in Neuroradiology
National Hospital for Neurology and Neurosurgery, London, UK

Paul S Sidhu, MRCP FRCR, Consultant Radiologist and Honorary Consultant Neuroradiologist
Kings College Hospital and the National Hospital for Neurology and Neurosurgery, London, UK

Introduction

The first description of an extracranial internal carotid artery (ICA) dissection as a cause of ischaemic stroke was reported by Jentzer in 1954 [1]. The incidence of ICA dissection is 2-3 per 100,000 per year [2] and of vertebral artery (VA) dissection, approximately 1-1.5 per 100,000 [3]. Although ICA dissection is the cause of less than 1% of all strokes, it is recognised as an important cause of stroke in young adults (mean age of occurrence, 25-45 years), with an incidence estimated at 10-25% [4,5]. The increased diagnosis of carotid artery dissection as a cause of stroke is almost entirely due to the availability of newer sophisticated diagnostic imaging techniques such as colour Doppler ultrasound (US), CT and MR imaging as well as increased awareness of the diverse clinical spectrum of an ICA/VA dissection [6].

Types of dissection

Carotid artery dissections are described either as traumatic or spontaneous. Traumatic dissections occur when preceded by an identifiable external force which may be penetrating (stab wound) or blunt (severe hyperextension) trauma. Blunt trauma accounts for 3-10% of carotid artery dissections [7].

The 'spontaneous' group of dissections may have an underlying disorder associated with increased risk, such as Ehlers-Danlos type 4, Marfan's syndrome, Adult Polycystic Kidney Disease and osteogenesis imperfecta type 1 [6]. In 15% of patients with a spontaneous dissection of the ICA/VA, changes of fibromuscular dysplasia are found at angiography and cystic medial necrosis demonstrated at post-mortem [6]. Patients with underlying fibromuscular dysplasia are usually older than those with spontaneous carotid artery dissections, often with a history of a minor precipitating event such as sneezing, nose blowing or sudden neck movements [8]. In 5% of patients with a spontaneous dissection of the ICA/VA, there is at least one family member who has had a history of spontaneous dissection. Studies have demonstrated that carotid artery dissection is associated with infections (viral upper respiratory tract) and migraine [9]. These patients have an elevated serum elastase level, suggesting an increase in extra-celluar matrix degradation [10].

Sites of dissection

In a series of 200 patients with spontaneous cervical artery dissections, the ICA was affected in 76% (unilateral in 62%, bilateral in 14%), the VA in 18% and both in 6% [11]. In VA dissections, lesions are most common in the distal segment of the artery at the level of the first and second cervical vertebrae [12]. An estimated 10% of VA dissections extend intra-cranially [11]. The commonest location for a spontaneous ICA dissection is the cervical segment about 2-3cm distal to the carotid bulb, an area that is probably subject to the most stretch with extension or rotation of the neck [6]. Atherosclerotic plaque lesions are more common at the carotid bifurcation, and traumatic carotid artery dissections more commonly involve the common carotid rather than the ICA. Carotid artery dissection may also be secondary to an extension of an aortic arch dissection. This involves the common carotid artery in up to 15% of patients [13].

Clinical spectrum

The classic triad of presentation of extra-cranial carotid artery dissection is unilateral headache, partial Horner's syndrome and ipsilateral cerebral ischaemia, which may occur some time after the dissection episode. However, this triad is found in less than 1/3 of patients. If any two of the triad are present, the diagnosis should be strongly suspected. Other presentations include amaurosis fugax, syncope, neck swelling, pulsatile tinnitus and cranial nerve dysfunction [6]. Dissection of the extra-cranial VA segment may be asymptomatic or present with ipsilateral head or neck ache. Other non-specific complaints may occur. These include dizziness and vertigo, amnesia, nausea and vomiting, or posterior circulation transient ischaemic attacks (TIA) [14]. Cerebral infarction is reported in approximately 40-60% of patients with carotid artery dissection and TIA in 20-30% [15]. Up to 5% of ischaemic strokes remain asymptomatic and are diagnosed coincidentally.

A less favourable picture is seen in intracranial ICA dissections which occur in a younger age group (mean age 25 years) with a mortality rate of 75% [16]. The onset of symptoms is usually rapid, more often associated with subarachnoid haemorrhage and

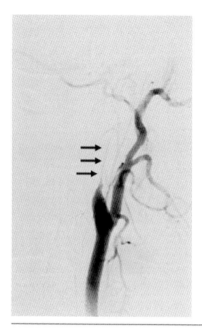

Figure 1. A selective right common carotid artery angiogram in a patient with an internal carotid artery dissection, demonstrating a narrowed 'true' lumen (arrows) compressed by thrombus in the 'false' lumen.

massive stroke with death [5]. Dissection of the intracranial VA is less common and is almost exclusively spontaneous [14,17]. Intracranial VA dissections present with posterior circulation infarctions or subarachnoid haemorrhage due to rupture of the adventitia. They are never asymptomatic [18].

Pathophysiology

The mechanism of dissection is thought to be the development of a tear of the intima of the vessel which allows blood to dissect between the layers of the media or between media and adventitia [19]. Haemorrhage from the vasa vasorum may occur directly into the media of the arterial wall. In both instances, the resulting haematoma dissects through the media resulting in luminal narrowing or total occlusion of the true vessel lumen following compression from the false lumen. Pseudoaneurysm formation occurs when the dissection plane is under the adventitial layer. At the same time, the thrombosed dissection may result in embolisation of fragments and subsequent stroke/TIA [20].

Imaging

Angiography

Carotid artery

Traditionally, the reference standard for diagnosis of carotid artery dissections has been conventional angiography [21]. Angiography demonstrates the arterial lumen, allows characterisation of the dissection, detection of fibromuscular dysplasia and other irregularities of the vessel wall [6]. Three main angiographic patterns have been described: stenotic, aneurysmal and occlusive types [8,22]. The pathognomonic features of carotid artery dissection are the findings of either an intimal flap or, in 10% of cases, a double lumen. A more common finding is an irregular stenosis, which starts about 2 to 3cm distal to the carotid bulb and extends for various lengths along the artery, but not past the entry into the petrous temporal bone (Figure 1). A tapered narrowing of the ICA ('rat's-tail' or 'string sign'), a flame-shaped occlusion or an aneurysm most commonly affecting the distal sub-cranial segment, are also described. Although these appearances are indicative of dissection, they are non-specific. Tapering or abrupt occlusion is the least specific angiographic feature [14,23]. The most common appearance is a tapered stenosis. Complete occlusion or an isolated aneurysm are seen less often.

Vertebral artery

The angiographic appearances of VA dissections are less specific than those seen in carotid artery dissection. In up to 20% of patients with spontaneous vertebral artery dissection, four-vessel arteriography reveals concurrent dissection of the ICA or contralateral VA [24].

Follow-up angiography

Carotid artery

Serial angiography demonstrates the changing patterns with the lumen often returning to normal over time. In one series of 42 patients with spontaneous dissection of the extra-cranial carotid artery, 59% of cases with a tapered stenosis and 25% of those with an isolated aneurysm demonstrated complete resolution over a mean time of 11 months [8]. Progression to occlusion was reported in 14% of stenotic dissections, 50% of aneurysms reduced in size and 25% remained unchanged.

Vertebral artery

Follow-up angiographic studies show resolution of VA abnormalities in 70% of cases [14,25]. Aneurysmal forms of cervical VA dissection resolve in 80% of cases and seem to have a better outcome than aneurysmal forms of ICA dissections [26].

Limitations of angiography

Angiography has limitations in the imaging of cervical artery dissections. Angiography is invasive and is not without risk [27]. A dissection may be missed by angiography alone when filling of the false lumen does not occur [28]. Angiography does not permit the visualisation of any arterial wall abnormalities which may occur at the site of thrombus formation.

As ICA dissection is not a stable condition, serial monitoring is required for the detection of possible recanalisation or progression to occlusion [29]. In recent years alternative non-invasive diagnostic modalities have been introduced both for initial diagnosis and follow-up of ICA dissections.

Magnetic Resonance (MR) Imaging

Appearances

Magnetic resonance techniques are replacing conventional angiography as the reference standard in the assessment of carotid and vertebral artery dissections [30,31]. MR imaging is non-invasive and is able to demonstrate both the vascular lumen and importantly, the artery wall haematoma to establish the presence of dissection. In addition, MR imaging

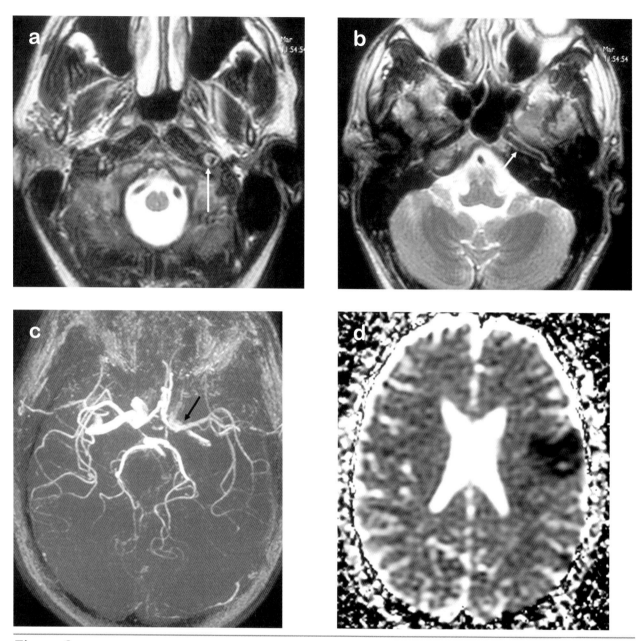

Figure 2. a) Axial T2-weighted MRI through the skull base demonstrates a crescent-shaped high signal intensity mural haematoma expanding the left internal carotid artery (ICA) as it enters the skull base (arrow). A low signal intensity flow void within the high signal area indicates patency of the left ICA. The flow void is however, much smaller than that of the normal contralateral ICA. b) Axial T2-weighted MRI through the skull base demonstrates extension of the mural haematoma into the horizontal segment (petrous portion) of the left ICA (arrow). c) Axial 3D time-of-flight MRA of the intracranial vessels. There is a marked reduction in calibre of the intracranial left ICA (arrow). The intramural haematoma is not visualised on this maximum intensity projection. Please note that there is also reduced flow signal in the left middle cerebral artery (MCA) compared to the right MCA. d) ADC map of a diffusion-weighted sequence. This demonstrates an acute infarct in the left MCA territory, which shows restricted water diffusion due to cytotoxic oedema (dark area).

enables precise delineation of the extent of the dissection and documents any ischaemic damage to the brain (Figure 2) [21,32,33].

Artery wall haematoma is characterised by a crescenteric shape adjacent to the vessel lumen, which is hyperintense on T1- and T2-weighted images between three days and several months after the dissection [34,35]. The hyperintensity is due to T1 shortening from methaemoglobin in the mural haematoma. Fat suppression techniques help to differentiate a small mural haematoma from surrounding soft tissue. Slow flow in the venous plexus surrounding the vertebral arteries, which is not eliminated by fat suppression, can however, also mimic an intramural haematoma. In the very early and chronic stage, the intramural haematoma is usually iso-intense to surrounding structures on T1-weighted images, with thickening of the vessel and narrowing of the patent lumen, the only indication of dissection. A mural haematoma can also be demonstrated on time-of-flight (TOF) MR angiography, as this technique does not completely suppress stationary tissue with short T1 values. Mural haematomas are, however, not detectable on phase-contrast or contrast-enhanced techniques, both of which are only able to visualise the vascular lumen [21,33,36]. On TOF MR angiography, flow within a residual vascular lumen can usually be distinguished from the mural haematoma as it gives a more intense signal [30]. This is particularly obvious on the source data. On maximum intensity projections the hyperintense haematoma can sometimes be indistinguishable from flow signal, giving the appearance of an enlarged vessel or vascular segment. Levy *et al* described an increase in the external diameter of the vessel in 18 out of 19 (95%) cases on TOF MR angiography and found it represented the most sensitive feature of dissection [32].

Accuracy and limitations

The quoted sensitivity and specificity for MR imaging in carotid artery dissection is 84% and 99% and for MR angiography, 95% and 99%. With the VA, the sensitivity and specificity is quoted at 60% and 58% for MR imaging and 20% and 100% for MR angiography [32]. MR imaging was found to be superior to MR angiography in the diagnosis of VA dissections, MR angiography having a limited role. In isolation, MR imaging has certain limitations. Both the degree of a stenosis and the longitudinal extension may be difficult to assess. This is due to the low blood flow velocities distal to a high-grade stenosis, which may cause flow-related enhancement problems. In addition, arteriopathies such as fibromuscular dysplasia may be missed.

Advanced MR techniques

Recently, with the development of faster, stronger gradients and with improved software, fast acquisition techniques have become available [37]. These newer techniques include, diffusion-weighted MR imaging (DWI), perfusion-weighted MR imaging (PWI) and ultra-fast contrast-enhanced MR angiography (CE-MRA).

CE-MRA has been demonstrated to be a feasible alternative to conventional angiography in patients with a variety of disease of the carotid artery [38]. Images are acquired within 30 seconds in the arterial phase of the first pass of a contrast bolus. In order to combine PWI and CE-MRA information in a single examination, it may be necessary to use a neck coil (for CE-MRA) in addition to a head coil. Leclerc *et al* have successfully used contrast-enhanced MRA in vertebral artery dissection to demonstrate vascular changes over time. These include the formation of pseudoaneurysms and the progression of stenoses to complete occlusion [39].

PWI also requires the injection of a contrast bolus and should be performed after CE-MRA. This avoids the potential to obscure an arterial abnormality by the venous hyper-intensity which may persist following a previous contrast injection. The amount of gadolinium administered as contrast in this scenario does not exceed safety limits. PWI may qualitatively demonstrate an area of vascular compromise. This may potentially be at risk of infarction with any further deterioration in its vascular supply.

In the context of arterial dissection, the combined use of new and conventional MR techniques provides information on a number of parameters:-

◆ Carotid artery obstruction and the shape of the stenosis (CE-MRA and TOF-MR angiography).
◆ The presence of vessel wall haematoma and the demonstration of a residual vessel lumen (T2-weighted MR imaging, TOF-MR angiography source images).
◆ The extent of the acute ischaemic tissue change (DW).
◆ The extent of the area of haemodynamic compromise (PW).
◆ The extent of chronic brain lesions (T2-weighted MR imaging).

Whilst vessel wall haematoma may be the only definite abnormality that can be demonstrated in a distal short-segment ICA dissection, the use of MR angiography, DWI and PWI can exclude or confirm the presence of high-grade vessel obstruction, recent ischaemic lesions and haemodynamic alterations caused by narrowing of the vessel. Multi-parametric MR imaging in conjunction with ultrasound studies may eliminate the need for conventional angiography in many patients and may be used to monitor the course of the disease follow-up [37].

Ultrasound

Ultrasound (US) provides a non-invasive, cost-effective, rapid and accurate method for assessing the presence of carotid dissections as well as for follow-up of patients [40,41]. As well as providing direct visualisation of the pathological findings related to an ICA dissection, US gives haemodynamic information, documents the extension of previously undiagnosed dissection, assesses patency of the true lumen and demonstrates the direction of flow within the true and false lumens [40-42].

Appearances

The gray-scale US findings may be divided into three categories:-

◆ Normal.
◆ Luminal flap with or without thrombus formation.

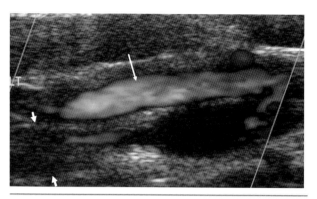

Figure 3. Longitudinal view through the carotid bulb, demonstrating echo-poor thrombus in the lumen of the internal carotid artery (short arrows) causing narrowing of the 'true' lumen with some colour Doppler flow seen. The long arrow indicates the external carotid artery which is hypertrophied to compensate for the narrowed internal carotid artery.

◆ Echo poor thrombus with or without lumen narrowing (Figure 3) [43].

The spectral Doppler US waveforms may be divided into four categories:-

◆ Normal.
◆ Damped or biphasic waveforms ('staccato' flow).
◆ Absent flow.
◆ High velocity flow [29,44].

These waveforms, however, are non-specific and also occur in high-grade stenosis and occlusions, but should raise the possibility of a dissection in the appropriate clinical setting (Figure 4) [40]. Two large series of ICA dissections have shown that the commonest spectral Doppler US findings in the affected ICA are either a bi-directional high resistance pattern ('staccato' flow) or absence of a signal in a total occlusion [29,41]. In an analysis of the value of US in spontaneous ICA dissection, a high accuracy in detecting dissections causing occlusion or high-grade stenosis was demonstrated, but the sensitivity of US was only 20% for low-grade stenosis [41].

Using colour and spectral Doppler US in spontaneous ICA dissections, different manifestations of flow haemodynamics have been documented. A high resistance, low velocity spectral Doppler signal corresponds to the angiographic appearance of a long narrowed segment of ICA ('string sign'), where a wall haematoma has arisen. Other findings include flow reversal with a to-and-fro spectral Doppler waveform pattern in the false lumen and a normal spectral Doppler waveform in the true lumen, forward high velocity flow with spectral broadening and low velocity flow reversal with some spectral broadening [44].

As the US appearances of ICA dissections have been reported in a limited number of patients, it is difficult to evaluate the diagnostic capabilities of colour Doppler US in the evaluation of ICA dissection. However, visualisation of intramural haematoma combined with 'staccato' (obstructive high resistance) flow, strongly indicates the presence of an ICA dissection. Such Doppler US findings in patients with clinical suspicion of spontaneous ICA dissection are sufficient to establish a definite diagnosis without the need for other imaging modalities. Patients with clinical suspicion of cervical artery dissection, having inconclusive or normal duplex scanning should be further investigated by MR imaging and MR angiography. A VA dissection is difficult to ascertain on colour Doppler US due to the nature of the position of the VA (between the transverse processes) and full interrogation is not possible. The same US features seen with a carotid artery dissection would apply, but is less likely to be clearly demonstrated [45].

Computed Tomography Angiography

Computed Tomography (CT) angiography is a minimally invasive technique which allows excellent visualisation of the carotid arteries and provides high-resolution images of the arterial lumen as well as the vessel wall. In addition, the data may be displayed using a MIP algorithm, which provides angiography-like images. CT has been shown to be valuable in the diagnosis of extra-cranial ICA dissections in the acute stage, providing results in close agreement with those obtained at conventional angiography [46]. The presence of a stenosis, mural thickening, occlusion, eccentric lumen, aneurysm formation and thin annular contrast enhancement are all signs of extra-cranial ICA dissections (Figure 5). The analysis of the residual arterial lumen and the measurement of the external diameter of the carotid artery at the dissection site compared to the diameter beyond the bulb are the most useful criteria for diagnosis [46]. Results similar to those of MR techniques have been reported for the detection and follow-up of carotid artery dissections, but experience with this technique remains limited. CT may also be employed in the follow-up of patients with dissection.

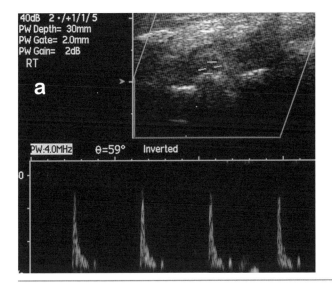
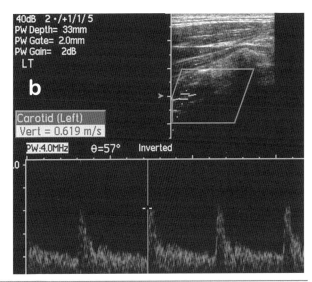

Figure 4. Spectral Doppler waveforms of the right and left vertebral arteries in a patient with a vertebral artery dissection. On the right VA a) the spectral Doppler waveform is of 'high-resistance' with low forward flow in diastole, whereas on the left VA b), the normal artery demonstrates a 'low-resistance' high forward flow in diastole.

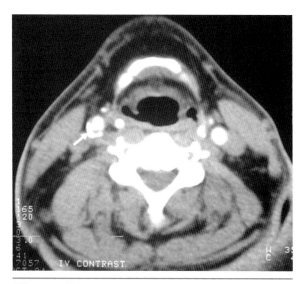

Figure 5. A contrast-enhanced arterial phase axial section through the upper neck at the level of the common carotid bifurcation, demonstrating a contrast-filled false lumen (arrow) of an internal carotid artery dissection. *Reproduced with the permission of The British Institute of Radiology. Sidhu PS, Jonker ND, Khaw KT, Patel N, Blomley MJ, Chaudhuri KR, et al. Spontaneous dissections of the internal carotid artery: appearances on colour Doppler ultrasound. Br J Radiol 1997; 70: 50-7.*

Clinical management

The risk of recurrent carotid artery dissection identified by angiography is approximately 2% in the first month and 1% annually thereafter [11,47]. The rate of recurrent events appears dependent upon the patient's age at the time of the first dissection, with an increased risk if the patient is under 45 years of age [47]. Dissection almost never occurs in the same artery at the same location [48]. About 80% of all strokes secondary to carotid artery dissection occur within one week of initial symptoms [6].

The aim of management is to prevent the development or perpetuation of neurological deficits and to abolish further ischaemic events by preventing thrombosis and embolisation. The cause of ischaemic events in patients with ICA dissection is usually thromboembolic or as a result of haemodynamic compromise [11,47]. Evidence to support this comes from a study of patients with any ischaemic stroke

secondary to a ICA dissection. In this study, a cortical or sub-cortical infarct was designated as embolic in origin, whereas small sub-cortical infarcts (<15mm), junctional or water-shed infarcts were designated as haemodynamic in origin. The study showed that of a total of 65 infarcts, 34 were cortical, 25 sub-cortical (one <15mm) and five junctional or watershed infarcts. This was thought to show that 92.2% of patients had an embolic infarct and only 7.7% of patients had a haemodynamic cerebral ischaemia event [2]. Recurrent events are probably also thromboembolic in nature, arising from fresh arterial tears [24]. Trans-cranial Doppler US of the middle cerebral artery detects cerebral micro-emboli in 46% to 56% of patients monitored in the immediate post-dissection period and may predict future ischaemic events [2].

Medical treatment

Despite the lack of controlled studies regarding the optimal treatment of cervical artery dissection, current medical management includes anti-thrombotic drugs and full dose anticoagulant therapy [6]. Anticoagulant therapy relies on evidence supporting the embolic nature of stroke complicating dissection. The majority of patients are treated with warfarin therapy for six months after initial treatment for 1-3 weeks with heparin. In patients with a residual aneurysm, persisting severe stenosis, or underlying arterial disease, long-term aspirin therapy is often used. Thrombolytic therapy, both intravenous and intra-arterial, is increasingly being employed in acute dissection, usually without significant complications or evidence of extension of the lesion. Nevertheless, this remains an unproven treatment method [49]. A therapeutic trial of anticoagulation versus aspirin has been suggested to ascertain optimal early management [50].

Early anticoagulation is recommended in extra-cranial VA dissection to reduce the risk of posterior circulation infarction. In intracranial VA dissection, anticoagulants are contraindicated because of the risk of precipitating a subarachnoid haemorrhage [6]. In patients with pseudoaneurysms, anticoagulation may be contraindicated because of risk of pseudoaneurysm rupture [20].

Surgery

Surgical options include resection of the diseased ICA with vein graft replacement, ICA ligation or clipping, gradual intra-luminal dilatation, thromboendarterectomy and 'patch' angioplasty, as well as extra-cranial-to-intracranial bypass procedures [51,52]. In the past, surgery was the sole method of carotid artery repair, but with the improvement in vascular stent technology, carotid artery stent insertion has made surgery to a large degree obsolete [53]. Surgery carries a risk of lower cranial nerve injury especially if a dissection aneurysm is located at the sub-petrous segment of the ICA [54].

Endovascular treatment

Endovascular techniques, such as percutaneous balloon dilatation and endovascular stent placement and coil embolisation of pseudoaneurysms, are low risk and have superseded surgery as the treatment of choice following failed medical management [55,56]. Endovascular stents provide the necessary centrifugal force to permit apposition of the dissected segment to the arterial wall in order to obliterate the false lumen and resolve the stenosis [57,58]. Endovascular stents also provide a mechanical support for coil embolisation of dissection-related wide-necked pseudoaneurysms [59,60].

The advantages of endovascular stenting are as follows:-

◆ It enables the identification of the true and false lumens by super-selective catheterisation.
◆ It allows immediate recanalisation of the artery with reperfusion of the ischaemic brain.
◆ It enables the simultaneous treatment of any coexisting pseudoaneurysm by coil embolisation.
◆ It eliminates the need for complicated carotid reconstructive procedures [61].

Routine anticoagulation is not indicated after endovascular stent insertion and the patient is maintained with anti-platelet agents only. Endovascular stent insertion may prove to be a suitable treatment alternative for patients in whom anticoagulation is contraindicated. Case series have shown a low complication rate [55,56]. The risk of distal embolisation of atheromatous debris, as occurs during balloon dilatation of the atherosclerotic carotid artery, is minimal in carotid artery dissection and the lesions are more compliant. Unlike atherosclerotic stenosis which requires higher pressure balloon dilatation to fracture the atheromatous plaque, stent deployment for dissection is less traumatic [61].

The major limitation to the use of endovascular stents for the treatment of carotid artery dissection involves difficulty in the selective micro-catheterisation of the true lumen of the dissected artery. The arterial segment to be treated is often long and frequently requires multiple stents correctly inter-positioned to avoid inter-stent arterial dissections. End-to-end stent implantation is often not successful [62].

Indications

There are as yet no guidelines as to which patients may benefit from an endovascular procedure. Nevertheless, the presence of objective evidence of cerebral ischaemia and salvageable tissue on MR imaging could help in selection of appropriate patients. The presence of a large ischaemic region, indicated by a diffusion-perfusion mismatch on MR imaging (with the perfusion deficit being larger than the diffusion deficit) [63] or the finding of delayed capillary filling (in areas known to be viable by diffusion MR imaging) during angiography may be an indication for endovascular therapy. Conversely, patients with irreversible ischaemic changes may not warrant endovascular treatment. If CT or MR imaging demonstrates an area of infarction that accounts for a neurological deficit, then restoring flow may not be useful and may increase haemorrhagic transformation of the stroke [53]. A description of the use of a combination of MR imaging (diffusion and perfusion) and angiography to identify potentially salvageable but at-risk brain tissue, and allow endovascular treatment, was successful in a small series of patients not responding to medical management [62].

Conclusions

The diagnosis of an extra-cranial dissection is readily achieved on non-invasive imaging, with the use of angiography reserved for cases where endovascular management is considered. A combination of MR imaging is the most useful adjunct to diagnosis, but US provides a practical method for follow-up of arterial patency. Endovascular treatment should be considered when medical treatment fails or there is progression of disease. Surgical management is rarely indicated.

Summary

- Incidence of ICA dissection is 2-3 per 100,000 per year.
- Increased diagnosis of dissection is attributable to improved imaging.
- Dissections may be spontaneous or traumatic.
- The classical triad of symptoms in an ICA dissection are unilateral headache, partial Horner's syndrome and cerebral ischaemia.
- Vertebral artery dissections may present with sub-arachnoid haemorrhage.
- Arteriography will demonstrate stenosis, occlusion or a pseudoaneurysm.
- MRI and MRA provide a useful overview of the extent of a dissection and documents cerebral ischaemia.
- US is useful for follow-up of arterial patency.
- Anticoagulation is the mainstay of medical treatment.
- Surgery has a limited role in management.
- Endovascular stent insertion and embolisation is the treatment of choice in failed medical management.

References

1. Jentzer A. Dissecting aneurysm of the left internal carotid artery. *Angiology* 1954; 5: 232-234.

2. Lucas C, Moulin T, Deplanque D, Tatu L, Chavot D. Stroke patterns of internal carotid artery dissection in 40 patients. *Stroke* 1998; 29: 2646-2648.

3. Bogousslavsky J, Regli F. Ischemic stroke in adults younger than 30 years of age: cause and prognosis. *Arch Neurol* 1987; 44: 479-482.

4. Ducrocq X, Lacour JC, Debouverie M, Bracard S, Girard F, Weber M. Accidents vasculaires cerebraux ischemiques du sujet jeune: etude prospective de 296 patients ages de 16 a 45 ans. *Rev Neurol (Paris)* 1999; 155: 575-582.

5. Hart RG, Easton JD. Dissections. *Stroke* 1985; 16: 925-927.

6. Schievink WI. Spontaneous dissection of the carotid and vertebral arteries. *N Engl J Med* 2001; 344: 898-906.

7. O'Sullivan RM, Raeb DA, Nugent RA, Robertson WD, Lapointe JS. Carotid and vertebral artery trauma: clinical and angiographic features. *Australas Radiol* 1991; 35: 47-55.

8. Houser OW, Mokri B, Sundt TM, Baker HL, Reese DF. Spontaneous cervical cephalic arterial dissection and its residuum: Angiographic spectrum. *Am J Neuroradiol* 1984; 5: 27-34.

9. Grau AJ, Brandt T, Buggle F, *et al*. Association of cervical artery dissection with recent infection. *Arch Neurol* 1999; 56: 851-856.

10. Tzourio C, El Amrani M, Robert L, Alperovitch A. Serum elastase activity is elevated in migraine. *Ann Neurol* 2000; 47: 648-651.

11. Schievink WI, Mokri B, O'Fallon WM. Recurrent spontaneous cervical-artery dissection. *N Engl J Med* 1994; 330: 393-397.

12. Fisher CM, Ojemann RG, Roberson GH. Spontaneous dissection of cervico-cerebral arteries. *Can J Neurol Sci* 1978; 5: 9-19.

13. Hirst AE, Johns VJ, Kime SW. Dissecting aneurysms of the aorta: a review of 505 cases. *Medicine (Baltimore)* 1958; 37: 217.

14. Mokri B, Houser OW, Sandok BA. Spontaneous dissections of the vertebral arteries. *Neurology* 1988; 38: 880-885.

15. Schievink WI, Mokri B, Whisnant JP. Internal carotid artery dissection in a community. Rochester. Minnesota. 1987-1992. *Stroke* 1993; 24: 1678-1680.

16. Schievink WI, Mokri B, Piepgras DG. Spontaneous dissections of the cervicocephalic arteries in childhood and adolescence. *Neurology* 1994; 44: 1607-1612.

17. Caplan LR, Baquis GD, Pessin MS, *et al*. Dissection of the intracranial vertebral artery. *Neurology* 1988; 38: 868-877.

18. Leys D, Moulin T, Stojkovic T, Begey S, Chavot D and the DONALD Investigators. Follow-up of patients with history of cervical artery dissection. *Cerebrovasc Dis* 1995; 5: 43-49.

19. Davies MJ, Treasure T, Richardson PD. The pathogenesis of spontaneous arterial dissection. *Heart* 1996; 75: 434-435.

20. Anson J, Crowell RM. Cervicocranial dissection. *Neurosurg* 1991; 29: 89-96.

21. Provenzale JM. Dissection of the internal carotid and vertebral arteries: imaging features. *Am J Roentgenol* 1995; 165: 1099-1104.

22. Hart RG, Easton JD. Dissections of cervical and cerebral arteries. *Neurol Clin* 1983; 1: 155-182.

23. Pelkonen O, Tikkakoski T, Leinonen S, Pyhtinen J, Lepojarvi M, Sotaniemi K. Extracranial internal carotid and vertebral artery dissections: angiographic spectrum, course and prognosis. *Neuroradiology* 2003; 45: 71-77.

24. Schievink WI. The treatment of spontaneous carotid and vertebral artery dissections. *Curr Opin Cardiol* 2000; 15: 316-321.

25. Hinse P, Thie A, Lachenmayer L. Dissection of the extracranial vertebral artery: a report of four cases and a review of the literature. *J Neurol Neurosurg Psych* 1991; 54: 863-869.

26. Touze E, Randoux B, Meary E, Arquizan C, Meder JF, Mas JL. Aneurysmal forms of cervical artery dissection. Associated factors and outcome. *Stroke* 2001; 32: 418-423.

27. Hankey GJ, Warlow CP, Sellar RJ. Cerebral angiographic risk in mild cerebrovascular disease. *Stroke* 1990; 21: 209-222.

28. Roome NS, Aberfeld DC. Spontaneous dissecting aneurysm of the internal carotid artery. *Arch Neurol* 1977; 34: 251-252.

29. Steinke W, Rautenberg W, Schwartz A, Hennerici M. Noninvasive monitoring of internal carotid artery dissection. *Stroke* 1994; 25: 998-1005.

30. Stringaris K, Liberopoulos K, Giaka E, *et al*. Three-dimensional time-of-flight MR angiography and MR imaging versus conventional angiography in carotid artery dissections. *Int Angiol* 1996; 15: 20-25.

31. Kirsch E, Kaim A, Engelter S, *et al*. MR angiography in internal carotid artery dissection: improvement of diagnosis by selective demonstration of the intraluminal haematoma. *Neuroradiology* 1998; 40: 704-709.

32. Levy C, Laissy JP, Raveau V, *et al*. Carotid and vertebral artery dissections: three-dimensional time-of-flight MR angiography and MR imaging versus conventional angiography. *Radiology* 1994; 190: 97-103.

33. Ozdoba C, Sturzenegger MN, Schroth G. Internal carotid artery dissection. MR imaging features and clinical-radiologic correlation. *Radiology* 1996; 199: 191-198.

34. Fiebach J, Brandt T, Nauth M, Jansen O. MRI with fat suppression in the visualization of wall hematoma in spontaneous dissection of the internal carotid artery. *Rofo Fortschr Geb Rontgenstr Neuen Bildgeb Verfahr* 1999; 171: 290-293.

35. Hirai T, Korogi Y, Ikushima I, Shigematsu Y, Morishita S, Yamashita Y. Intracranial artery dissections: serial evaluation with MR imaging, MR angiography, and source images of MR angiography. *Radiat Med* 2003; 21: 86-93.

36. Kitanaka C, Tanaka J, Kuwahara M, Teraoka A. Magnetic resonance imaging study of intracranial vertebrobasilar artery dissections. *Stroke* 1994; 25: 571-575.

37. Gass A, Szabo K, Lanczik O, Hennerici MG. Magnetic resonance imaging assessment of carotid artery dissection. *Cerebrovasc Dis* 2002; 13: 70-73.

38. Parker DL, Goodrich KC, Alexander AL, Buswell HR, Blatter DD, Tsuruda JS. Optimized visualization of vessels in contrast-enhanced intracranial MR angiography. *Magn Reson Med* 1998; 40: 873-882.

39. Leclerc X, Lucas C, Godefroy O, *et al.* Preliminary experience using contrast-enhanced MR angiography to assess vertebral artery structure for the follow-up of suspected dissection. *Am J Neuroradiol* 1999; 20: 1482-90.

40. Bluth EI, Shyn PB, Sullivan M, Merritt CR. Doppler color flow imaging of carotid artery dissection. *J Ultrasound Med* 1989; 8: 149-153.

41. Sturzenegger M, Mattle HP, Rivoir A, Baumgartner RW. Ultrasound findings in carotid artery dissection: analysis of 43 patients. *Neurology* 1995; 45: 691-698.

42. Logason K, Hardemark HG, Barlin T, Bergqvist D, Ahlstom H, Karacagil S. Duplex scan findings in patients with spontaneous cervical artery dissections. *Eur J Vasc Endovasc Surg* 2002; 23: 295-298.

43. Gardner DJ, Gosink BB, Kallman CE. Internal carotid artery dissections: Duplex ultrasound imaging. *J Ultrasound Med* 1991; 10: 607-614.

44. Sidhu PS, Jonker ND, Khaw KT, *et al.* Spontaneous dissections of the internal carotid artery: appearances on color Doppler ultrasound. *Br J Radiol* 1997; 70: 50-57.

45. Sturzenegger M, Mattle HP, Rivoir A, Rihs F, Schmid C. Ultrasound findings in spontaneous extracranial vertebral artery dissection. *Stroke* 1993; 24: 1910-1921.

46. Leclerc X, Godefroy O, Salhi A, Lucas C, Leys D, Pruvo JP. Helical CT for the diagnosis of extracranial internal carotid artery dissection. *Stroke* 1996; 27: 461-466.

47. Bassetti C, Carruzzo A, Sturzenegger M, Tuncdogan E. Recurrence of cervical artery dissection. *Stroke* 1996; 27: 1804-1807.

48. Brandt T, Orberk E, Weber F, *et al.* Pathogensis of cervical arterial dissections. Association with connective tissue diseases. *Neurology* 2001; 57: 24-30.

49. Arnold M, Nedeltchev K, Sturzenegger M, Schroth G, Loher TJ. Thrombolysis in patients with acute stroke caused by cervical artery dissection: analysis of 9 patients and review of the literature. *Arch Neurol* 2002; 59: 549-553.

50. Beletsky V, Nadareishvili Z, Lynch J, Shuaib A, Woolfenden A, Norris JW. Cervical arterial dissection. Time for a therapeutic trial? *Stroke* 2003; 34: 2856-2860.

51. Treiman GS, Treiman RL, Foran RF, *et al.* Spontaneous dissection of the internal carotid artery: a nineteen-year clinical experience. *J Vasc Surg* 1996; 24: 597-605.

52. Coffin O, Maiza D, Galateau-Salle F, *et al.* Results of surgical management of internal carotid artery aneurysm by the cervical approach. *Ann Vasc Surg* 2004; 24: 597-605.

53. Bejjani GK, Monsein LH, Laird JR, Satler LF, Starnes BW, Aulisi EF. Treatment of symptomatic cervical carotid dissections with endovascular stents. *Neurosurgery* 1999; 44: 755-761.

54. Muller BT, Luther B, Hort W, Neumann-Haefelin T, Aulich A, Sandmann W. Surgical treatment of 50 carotid dissections: indications and results. *J Vasc Surg* 2000; 31: 980-988.

55. Lylyk P, Cohen JE, Ceratto R, Ferrario A, Miranda C. Combined endovascular treatment of dissecting vertebral artery aneurysms by using stents and coils. *J Neurosurg* 2001; 94: 427-432.

56. Lylyk P, Cohen JE, Ceratto R, Ferrario A, Miranda C. Angioplasty and Stent Placement in Intracranial Atherosclerotic Stenoses and Dissections. *Am J Neuroradiol* 2002; 23: 430-436.

57. Hong MK, Salter SF, Gallino R, Leon MB. Intravascular stenting as a definitive treatment of spontaneous carotid artery dissection. *Am J Cardiol* 1997; 79: 538.

58. DeOcampo J, Brillman J, Levy DI. Stenting: a new approach to carotid dissection. *J Neuroimaging* 1997; 7: 187-190.

59. Mericle RA, Lanzino G, WAkhloo AK, Guterman LR, Hopkins LN. Stenting and secondary coiling of intracranial internal carotid artery aneurysm: technical case report. *Neurosurgery* 1998; 43: 1229-1234.

60. Higashida RT, Smith W, Gress D, *et al.* Intravascular stent and endovascular coil placement for a ruptured fusiform aneurysm of the basilar artery. Case report and review of the literature. *J Neurosurg* 1997; 87: 944-999.

61. Malek AM, Higashida RT, Phatouros CC, *et al.* Endovascular Management of Extracranial Carotid Artery Dissection Achieved Using Stent Angioplasty. *Am J Neuroradiol* 2000; 21: 1280-1292.

62. Cohen JE, Leker RR, Gotkine M, Gomori M, Ben-Hur T. Emergent stenting to treat patients with carotid artery dissections. Clinically and radiologically directed therapeutic decision making. *Stroke* 2003; 34: e254-e257.

63. Schlaug G, Benfield A, Baird AE, *et al.* The ischemic penumbra: Operationally defined by diffusion and perfusion MRI. *Neurology* 1999; 53: 1528-1537.

Chapter 17

The asymptomatic carotid surgery trial (ACST): implications for intervention

Joanna Marro, BSc, ACST Trial Co-ordinator
Alison Halliday, MS FRCS, Consultant Vascular Surgeon
On behalf of the Asymptomatic Carotid Surgery Trial collaborators
St George's Hospital Medical School, London, UK

Introduction

In 1991, the European Carotid Surgery Trial (ECST)[1] and the North American Symptomatic Carotid Surgery Trial (NASCET) [2] demonstrated the net benefits of endarterectomy for patients who had tight (70-99%) carotid artery narrowing and were 'symptomatic' i.e. had already had some neurological symptom (transient cerebral or retinal ischaemia or minor stroke) in the relevant carotid territory within the past six months. In particular, these studies have shown that CEA prevents disabling and fatal stroke in men and women, including those over 80 years of age. A recent meta-analysis of all such trials in symptomatic patients has further supported CEA being of substantial net value in these patients [3].

There remained, however, much uncertainty about the net benefits among 'asymptomatic' patients with similar degrees of carotid artery narrowing but no such neurological symptoms within the past few months. In 1993, the Veterans' Administration (VA) trial [4], which randomised 444 men, showed that CEA reduced the risk of transient ischaemic attack (TIA) and stroke, but not of stroke alone. The Asymptomatic Carotid Surgery Trial (ACST) was therefore started in 1993 to determine whether, in neurologically asymptomatic patients with appropriate carotid stenosis, CEA would reduce the 5-year risk of stroke and death, and particularly of disabling stroke and death [5]. The trial would also enable any high-risk group to be identified. In 1995, the Asymptomatic Carotid Atherosclerosis Study (ACAS) trial [6] of 1659 patients showed that CEA reduced 5-year stroke risk. However, ACST continued randomising patients as considerable uncertainty remained about the place of endarterectomy in these asymptomatic patients.

Methods

ACST is a prospective international multicentre randomised trial (level Ia evidence) which had a recruitment target of just over 3000 'asymptomatic' patients. At each centre there was to be at least one vascular surgeon or neurosurgeon and one neurologist or stroke physician collaborating in the trial. Prospective surgical collaborators were asked to submit a record of their last 50 carotid endarterectomies. The number of strokes or deaths occurring within 30 days of surgery was not to exceed 3/50 (6%) for symptomatic CEA.

Patients were allocated (by 'minimised' randomisation [7]) either to immediate surgery, or to deferral of any carotid surgery until a definite need for it was thought to have arisen eg. if relevant carotid territory symptoms occurred. The protocol specified that for patients randomised to surgery, carotid endarterectomy was to be carried out routinely as soon as possible. Surgeons used their normal operative techniques and anaesthetic technique was also at the discretion of the individual centres. Patients in both arms of the trial were to receive appropriate medical treatment, which generally included anti-platelet therapy, antihypertensive therapy and lipid-lowering therapy. Information collected at the time of randomisation included: age; sex; hypertension; diabetes; previous contralateral symptoms/CEA; previous ipsilateral symptoms over six months before; percentage carotid stenosis on each side; estimate of plaque echolucency; total cholesterol; blood pressure and current drug therapy.

Patients were eligible for ACST if they were 'asymptomatic' i.e. their carotid stenosis had not caused symptoms for at least six months, they had unilateral or bilateral carotid artery stenosis that was severe (which, in practice, generally meant 60-99% carotid artery diameter reduction on ultrasound) and had not been operated on, and both doctor and patient were substantially uncertain [8,9] whether the patient should undergo immediate CEA or deferral of any CEA. In addition, patients were to have no past history of ipsilateral disabling or severe contralateral stroke, no indications for, or contraindications to carotid endarterectomy and no known circumstance or condition likely to preclude long-term follow-up, in particular, no other severe life-threatening disease. Exclusion criteria included previous ipsilateral CEA, high risk of adverse effects from surgery, some likely cardiac source of emboli, or any major life-threatening condition other than carotid stenosis.

Patients were seen at four months after randomisation, 12 months, and yearly thereafter for at least five years, chiefly to record any CEAs, their operative morbidity, and the details of any strokes or deaths. Randomisation was based on duplex (not angiographic) stenosis (angiograms were optional in ACST and in later years were generally not done) and collaborators were also asked to perform a duplex Doppler ultrasound examination of both carotid arteries at each visit up to five years. In addition, blood pressure and use of antiplatelet, anticoagulant, lipid-lowering and antihypertensive drugs were recorded at every follow-up.

The main stroke outcomes were the perioperative hazards of stroke or death, and the incidence of non-perioperative strokes. The causes of all non-stroke deaths were also recorded. Strokes were classified according to their nature, location and consequences (fatal, disabling or non-disabling). A fatal stroke was one considered by the clinical endpoint review committee to have caused the death of the patient, either directly or by some non-neurological complication (eg. pneumonia). A disabling stroke was one that had a modified Rankin score [10] of 3, 4, 5 at six months (a Rankin score of 3 involves moderate neurological disability from the index stroke that involves the need for some help in daily affairs). A non-disabling stroke was one that had a modified Rankin score of 0, 1, 2 at six months (a Rankin score of 2 involves only slight disability from the index stroke, with the patient perhaps unable to carry out some previous activities but still able to look after their own daily affairs without assistance). Surgical events were all strokes and deaths occurring within 30 days of CEA.

Patient characteristics

3120 patients were randomised between April 1993 and July 2003 and followed-up for at least five years (mean 3.4 years). A total of 126 centres randomised patients in 30 countries. Thirty centres randomised more than 30 patients and 18 centres randomised more than 50 patients. Overall, an average of 25 patients were randomised per centre. A third of patients (1069) were randomised from the UK. The remaining two thirds were mainly randomised from Europe.

1560 patients were allocated to immediate surgery and 1560 to deferred surgery (Figure 1). Patient characteristics were very similar to those of the ACAS trial. At randomisation, average age was 68 years (range 40-91 years). 66% of patients were male. Hypertension was being treated in 65% of patients and mean systolic blood pressure was 153 mmHg.

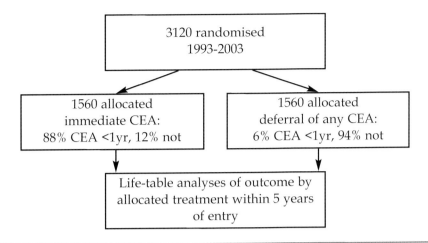

Figure 1. Randomisation and 'intention-to-treat' analysis of events within five years of entry into ACST.

Mean cholesterol was 5.8mmol/L and 20% of patients were reported to have diabetes. 24% of patients had had a previous contralateral CEA, 8% had an ipsilateral CT infarct and 9% had contralateral occlusion. Mean ipsilateral carotid artery stenosis on duplex ultrasound was 80% at the time of randomisation (carotid artery narrowing on ultrasound was usually rounded to 70%, 80% or 90%). Use of antiplatelet, anticoagulant and lipid-lowering drugs as well as antihypertensive therapy was recorded. During the period of enrollment the use of lipid-lowering therapy and antihypertensive therapy at randomisation increased (17% to 58% and 61% to 72%,

respectively). The use of antiplatelet and anticoagulant treatment, however, remained approximately the same throughout the recruitment period (89% and 6%, respectively). Because minimised randomisation was used, there are no significant differences between the initial characteristics of the two treatment groups.

Compliance

Time from recruitment to ipsilateral surgery (compliance) is shown in Figure 2. On average during

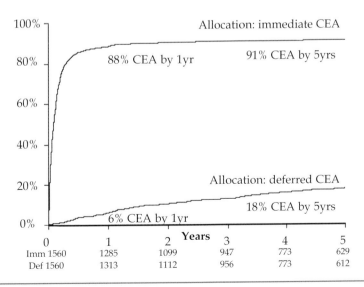

Figure 2. Proportion with ipsilateral CEA by time from randomisation, with number alive and still under observation at various times.

the first five years, ~90% patients allocated immediate surgery had ipsilateral CEA, 50% within one month and 88% by one year. Patients allocated surgery who did not have it generally changed their minds after further discussions with their family or physician. Alternatively, other circumstances, such as the surgeon deciding against surgery following the preoperative assessment, sometimes made early surgery difficult.

Approximately 10% (201) of patients allocated deferred surgery had ipsilateral CEA during the first five years. Half (101) of those in the deferred group who went on to have the operation did so because they became 'symptomatic' (92 ipsilateral TIAs or stroke, nine non-specific symptoms possibly vertebrobasilar). Other reasons for having the operation included in preparation for or in conjunction with other (eg. cardiac) surgery (7), because the patient or surgeon changed their mind after further discussion (61), or for other factors (eg. increasing carotid stenosis, change in plaque composition, new infarction on brainscanning [32]).

Analyses

Analysis of data was on an intention to treat basis. Among those in either group who underwent CEA, the risk per CEA of a perioperative 'event' (stroke or any death within 30 days) was recorded. The 5-year stroke risk (including perioperative events) of all patients allocated to immediate CEA has been compared to those allocated to deferral using Kaplan-Meier life table analysis.

Results

The 5-year results for this trial have now been published [11]. In asymptomatic patients younger than 75 years of age with carotid diameter reduction about 70% or more on ultrasound (many of whom were on aspirin, antihypertensive, and, in recent years, statin therapy), immediate CEA halved the net 5-year stroke risk from about 12% to about 6% (including the 3% perioperative hazard). Half this 5-year benefit involved disabling or fatal strokes. But, outside trials, inappropriate selection of patients or poor surgery could obviate such benefits. The longer-term effects are not yet known. For this reason, ACST will continue to follow-up patients until 2008 (10-year results).

Implications for intervention

ACST is currently the largest vascular surgery trial in the world. It will provide reliable information on the first five years of follow-up, but it is imperative that this follow-up continues in order to determine the 10-year results. This will enable the effect of surgery on stroke prevention to be accurately assessed in this patient group. ACST is a 'real life' trial and the results are generalisable. One third (1069) of patients are from the UK (the largest contributor) and the remaining patients are from mainly European countries.

ACST is nearly twice the size of the next largest similar trial (ACAS, 1659 patients). A meta-analysis of the ACST 5-year results with prior randomised trials will more than double the size of the currently published meta-analyses making the results much more reliable and informative (two meta-analyses have been published in recent years [12,13]; both showed that there is some evidence favouring CEA in patients with asymptomatic carotid stenosis; neither routinely recommended CEA in these patients). A combination of the results of the two major trials (ACST and ACAS) has been published [11] as part of the 5-year results paper and an individual patient data meta-analysis of all trials is planned. Continuation of follow-up of ACST patients to ten years will be essential as ACAS discontinued follow-up in 1995.

The recent Heart Protection study results [14] showed that statins and aspirin reduced risk of stroke and myocardial infarction and halved the need for carotid interventions caused by stroke and transient ischaemic symptoms. ACST routinely collects information on drug therapy at every follow-up and, as ACST continues to 2008, important information will be gained about how compliance with drug therapy (statins, aspirin and antihypertensive treatment) may affect stroke risk.

The interim 5-year results of ACST will improve understanding of the outcomes and appropriate use of surgery. The 10-year results of this study will inform medical practice about long-term life expectancy after surgery, stroke-free life expectancy, the impact of medical treatment and the impact on stroke costs following surgery.

Summary

◆ ACST is currently the largest vascular surgery trial in the world.

◆ 3120 patients have been randomised either to immediate carotid endarterectomy or deferral of any carotid surgery until a definite need for it was thought to have arisen.

◆ Patient characteristics at randomisation were similar to those in ACAS.

◆ Because minimised randomisation was used, there were no significant differences between the initial characteristics of the two treatment groups.

◆ On average during the first five years, ~90% patients allocated immediate surgery and ~10% allocated deferral of surgery, had ipsilateral CEA.

◆ In asymptomatic patients younger than 75 years of age with carotid diameter reduction about 70% or more on ultrasound, immediate CEA halved the net 5-year stroke risk from about 12% to about 6% (including the 3% perioperative hazard). Half this 5-year benefit involved disabling or fatal strokes.

◆ Subsidiary analyses to identify any 'high-risk group' that might benefit from intervention have also been published.

References

1. European Carotid Surgery Trialists' Collaborative Group. MRC European Carotid Surgery Trial: interim results for symptomatic patients with severe (70-99%) or with mild (0-29%) carotid stenosis. *Lancet* 1991; 337: 1235-43.

2. North American Symptomatic Carotid Endarterectomy Trial Collaborators. Beneficial effect of carotid endarterectomy in symptomatic patients with high-grade stenosis. *N Engl J Med* 1991; 325: 445-53.

3. Rothwell PM, Eliasziw M, Gutnikov SA, *et al.* for the Carotid Endarterectomy Trialists' Collaboration. Analysis of pooled data from the randomised controlled trials of endarterectomy for symptomatic carotid stenosis. *Lancet* 2003; 361: 107-16.

4. Hobson RW II, Weiss DG, Fields WS for the VA Co-operative Study Group. Efficacy of carotid endarterectomy for asymptomatic carotid stenosis. *N Engl J Med* 1993; 328: 221-7.

5. Halliday AW, Thomas D, Mansfield A. The Asymptomatic Carotid Surgery Trial (ACST) Rationale and Design. *Eur J Vasc Surg* 1994; 8: 703-10.

6. Executive Committee for the Asymptomatic Carotid Atherosclerosis Study. Endarterectomy for asymptomatic carotid artery stenosis. *JAMA* 1995; 273: 1421-8.

7. Pocock SJ, Simon R. Sequential treatment assignment with balancing for prognostic factors in the controlled clinical trial. *Biometrics* 1975; 31: 103-15.

8. Peto R, Baigent C. Trials: the next 50 years. Large scale randomised evidence of moderate benefits. *Lancet* 1998; 317: 1170.

9. Collins R, Peto R, Gray R, *et al.* Large-scale randomised evidence: trials and overviews. In: *Oxford textbook of medicine*, 4th ed. Warrell DA, Cox TM, Firth JD, Benz EJ Jr, Eds. Oxford University Press, Oxford, 2003: pp24-36.

10. Van Swieten JC, Koudstaal PJ, Visser MC, *et al.* Interobserver agreement for the assessment of handicap in stroke patients. *Stroke* 1988; 19: 604-7.

11. MRC Asymptomatic Carotid Surgery Trial (ACST) Collaborative Group. Prevention of disabling and fatal strokes by successful carotid endarterectomy in patients without recent neurological symptoms: randomised controlled trial. *Lancet* 2004; 383: 1491-502.

12. Benevente O, Moher D, Pham B. Carotid endarterectomy for asymptomatic carotid stenosis: a meta-analysis. *British Medical Journal* 1998; 317: 1477-80.

13. Chambers BR, You RX, Donnan GA. Carotid endarterectomy for asymptomatic carotid stenosis (Cochrane Review). In: *The Cochrane Library*, Issue 3, 2003. Update Software, Oxford.

14. Heart Protection Study Collaborative Group. MRC/BHF Heart Protection Study of cholesterol lowering with simvastatin in 20 536 high-risk individuals: a randomised placebo-controlled trial. *Lancet* 2002; 360: 7-22.

Chapter 18

The evolution of peripheral arterial stents: are we winning?

Ralph W Jackson, MRCP FRCR, Consultant Vascular and Interventional Radiologist
Northern Vascular Centre, Freeman Hospital, Newcastle-upon-Tyne, UK

Introduction

Basic stent designs and delivery systems have not changed dramatically since the first clinical experiments in the early 1980s. Whilst there have been numerous technical developments, the main advances have been in understanding the biological environment in which stents are placed and the subsequent processes that lead to failure. In addition, the clinical applications for stents have been both hugely expanded and then refined. Indeed, there is barely a system in the body in which stents have not been inserted. This chapter will discuss the use of stents in peripheral vascular disease with particular reference to the femoropopliteal segment.

The idea of using a device to maintain arterial patency following dilatation has been around almost as long as angioplasty itself. In 1969, Dotter was of the opinion that 'transluminal catheter dilatation offers a simple, rational and effective alternative to conventional vascular surgery in the relief of primary atheromatous narrowing... While spectacular and lasting successes have been achieved by catheter recanalisation, vein grafting remains the treatment of choice for long-segment femoropopliteal occlusion'. He published his first experience of using a stainless steel coilspring in six normal canine femoral or popliteal arteries. The three coilsprings coated in silicone occluded within 24 hours but two out of three non-coated devices remained patent at two years [1]. This chapter aims to address the question, 'has the potential of the stent been realised and what do we know about its evolution?'

Stent basics

The majority of stents in current clinical use are made from stainless steel, nitinol or elgiloy (Wallstent), a chromium-cobalt alloy. Tantalum stents are less commonly used. Stents can be either delivered on a balloon catheter for passive dilatation or be self-expanding. Combinations of metal stent with coatings, coverings and attached material (stent grafts) have also been developed.

More information regarding stent properties, materials and designs is provided in chapters written by Schild and Strunk [2] and Dyet and Schurmann [3]. The article by Stoeckel [4] is particularly good at explaining different stent designs and configurations. Whilst many stents are individually named, there has been no attempt to describe all stents currently and previously available.

Stent properties

Ideally, a metal stent should be non-corrodible, inert and have low thrombogenicity (biocompatible). It should also be radio-opaque, easily positioned, flexible and have elastic radial force (crush resistance) and hoop strength to resist recoil. In addition, the stent should be well apposed to the vessel wall, be quickly covered by endothelium and maintain vessel compliance. As little metal as possible should be in contact with the vessel wall. The delivery system should be low profile and allow the stent to track through tortuous vessels. It would be desirable to have a large number of lengths and sizes available for use and at low cost.

Stent materials

316L stainless steel is an alloy of predominantly iron, chromium and nickel. The surface of the stent is formed by chromium oxide and is highly electropolished to produce a smooth, non-thrombogenic surface. Stainless steel stents are relatively rigid and have high radial force, but are susceptible to crushing.

Nitinol is an alloy of nickel and titanium which has thermal memory and super-elastic properties. This renders the stents highly crush-resistant with good radial force at body temperature. The surface layer is made up of titanium oxide. Nitinol is less radio-opaque than stainless steel, but has the advantage over stainless steel of being non-paramagnetic and therefore, causing less of a susceptibility artifact during magnetic resonance imaging.

Wallstents (Boston Scientific) are made from individual wires, braided to form a cylinder. The braiding angle determines the radial force and degree of shortening during deployment. The stents are flexible and reasonably radio-opaque. Whilst the degree of shortening of the stent is predictable, this only applies if the stent achieves its nominal unconstrained diameter.

The only tantalum stent that has been used in the periphery is the Strecker (Boston Scientific) stent, which is a balloon-expanded knitted wire design. This is a very flexible stent and is highly radio-opaque.

Stent designs

The majority of stents in peripheral vascular usage are manufactured from wires or tubes of their raw material and come in coil, woven and sequential ring forms. The latter can be divided into open- or closed-cell (see below) configuration.

The simplest wire form is the nitinol coil (Intracoil, Intratherapeutics). In addition to the Wallstent and the Strecker stent, other wire designs include the Symphony (Boston Scientific, welded nitinol, closed-cell), the ZA (Cook, knitted nitinol) and the Bridge (Medtronic AVE, sequential, stainless steel, welded rings, open-cell) stents.

The majority of other peripheral vascular stents are laser cut from tubes. Most stents are essentially a series of Z-shaped rings connected by longitudinal bridging elements. Depending on the distribution of the longitudinal elements, closed or open cells are described. A closed-cell design is where every point of each sequential ring is connected. The original stents, developed by Palmaz and colleagues in the 1980s, were stainless steel tubes, laser cut with longitudinal slots which on expansion gave a diamond shaped lattice; a closed-cell design. These had excellent radial strength but were rather inflexible and shortened on expansion. Subsequent developments of this design, such as the Corinthian (Cordis), incorporated flexible bridging points which allowed more flexibility and minimal shortening. The advantage of the closed-cell design is a uniform surface irrespective of the degree of bending. Open-cell designs are more flexible due to the fact that not all points between rings are connected. Common examples of this design include the SMART (Cordis), Luminexx (Bard) and SelfX (Jomed).

To increase the radio-opacity of stainless steel and nitinol stents, markers have been attached to their ends. These additions are typically made from gold, platinum or tantalum, and can be sleeves crimped around a strut, rivets coined into tabs at the end of the stent, integrated in a strut, or welded-on tabs.

Originally most balloon inflated stents had to be mounted and then secured either by hand or using a specific crimping device. Now, almost all stents are available pre-mounted. Theoretically, at least, this should reduce stent displacement, a very tedious and sometimes serious complication.

Whatever the stent configuration it has to be able to withstand the forces of compression and flexion commonly found in peripheral arteries, particularly in the external iliac and popliteal segments where stent fractures have been reported [5].

Covered stents and stent grafts

A number of both balloon mounted and self-expanding stents are available with coverings and attached graft material. The two main graft materials are polyester (Dacron) and polytetrafluoroethylene (PTFE). The main indication for these devices has been to seal arterial ruptures and fistulae and exclude aneurysms. Whilst they have been used to treat atherosclerotic stenoses and occlusions, their role for these indications is not yet proven. The graft material itself may slow the rate of endothelialisation when compared with bare stents. A novel spiral ribbon stent graft employing PTFE supported by nitinol (aSpire, Vascular Architects) has been developed so that half the stented length of vessel is uncovered. This allows side-branches and collaterals to be uncovered and may help with endothelialisation. A non-randomised observational trial is on-going.

Coated stents

Coatings have been applied to stents both to reduce thrombus formation and to prevent neointimal hyperplasia. There are basically two types of coatings, biocompatible and drug eluting. Drugs used primarily in the coronary arteries have included anticoagulants such as heparin and hirudin, corticosteroids and antimitotic agents. Heparin-bonded stents may not only reduce immediate thrombus formation but also inhibit smooth muscle proliferation. Whilst this has been demonstrated in animal experiments, human studies are lacking [6]. The antimitotic drug eluting stents are the topic of Chapter 19.

The biocompatible coatings include carbon, silicon carbide and phosphorylcholine. These coatings render the stent surface smoother and less thrombogenic and have been shown to be well tolerated in human coronary artery trials and in porcine iliac and renal arteries [7]. Trials for their use in the periphery have not yet reported.

Delivery systems

There has been a gradual diminution in the shaft size of stent systems over the years. Increased flexibility of both the stents and their delivery systems has allowed stenting to be performed from a contralateral femoral approach. This approach is associated with fewer serious bleeding complications but longer catheters, wires and delivery systems are needed and occlusions may be less easily dealt with, particularly in the distal femoropopliteal segment. Typically, for peripheral vascular interventions a 6 French sheath will suffice. Covered stents and stent grafts commonly require 8 to 10 French sheaths.

Stent interactions with the body

Stents work by preventing immediate elastic recoil and holding back dissection flaps after balloon dilatation. In the longer term they may prevent constrictive remodelling. Ideally, a stent will return laminar flow to the treated segment of artery and the stent will be quickly incorporated into the vessel and covered by endothelium. Because this is not usually the case, all stents in the vascular tree suffer from the same problems of immediate thrombosis and later restenosis due to neointimal hyperplasia. The understanding of these mechanisms and methods to counteract them has been the main area of research and development.

Stents are inherently thrombogenic and incite an inflammatory response within the vessel in which they are implanted. The positive electrical charge found on the stent surface attracts plasma proteins unlike the negative surface charge of a healthy endothelium. Unfortunately, there are no stents that maintain an electronegative surface charge when placed in the body [2]. A thin layer of proteins, rich in fibrinogen, immediately forms on the stent surface. Fibrinogen has a number of ligands for platelets, monocytes and possibly endothelial cells. The configuration of the fibrinogen on the stent surface may determine these cellular interactions. Certain materials, such as 316L stainless steel, induce a favourable conformation of fibrinogen with a relatively higher concentration of adhesive sites for endothelial cells than for platelets and monocytes [8]. The activation of platelets and monocytes by fibrinogen is central to the coagulation cascade and is not only caused by fibrinogen, but also by sub-endothelial tissues exposed during dilatation and stent placement. In addition to aspirin, drugs have been developed to prevent platelet aggregation. These include the thienopyridines, clopidogrel and ticlopidine, which work synergistically with aspirin and the glycoprotein IIb/IIIa receptor antagonists, abciximab, eptifibatide and tirofiban. Although these drugs are widely used in coronary applications, they are not yet routinely used in peripheral arterial interventions [9]. Platelet activation and inflammatory responses to the stents release cytokines, mitogens and chemotactic factors which activate vascular smooth muscle cells. The thrombus acts as a scaffold into which the smooth muscle cells migrate and proliferate.

Patches of viable endothelium protrude through stent interstices. Endothelialisation starts from these areas and adjacent vascular segments. This process could be promoted by stents covered with agents that attract endothelial cells and their precursors resulting in a viable endothelial surface which would reduce thrombus and neointimal hyperplasia. Certainly, surface engineering to promote endothelialisation is a major area of clinical research.

Stent apposition with the vessel wall is important for a number of reasons. The better embedded the stent the less metal is in contact with blood. A correctly sized and fully expanded stent will also reduce turbulent flow. Decreased flow velocities in areas of turbulence promote thrombus formation. Most stent manufacturers therefore recommend over sizing the stent by 10-15% with respect to the vessel diameter. Further over sizing causes wall trauma and may predispose to spasm and eventually increased neointimal hyperplasia. Unfortunately, stents also increase the vessel wall stiffness and reduce compliance. This leads to increased mechanical stress at the junction with the non-stented artery and endothelial damage [2].

Evidence for stents in the peripheral arteries

Since the 1980s many papers have addressed the role of stents within the peripheral arteries. Evidence, however, is hampered by the lack of randomised controlled trials examining balloon angioplasty versus primary stenting and different stents against each other. There has also been a lack of uniformity in reporting both demographic details and clinical and radiological outcomes. Very different anticoagulant and antiplatelet regimes have been employed reflecting the change in clinical practice that the newer antiplatelet agents have brought about. Follow-up may have been purely clinical (walking distance, ankle-brachial pressure index, ulcer healing) or involved arterial imaging with angiography, duplex ultrasound or both. In an effort to standardise these factors, the Society of Interventional Radiologists has published reporting standards [10].

In January 2000, the TransAtlantic Intersociety Consensus (TASC) document on the management of peripheral vascular disease was published as a supplement to the *Journal of Vascular Surgery* [11]. Iliac and femoropopliteal lesions were categorised as to whether endovascular or surgical treatments were recommended as first line treatment. What could be decided was that short (less than 3cm) focal stenoses should be treated endovascularly and that complete segmental occlusions should be treated surgically. However, all the other combinations of stenoses or occlusions could be treated either way and there were differences in opinion across the Atlantic on exactly how to categorise these lesions. From the available literature, weighted average outcomes of endovascular interventions were also derived. These are shown in Table 1. A number of recommendations were made and critical issues were recognised. Amongst these are:-

◆ Recommendation 33. Stenting improves the technical and initial clinical success in cases of residual pressure gradient or dissection after angioplasty, or in cases of elastic recoil.
◆ Recommendation 36. Femoropopliteal stenting as a primary approach to the interventional treatment of claudication or critical limb ischaemia is not indicated. However, stents may

Table 1. TASC outcomes after iliac and femoropopliteal interventions [11].

		Patients	Limbs	IC (%)	Success (%)	Primary patency (%)			Complication (%)
						1yr	3yr	5yr	
Iliac	Stenosis	-	1264	77	95	78	66	61	3.6
PTA	Occlusion	-	291	82	83	68	61	-	6
Iliac	Stenosis	1365	1430	78	99	90	74	72	6.3
stent	Occlusion	187	-	86	82	72	64	-	5.6
Fempop	PTA	1241	1469	72	90	61	51	48	4.3
	Stent	585	600	80	98	67	58	-	-

have a limited role in the salvage of acute percutaneous transluminal angioplasty failures or interventions.

◆ Critical Issue 13. Primary stenting is widely used to optimize procedural results in iliac artery occlusions. This practice needs to be subjected to rigorous clinical evaluation.

In 2001, Muradin and colleagues published a meta-analysis of long-term results of balloon dilatation and stent implantation in the treatment of femoropopliteal arterial disease [12]. They found 19 studies that met the inclusion criteria, representing 923 balloon dilations and 473 stent implantations. Combined 3-year patency rates are shown in Table 2. The patency rates after stent implantation were independent of clinical

Table 2. Meta-analysis of long-term results of balloon dilatation and stent implantation in the treatment of femoropopliteal arterial disease [12].

	Indication	3-yr patency (%)
PTA	Stenosis and IC	61
	Occlusion and IC	48
	Stenosis and CLI	43
	Occlusion and CLI	30
Stent	All	63-66

indication and lesion type. Whilst there appeared to be improved patency after stenting, they could not rule out publication bias favouring stenting outcomes.

Since then, Cejna *et al* have published a study evaluating stent placement versus angioplasty in the treatment of chronic symptoms in short (up to 5cm) femoropopliteal lesions [13]. The study randomised 154 limbs in 141 patients, of whom 108 (77%) were claudicants. After Palmaz stent placement, the primary success rate was significantly higher than after PTA (99% vs 84%). The cumulative 1- and 2-year angiographic primary patency rates were 63% and 53%, respectively, for both groups and clinical and haemodynamic success was not improved by placing a stent.

In 2004, Bachoo and Thorpe published a Cochrane Review entitled *Endovascular Stents for Intermittent Claudication* [14]. They discovered only two studies that satisfied the inclusion criteria. There were a total of 104 subjects only with femoropopliteal disease. Angioplasty and stenting with the Palmaz stent was compared with angioplasty alone. When combining the two papers there were no differences in the patency rates or secondary outcomes. They concluded that 'the small number of relevant trials identified, together with the small sample sizes and methodological weaknesses, severely limit the usefulness of this review in guiding practice. Larger multicentre trials are needed'.

Most of the studies included in the meta-analyses and Cochrane review involved the use of the Palmaz, Strecker and Wallstent. We do not know if these results can be generalised to include the more recent nitinol stents.

The patient populations have been primarily claudicants and not those with critical limb ischaemia. In this latter group the treatment aims are to alleviate rest pain, prevent tissue loss and heal ulcers. These patients usually have multi-level disease and occlusions. The improved immediate technical success rates and superior short-term patency of stenting may therefore be justified.

Is the evidence any different for stent grafts? Disappointing results were found with a Dacron covered nitinol stent graft (Cragg Endo-Pro, now Passager, Boston Scientific) used to treat recurrent femoropopliteal stenoses. Primary patency rates at one and seven years were 23% and 17% respectively [15]. Recently, however, there have been encouraging results with the Hemobahn stent graft, made from expanded PTFE with external nitinol support (WL Gore). In 2000, Lammer *et al* showed that this stent graft could be used safely in 80 femoral arteries with 79% 12-month primary patency [16]. Two trials, published last year, reported 74-87%, 2-year primary patency rates after treatment of relatively long femoropopliteal lesions [17,18].

Conclusions

In response to the question 'are we winning?' the answer would seem to be 'not yet'. Undoubtedly, more is known about why we have not yet won but whether recent advances, such as drug elution, hold the key is debatable.

Summary

◆   Routine stenting is not justified in peripheral arterial interventions.
◆   Stents do, however, have a role in salvaging failed angioplasty.
◆   No one stent is clearly superior to another.
◆   More trials are needed.

References

1. Dotter CT. Transluminally-placed coilspring endarterial tube grafts: long-term patency in canine popliteal artery. *Invest Radiol* 1969; 4: 329-332.

2. Schild HH, Strunk H. Biological effects of metallic stents. In: *Textbook of Metallic Stents*. Adam A, Dondelinger RF, Mueller PR, Eds. Isis Medical Media Ltd, Oxford, 1997.

3. Dyet JF, Schurmann K. The physical and biological properties of metallic stents. In: *Textbook of Endovascular Procedures*. Dyet JF, Ettles DF, Nicholson AA, Wilson SE, Eds. Churchill Livingstone, The Curtis Center, Independence Square West, Philadelphia, USA, 2000.

4. Stoeckel D, Bonsignore C, Duda S. A survey of stent designs. *Min Invas Ther & Allied Technol* 2002; 11(4): 137-147. Available at www.nitinol-europe.com/pdf/stoeckelfinal.pdf.

5. Babalyk E, Gülbaran M, Gürmen T, *et al*. Fracture of popliteal artery stents. *Circ J* 2003; 67: 643-645.

6. Lin PH, Chronos NA, Marijianowski MM, *et al*. Heparin-coated balloon-expandable stent reduces intimal hyperplasia in the iliac artery in baboons. *J Vasc Intervent Radiol* 2003; 14: 603-611.

7. Galloni M, Prunotto M, Santarelli A, *et al*. Carbon-coated stents implanted in porcine iliac and renal arteries: histologic and histomorphometric study. *J Vasc Intervent Radiol* 2003; 14: 1053-1061.

8. Palmaz JC. Stents from the past, present and future. *Endovascular Today* 2004; 37-41.

9. Shlansky-Goldberg R. Platelet aggregation inhibitors for use in peripheral vascular interventions: what can we learn from the experience in the coronary arteries? *J Vasc Intervent Radiol* 2002; 13: 229-246.

10. Guidelines for Percutaneous Transluminal Angioplasty Society of Interventional Radiology. Standards of Practice Committee. *J Vasc Intervent Radiol* 2003; 14: S209-S217.

11. TASC (2000) TransAtlantic Intersociety Consensus document on management of peripheral arterial disease. *J Vasc Surg* 31: S1-S296.

12. Muradin GS, Bosch JL, Stijnen T, *et al*. Balloon dilation and stent implantation for treatment of femoropopliteal arterial disease: meta-analysis. *Radiology* 2001; 221: 137-145.

13. Cejna M, Thurnher S, Illiasch H, *et al*. PTA versus Palmaz stent placement in femoropopliteal artery obstructions: a multicenter prospective randomized study. *J Vasc Intervent Radiol* 2001; 12: 23-31.

14. Bachoo P, Thorpe P. Endovascular stents for intermittent claudication (Cochrane Review). In: *The Cochrane Library*, Issue 1, 2004. John Wiley & Sons Ltd, Chichester, UK.

15. Ahmadi R, Schillinger M, Maca T, *et al*. Femoropopliteal arteries: immediate and long-term results with a Dacron-covered stent-graft. *Radiology* 2002; 223: 345-350.

16. Lammer J, Dake MD, Bleyn J, *et al*. Peripheral arterial obstruction: prospective study of treatment with a transluminally placed self-expanding stent-graft. International Trial Study Group. *Radiology* 2000; 217(1): 95-104.

17. Jahnke T, Andresen R, Müller-Hülsbeck S, *et al*. Hemobahn stent-grafts for the treatment of femoropopliteal arterial obstructions: midterm results of a prospective trial. *J Vasc Intervent Radiol* 2003; 14: 41-51.

18. Saxon RR, Coffman JM, Gooding JM, *et al*. Long-term results of ePTFE stent-graft versus angioplasty in the femoropopliteal artery: single center experience from a prospective, randomized trial. *J Vasc Intervent Radiol* 2003;14: 3.

Chapter 19

Drug eluting and biodegradable stents

Dominic Fay, MRCP FRCR, Specialist Registrar, Interventional Radiology

Philip Davey, MRCS, Research Fellow, Vascular Surgery

Michael G Wyatt, MSc MD FRCS, Consultant Vascular Surgeon

John Rose, FRCP FRCR, Consultant Vascular Radiologist

Northern Vascular Centre, Freeman Hospital, Newcastle-upon-Tyne, UK

Introduction

Since the introduction of balloon angioplasty, practitioners and patients have been impressed by the technique's immediate success only to be later disappointed by the limited durability in certain territories. The complication of restenosis and re-occlusion is of relevance in all vascular regions but is of particular interest in the highly susceptible femoropopliteal segments. Over the last decade the experimental use of drug eluting and biodegradable stents has attracted almost unprecedented interest amongst interventional cardiologists and more recently, peripheral vascular interventionists. This has been due to the impressive early clinical data resulting from the latest iterations of drug eluting stents in the coronary vasculature and the hope that, in the battle against restenosis, the cavalry may finally have arrived.

The need for drug eluting stents

While percutaneous transluminal angioplasty (PTA) has become an established technique for the treatment of intermittent claudication, most practitioners in the UK remain concerned by the poor longer-term results in long segment femoropopliteal disease. Many would therefore restrict the use of angioplasty in claudicants to short segment disease of the iliac or femoral vessels where patency rates appear better, only treating occlusive iliac or extensive infra-inguinal disease in the event of critical limb ischaemia (CLI). A randomised study comparing PTA and exercise in 62 patients demonstrated no difference in symptoms, ankle brachial pressure index or overall quality of life at two years[1]. The high incidence and rapid onset of restenosis and re-occlusion is likely to partly explain these results. An analysis of pooled data from eight studies of femoropopliteal PTA with 1469 treated limbs in 1241 patients gave a weighted average of 61% primary patency at 12 months, declining to 51% at three years [2]. The use of bare metal stents (BMS) provides little improvement, with early lumen gain being offset by restenosis to provide similar long-term results. Two randomised studies comparing PTA and BMS showed improved primary success rates with stents but no difference in angiographic, haemodynamic or clinical results in the longer-term [3,4]. With these findings in mind, most UK practitioners currently restrict the use of stents in the femoropopliteal arteries to those cases where there has been an initial suboptimal result.

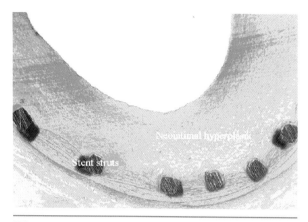

Figure 1. Neointimal hyperplasia in response to stent implantation in porcine coronary artery.

The cardiology community has embraced bare metal stents more enthusiastically, encouraged by large trials in the 1990s showing clinical and angiographic benefits from their use [5,6]. Nevertheless, early gains are to a degree offset by restenosis within the early implantation period [7].

Restenosis is incompletely understood but is considered to be the result of a combination of elastic vessel wall recoil, vessel wall remodelling and neointimal hyperplasia, i.e. overgrowth of vessel intima through the stent interstices (Figure 1). Stent placement excites a local inflammatory reaction greater than that produced by angioplasty alone and

the result is that neointimal hyperplasia is provoked rather than prevented by stents. It is this process that is largely responsible for in-stent restenosis [8].

Several avenues have been or are being explored in an attempt to diminish restenosis including brachytherapy, sonotherapy, photoangioplasty, gene therapy and the use of systemic pharmacological agents such as anti-platelets and anti-oxidants. Inert stent coatings such as gold, chromium and titanium have been employed to resist corrosion and there has been interest in the use of antithrombotic coatings such as heparin and hirudin. Brachytherapy, the use of stents that apply low energy radiotherapy at the implantation site, has been partially successful but dogged by 'edge effects' or 'candy wrapper' restenosis, i.e. excessive restenosis just beyond the margins of the stent. Photoangioplasty and sonotherapy are to date experimental and none of the aforementioned techniques have provoked the same level of interest as anti-proliferative drug eluting stents.

Principles of drug eluting stents

The use of systemic anti-proliferative agents to inhibit neointimal hyperplasia has severe limitations, largely because of the narrow therapeutic index of the agents employed and the difficulty of consistently and

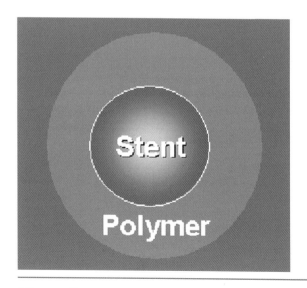
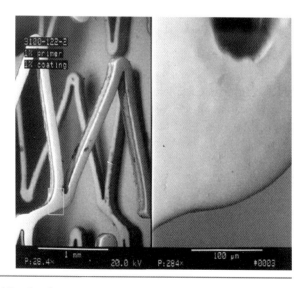

Figure 2. Polymer coating of a sirolimus eluting 'Cypher' stent (Cordis).

accurately achieving the required drug concentrations at the site of stent deployment. Using a stent for drug delivery allows high local concentrations of the drug while minimising systemic levels. This is usually achieved by binding the drug within a polymer matrix in which the stent can then be coated to a thickness of a few microns (Figure 2), although paclitaxel has been applied directly to stent surfaces. Once the stent is deployed, the drug is usually released over a few weeks, exerting its effects at the time when the inflammatory response to stent implantation would be maximal. If a polymer coating is utilised, then this should remain intact during stent deployment without compromising the mechanical properties of the stent. Ideally, the polymer coating should then either dissolve as the drug is released or remain intact and inert after final drug clearance from the stent. Thus, the three basic aspects to consider in the construction of a drug eluting stent are the pharmacological agent, the method of binding the drug and the stent platform.

Suitable pharmacological agents (Table 1)

Anticancer agents such as paclitaxel, actinomycin D and vincristine, and immunosuppressants such as sirolimus, tacrolimus and everolimus have been employed [8, 9]. These agents act via either cytotoxic or cytostatic mechanisms (Figure 3), but work has also been done using more conventional anti-inflammatories such as dexamethasone [10]. Only sirolimus eluting stents have been subjected to clinical trials in the peripheral arteries of humans.

Sirolimus

Sirolimus was isolated from soil samples containing *Streptomyces hygroscopicus* in the 1970s and originally was examined as a potential antimicrobial agent. The soil samples had been removed from Easter Island, 'Rapa-Nui' to its inhabitants, hence the alternative name rapamycin and the trade name, Rapamune. Later work showed its greater potential as an immunosuppressant and it was approved by the United States Food and Drug Administration in 1999 as an anti-rejection agent in renal transplantation. It acts in a similar manner to tacrolimus and cyclosporin A to cause cell cycle arrest and inhibition of cell proliferation [8].

Paclitaxel

Paclitaxel is a member of the taxane group of cytotoxic drugs and in the UK is indicated, in conjunction with platinum agents, for the treatment of metastatic ovarian cancer, breast cancer and some cases of non-small cell lung cancer [11]. It acts via alteration of cellular microtubule function and suppresses migration and proliferation of vascular smooth muscle cells. While these effects combine to reduce neointimal hyperplasia, endothelisation is also delayed for up to three months with the important consequence of necessitating dual antiplatelet therapy for this period [8].

Table 1. Pharmacological agents studied in the prevention of restenosis.

Immunosupressives	Anti-proliferatives	Healing & Re-endothelialisation
Dexamethasone	Paclitaxel	BCP 671
Prednisolone	Actinomycin	VEGF
γ Inteferon	Mitomycin	Estradiols
Sirolimus	Sirolimus	Nitric oxide donors
Tacrolimus	Methotrexate	
Everolimus	Vincristine	
Cyclosporine	Statins	

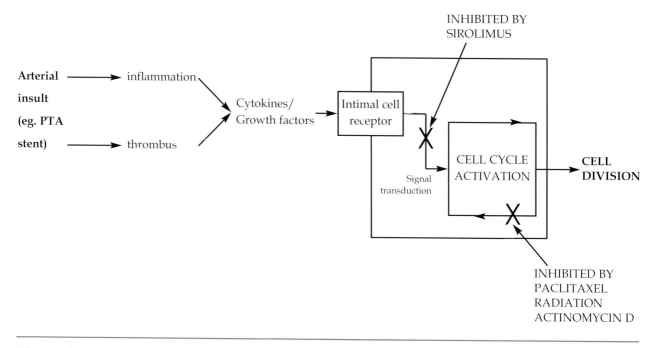

Figure 3. Mechanisms of action of common anti-proliferative agents.

Polymer coatings

Covering vascular stents with a polymer coating has been suggested for some years as a method of both improving the surface characteristics of the metal and for targeted delivery of pharmacotherapy [12]. Despite a prolonged search for safe and efficacious polymers for targeted drug delivery in many different parts of the human body, the ideal endovascular polymer matrix has yet to be found. Polymer-based coatings may be non-degradable or biodegradable [9] and a covering that enables predictable surface erosion could produce the desired consistency of drug release [13]. Rigorous testing of such biomaterials is required to exclude the possibility of local or systemic toxic effects of the breakdown products.

Basic stent platforms

Many different combinations of stent design and pharmacotherapy have been tried experimentally and discarded over the last decade. An outline of selected stents currently undergoing clinical trials is given in Table 2.

Current drug eluting stent data

Coronary trials

After encouraging results from smaller studies [14,15], large randomised trials have now been published comparing bare metal and drug eluting stents in human coronary arteries [16,17]. A 1,314 patient multicentre randomised controlled trial of bare metal versus paclitaxel eluting stents[17] showed significant reductions in angiographic in-stent restenosis and major adverse cardiac events at nine months follow-up in the paclitaxel eluting group. A 1,058 patient randomised controlled trial of sirolimus eluting versus bare metal stents[16] reported similar findings. Shortly after the publication of this trial, the National Institute for Clinical Excellence (NICE) issued guidelines which recommended the use of sirolimus or paclitaxel eluting stents in coronary artery lesions greater than 15mm length or in target vessels less than 3mm diameter [18]. When one considers the cost of drug eluting stents compared to bare metal coronary stents (around 2,400 Eu. versus 500 Eu.)[19], this is an important endorsement.

Table 2. Drug eluting stents currently under clinical evaluation.

Proprietary name	Target vessel(s)	Active agents	Stent/Material
Manufacturer			Balloon Mounted (BM) Self-expanded (SE)
Cypher			
Cordis	Coronary	Sirolimus (Rapamycin)	BXVelocity /steel BM
	Renal	Sirolimus	Genesis / nitinol BM
	Peripheral	Sirolimus	Smart / nitinol SE
Taxus			
Boston Scientific	Coronary	Paclitaxel	Express 2 /steel BM
V-Flex Plus PTX			
Cook	Coronary	Paclitaxel	V-Flex /steel BM
Dexamet			
Medtronic	Coronary	Dexamethasone	Driver / cobalt-chromium BM

Peripheral arteries

With poor long-term results from angioplasty and bare metal stent placement in the femoropopliteal arteries, potential solutions excite much interest. While cardiological data and techniques may occasionally be applicable to peripheral vascular work, there needs to be caution in extrapolating the findings of coronary studies to peripheral vessels. This is perhaps illustrated best by the behaviour of bare metal stents in the coronary versus the femoropopliteal arteries. Large studies have associated coronary stents with better angiographic and clinical outcomes [5,6] than those following coronary angioplasty. In the femoropopliteal segments, despite enjoying better initial angiographic results, stented patients have not fared better than those treated with angioplasty after 12, 24 or 36 months [3,4].

Sirocco data

To date, there has been only one published controlled study examining the use of drug eluting stents in the peripheral arteries of humans. This was the Sirocco trial, a multicentre double blind randomised prospective trial supported by Cordis [20]. Patients with chronic limb ischaemia (Rutherford stage 2 to 4) were randomised to receive either bare metal or sirolimus eluting nitinol self-expandable SMART stents (Cordis products). The inclusion criteria deliberately included complex lesions (stenosis over 7cm to 20cm or occlusion over 4cm to 20cm) in the hope that these 'difficult' lesions would allow the greatest differences to be shown. Eighteen patients were randomised to each arm, with the primary endpoint being in-stent mean percentage diameter stenosis after six months measured by quantitative angiography. Secondary endpoints included duplex ultrasound findings, ankle-brachial pressure indices, haemodynamic failures, prolonged hospital stay or death. The systemic levels of sirolimus were also assessed.

Both groups had similar baseline demographics although there was a significantly higher incidence of moderate to severely calcified lesions in the sirolimus eluting group, which also contained a non-significant preponderance of smokers, diabetics and severely ischaemic limbs. The authors state that the sirolimus eluting stent group were therefore at greater risk of restenosis than the controls.

All patients enjoyed a technically successful procedure employing up to three stents (mean 2.2 per patient) to treat lesions of mean length 85mm, slightly over half of which (57%) were full occlusions. Follow-up angiography was performed in 33 patients after six months.

While there were trends towards an improvement in the sirolimus eluting group with respect to the primary endpoint and a number of further measures of vessel patency, only the difference in in-stent mean lumen diameter (4.95mm in the sirolimus group versus 4.31mm in the bare stent group) achieved statistical significance (p=0.047). Taking 'restenosis' to mean binary in-lesion or in-stent restenosis of greater than 50%, no patients in the sirolimus group suffered restenosis to this degree compared to seven in the bare metal group, although this observation was not statistically significant. Claims of 'zero restenosis' have been based on this data.

Late Sirocco follow-up

Duplex ultrasound data from 18 month follow-up in these patients was presented at the 2003 Cardiovascular & Interventional Radiological Society of Europe (CIRSE) annual meeting. This showed a continued trend towards lower levels of restenosis in the sirolimus eluting group [21]. This paper also described parallel work examining the effect of different rates of drug release from the stents which appeared to show a benefit in using preparations that eluted sirolimus more gradually (greater than 28 days versus less than 15 days for fast elution).

Bare metal stents

With a total occlusion rate of 5.9% at six months the bare metal SMART stents in the control arm of the

Sirocco trial performed much better than the previously reported series of bare metal stents used in the femoropopliteal segments [2,3,4]. It may be that with further development, the potential of bare metal femoropopliteal stents is better than originally believed.

Biodegradable stents

The rationale for using fully biodegradable stents for endovascular applications is based on the belief that the benefits of stent usage are greatest during the early post-deployment period. Thus, stents are at best, unnecessary and at worst, harmful if they remain in situ beyond this time.

The materials employed to create biodegradable stents include polyhydroxybutyrate (PHB) and poly-L-lactic acid (PLLA). PHB stents have been shown to undergo complete degradation in vivo at 12-24 months [22].

Biodegradable stents have been used in the coronary arteries and urinary tracts [23,24] and there has also been interest in their potential use in the treatment of benign oesophageal strictures [25]. Preliminary small studies have shown PLLA biodegradable stent placement to be safe and feasible in human coronary arteries in the short-term [23]. However, the authors concede that their examination of the data at six months follow-up excludes the important period when the stents might be expected to dismantle having undergone partial dissolution.

No human data has yet been published on the use of biodegradable stents in the peripheral arteries but an animal study, using PHB stents in rabbit iliac arteries, showed excessive inflammatory reactions to stent placement and concluded that clinical use of these stents was not feasible [22]. A current trial is examining the use of fully absorbable magnesium alloy femoropopliteal stents in humans and early reports are encouraging [26]. It may be that future peripheral artery studies using different biodegradable stent materials may yield better results but this seems likely to be some time away.

Conclusions

In the quest for a minimally invasive solution to femoropopliteal arterial disease there may in future be a role for drug eluting stents to play. Currently, however, the peripheral vascular data is limited to relatively short-term follow-up in small numbers of patients and does not show the clear benefit of drug elution that was widely anticipated. The coronary trials are more persuasive but still short-term and there are hazards in extrapolating data from one vascular territory to clinical practice in another. In addition, biodegradable stents remain experimental both in coronary and peripheral vascular work.

Acknowledgements

We are grateful to Cordis for permission to reproduce Figures 1 and 2.

Summary

◆ Re-stenosis is a complex multifactorial process and is a major limiting factor in the long-term durability of angioplasty.

◆ Drug eluting stents act to inhibit restenosis by using the stent as a platform for local delivery of (commonly) anti-proliferative drugs.

◆ The coronary use of drug eluting stents is supported by large prospective trials and has been endorsed by NICE.

◆ In the peripheral vascular system only much smaller trials have been published to date and clear benefits have not yet been shown.

◆ More peripheral drug eluting stents are expected to arrive on the market shortly and the results of further trials are eagerly awaited.

◆ Biodegradable peripheral arterial stents using absorbable polymers or alloys are under current evaluation but their clinical use seems distant.

References

1. Whyman MR, Foukes FGR, Kerracher EMG, *et al.* Is intermittent claudication improved by percutaneous transluminal angioplasty? A randomized controlled trial. *J Vasc Surg* 1997; 26(4): 551-7.

2. Lammer J. Femoropopliteal artery obstructions: from the balloon to the stent graft. *Cardiovasc Intervent Radiol* 2001; 24: 73-83.

3. Cejna M, Thurnher S, Illiasch H, *et al.* PTA versus Palmaz Stent Placement in Femoropopliteal Artery Obstructions: A Multicenter Prospective Randomized Study. *J Vasc Intervent Radiol* 2001; 12: 23-31.

4. Grimm J, Muller-Hulsbeck S, Jahnke T, *et al.* Randomized study to compare PTA alone with Palmaz stent placement for femoropopliteal lesions. *J Vasc Intervent Radiol* 2001; 12: 935-51.

5. Serruys PW, de Jaegere P, Kiemeneij F, *et al.* A comparison of balloon-expandable stent implantation with balloon angioplasty in patients with coronary artery disease. *N Eng J Med* 1994; 331: 489-95.

6. Fischman DL, Leon MB, Baim DS, *et al.* A randomised comparison of coronary-stent placement and balloon angioplasty in the treatment of coronary artery disease. *N Eng J Med* 1994; 331: 496-501.

7. Kimura T, Yokoi H, Nakagawa Y, *et al.* Three-year follow-up after implantation of metallic coronary-artery stents. *N Eng J Med* 1996; 334: 561-6.

8. Duda SH, Poerner TC, Wiesinger B, *et al.* Drug eluting stents: potential applications for peripheral arterial occlusive disease. *J Vasc Intervent Radiol* 2003; 14: 291-301.

9. Regar E, Sianos G, Serruys PW. Stent development and local drug delivery. *Br Med Bull* 2001; 59(1); 227-48.

10. Strecker EP, Gabelmann A, *et al.* Effect on intimal hyperplasia of dexamethasone released from coated metal stents compared with non-coated stents in canine femoral arteries. *Cardiovasc Intervent Radiol* 1998; 21: 487-496.

11. British National Formulary 46th Edition. 2003 (Sep). http://www.bnf.org.

12. Dyet JF, Schurmann K. Improving the Biocompatability of Endovascular Prostheses. In: *Textbook of Endovascular Procedures*. Dyet, Ettles, Nicholson, Wilson, Eds. Churchill Livingstone 2000; Chapter 2: pp24-26.

13. Langer R. Drug delivery and targeting. *Nature* 1998 Apr 30; 392 (6679 Suppl): 5-10.

14. Sousa JE, Costa MA, Abiziad A, *et al.* Lack of neointimal proliferation after implantation of sirolimus-coated stents in human coronary arteries. A quantitative coronary angiography and three dimensional intravascular ultrasound study. *Circulation* 2001; 103: 192-195.

15. Sousa JE, Costa MA, *et al.* Sustained suppression of neointimal proliferation by sirolimus-eluting stents. One year angiographic and intravascular ultrasound follow-up. *Circulation* 2001; 104: 2007-2011.

16. Moses JW, Leon MB, Popma JJ, *et al.* Sirolimus-eluting stents versus standard stents in patients with stenosis in a native coronary artery. *N Eng J Med* 2003; 349(14): 1315-23.

17. Stone GW, Ellis SG, Cox DA, *et al.* A polymer-based, paclitaxel-eluting stent in patients with coronary artery disease. *N Eng J Med* 2004; 350(3): 221-31.

18. Guidance on the use of coronary artery stents. Technology appraisal 71. National Institute of Clinical Excellence 2003 (Oct). ISBN 1-84257-413-2. http://www.nice.org.uk

19. Fattori R, Piva T. Drug-eluting stents in vascular intervention. *Lancet* 2003; 361: 247-9

20. Duda SH, Puisch B, Richter G, *et al.* Sirolimus-eluting stents for the treatment of obstructive superficial femoral artery disease. Six-month results. *Circulation* 2002; 106: 1505-1509.

21. Duda SH, Wiesinger B, Richter GM, *et al.* Sirolimus-eluting stents in SFA obstructions: long-term SIROCCO trial results. (Abstract). CIRSE Annual Meeting Program and Abstracts 2003: p157.

22 Unverdorben M, Spielberger A, Schywalsky M, *et al.* A polyhydroxybutyrate biodegradable stent: preliminary experience in the rabbit. *Cardiovasc Intervent Radiol* 2002; 25: 127-32.

23. Tamai H, Igaki K, Kyo E, *et al.* Initial and 6-month results of biodegradable poly-l-lactic acid coronary stents in humans. *Circulation* 2000; 102(4): 399-404.

24. Knutson T, Pettersson S, Dahlstrand C. The use of biodegradable PGA stents to judge the risk of post-TURP incontinence in patients with combined bladder outlet obstruction and overactive bladder. *Eur Urol* 2002; 42(3): 267-7.

25. Morgan R, Adam A. Use of metallic stents and balloons in the oesophagus and gastrointestinal tract. *J Vasc Intervent Radiol* 2001; 12: 283-97.

26. Vascular News 2004; Issue 21 (Feb): 1.

Chapter 20

Thrombolysis for acute leg ischaemia: 20 years and out?

Jonothan J Earnshaw, DM FRCS, Consultant Vascular Surgeon

Gloucestershire Royal Hospital, Gloucester, UK

Introduction

It is 20 years since thrombolysis became available for routine clinical use. During this time it has become standard treatment for patients with acute myocardial infarction and selected patients with acute pulmonary embolism. Two decades of investigation into thrombolysis for acute leg ischaemia have produced a wealth of clinical and research experience, and several large randomised trials. It is a good time to take stock and explore whether an exact role for thrombolysis of acute leg ischaemia can be agreed. It has been claimed that lysis could replace surgical thromboembolectomy[1], whereas Porter has suggested the randomised trials show its role is limited as first line therapy [2]. These extreme views are not appropriate and there is likely to be a middle ground where there is consensus about the place of thrombolysis.

The natural history of any new technique is an initial enthusiasm followed by a degree of scepticism as its limitations become apparent. There is good evidence that this pattern has been followed with thrombolysis for acute leg ischaemia. In the early 1990s, enthusiastic surgeons and radiologists in the UK formed the Thrombolysis Study Group to investigate the outcome of intra-arterial thrombolysis for acute leg ischaemia. They created the NATALI database (National Audit of Thrombolysis for Acute Leg Ischaemia) and prospectively recorded all episodes of lysis in patients under their care from 1990 to 2000. They reported greater use of the technique in the mid 1990s, with a reduction since [3]. When questioned, members of the Group admitted a reduction in use, partly because of concerns about complications and partly because of doubts about long-term efficacy [4]. Industry figures from the UK, however, show that the sales of the doses of tissue plasminogen activator (tPA) used for acute leg ischaemia (10mg and 20mg) have continued to increase slowly (Figure 1). Likewise, a recent report from North America also suggests that a consistent 10% of episodes of acute leg ischaemia are treated by primary thrombolysis [5]. This is evidence that thrombolysis has now found a steady role in the management of acute leg ischaemia. It is possible that surgeons and radiologists have learned lessons from the data produced in the 1990s and are now using this information to select patients they think are likely to get the best possible results.

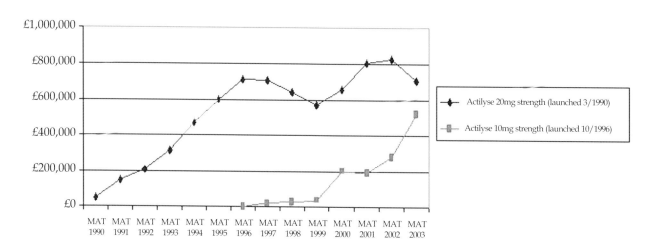

Source: Dataview and IMS Audits

Figure 1. Sales of Actilyse (tPA) monitored by International Medical Statistics (IMS), an industry standard, at the doses used for peripheral thrombolysis. MAT = moving annual total (each data point refers to a 12-month interval).

A history of thrombolysis

The first plasminogen activator was discovered in the 1930s and termed streptokinase because haemolytic streptococci produced it. It took 30 years for streptokinase of sufficient purity to be available for clinical trials that began in the 1960s. Charles Dotter first used the intra-arterial route to deliver streptokinase therapy for acute leg ischaemia in 1974, but at that stage the catheter delivery systems were relatively rudimentary [6]. As the specialty of interventional radiology was born in the 1980s and modern flexible thin-walled catheter delivery systems became available, the first large series of patients with acute leg ischaemia treated with low-dose intra-arterial streptokinase were described. New agents such as tissue plasminogen activator (tPA) and urokinase became available in the late 1980s and these agents have proved safer and probably more effective than streptokinase, which is now seldom used for acute leg ischaemia [7].

Many surgeons and radiologists explored the potential of thrombolysis for acute leg ischaemia in the 1980s and a large number of single centre series were published by enthusiasts with good results; others remained sceptical. Some were scarred by the significant side-effects of thrombolysis, such as bleeding and stroke, forgetting that the surgical alternative has its own complications. Indeed, the first randomised trial that compared surgery and thrombolysis done in New York showed a significant difference in early outcome directly related to the perioperative cardiorespiratory mortality following the surgery [8]. For some radiologists, this was their first experience of major clinical complications from an intervention.

The randomised trials

In the 1990s there was an attempt to prove once and for all whether surgery or thrombolysis was optimal for acute leg ischaemia (Table 1). The New York study was the first major trial to show an

Table 1. Results of randomised trials that compared surgery and thrombolysis for acute leg ischaemia. AFS = amputation-free survival.

Trial	Number randomised		Primary endpoints	
			AFS at 12 months	
New York study [8]	surgery	57	52%	
	lysis	57	75%	

Comment: the difference between the groups was attributed to a significant increase in cardiorespiratory deaths within 30 days after surgery.

Trial	Number randomised		*AFS at one month*	*AFS at six months*
STILE study [9]	surgery	144	88.8%	82.3%
	lysis	248	90.1%	82.9%

Comment: this study had methodological flaws (see text), but the authors reported that surgery was more effective and safer, because of the number of patients with ongoing ischaemia at the end of lysis.

Trial	Number randomised		*AFS at six months*	*AFS at one year*
TOPAS study [10]	surgery	272	74.8%	69.9%
	lysis	272	71.8%	65%

Comment: the differences between the groups were not significant. Lysis was associated with a higher risk of bleeding complications, but reduced the need for open surgical procedures.

advantage for thrombolysis in acute leg ischaemia [8]. Next came the STILE trial (Surgery versus Thrombolysis for Ischaemia of the Lower Extremity), a multicentre comparison that included almost 400 patients [9]. This trial was flawed by poor design, as it included patients with ischaemia for up to six months. It was also hampered by lack of expertise; many of the radiologists were unfamiliar with this new technique and failed to insert catheters into the arterial occlusion. The trial did, however, suggest that patients with ischaemia for less than 14 days had advantages from thrombolysis.

The TOPAS trial (Thrombolysis Or Peripheral Artery Surgery) was supposed to provide a definitive answer [10]. It was organised by Ken Ouriel, the surgeon who completed the initial New York study. The first phase of TOPAS was designed to find the optimal dose of intra-arterial urokinase for acute leg ischaemia; in the second phase this was compared in

a randomised trial against optimal surgery. In total, over 500 patients were included in this multicentre trial, but no major differences in outcome could be established between either method (Table 1). Some have taken this to mean there is no advantage from thrombolysis so it should not replace traditional vascular surgical techniques [2]. An alternative conclusion would be that surgery and thrombolysis are both effective and that surgeons and radiologists should take each patient with acute leg ischaemia and treat them individually.

Lessons from the trials

The big question remains how to decide which patients with acute leg ischaemia will benefit from thrombolysis. Evidence can be taken from the randomised trials and their systematic review [11,12]. Additional information has come from the NATALI

Table 2. Pre-treatment factors that affected outcome adversely in multivariate analysis of 1147 episodes of primary thrombolysis for acute leg ischaemia: The NATALI database [3].

Reduced 30-day amputation-free survival

Increasing age
Diabetes mellitus
Shorter duration ischaemia
Severity of ischaemia (presence of a
neurosensory deficit, Fontaine Grade)

Increased risk of amputation with survival

Male sex
Younger age
Graft occlusion
Thrombotic occlusion
Severity of ischaemia (Fontaine Grade)

Increased death rate within 30 days

Female sex
Increasing age
Ischaemic heart disease
Native vessel occlusion
Embolic occlusion

database maintained by members of the Thrombolysis Study Group, which contains details of over 1000 episodes of intra-arterial thrombolysis for acute leg ischaemia [3].

Data from the STILE study would suggest that the outcome is better from thrombolysis of vascular graft occlusions, especially prosthetic grafts, rather than native vessel occlusions [13]. This was also concluded by the systematic review [11]. Surgeons have traditionally been taught to differentiate between patients with thrombosis or embolism. It can be difficult to distinguish between these two and the trials suggest that it does not make a great deal of difference to outcome. Systematic review also suggests that the duration of ischaemia significantly affected outcome and advised against thrombolysis for ischaemia of longer than 14 days[11].

Data from the NATALI database suggests that elderly patients, especially women and those with more severe ischaemia have a worse outcome from intra-arterial thrombolysis [3]. Information from the NATALI database summarised in Table 2 can be used and taken into account when making decisions for individual patients.

Other possible ways of predicting outcome include risk-scoring systems such as the physiological score from the Physiological and Operative Severity Score for the enumeration of Morbidity and mortality (POSSUM)[14]. There is the prospect in future of using multivariate analysis, such as Bayes to provide risk prediction for individual patients.

The main problem is that identifying patients with acute leg ischaemia who are likely to do badly from intra-arterial thrombolysis, is only an advantage if the alternative (i.e. surgery) is likely to produce better outcomes. It might be the case that patients unlikely to do well with thrombolysis will also do badly with surgery, but this has never been tested scientifically.

In general, using the above information to assist, decisions are best made individually for patients with acute leg ischaemia. If there is an obvious surgical option available, then it should probably be used. For example, a local embolus at the common femoral bifurcation or within the superficial femoral artery, can often be retrieved by embolectomy under local anaesthetic. In this case the risks of intra-arterial thrombolysis are clearly inappropriate (Figure 2). There is a subgroup of elderly women with acute embolic ischaemia who have a high chance of flow restoration following embolectomy under local anaesthetic [15].

Standard vascular surgical factors should also be taken into account. For example, if a patient with a superficial femoral artery occlusion has no vein for a distal bypass, then the surgical option is a high-risk prosthetic graft and thrombolysis may therefore be a good alternative. A similar example is shown in Figure 3, in a patient with acute tibioperoneal trunk occlusion, where surgical options are limited.

On some occasions there is no surgical option, eg. thrombotic superficial femoral artery occlusion with no

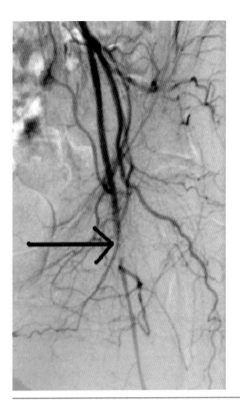

Figure 2. Embolic occlusion (arrow) of the superficial femoral artery suitable for embolectomy under local anaesthetic.

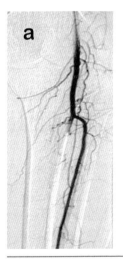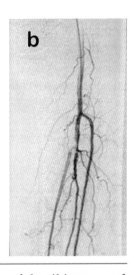

Figure 3. a) Acute occlusion of the tibioperoneal trunk, possibly due to embolism from an aortic aneurysm. b) After thrombolysis with low-dose tPA, the peroneal artery is recanalised although the posterior tibial artery still contains thrombus. The patient was anticoagulated and the leg remained viable.

run-off for a bypass. Lysis may be high-risk, with a low chance of success in this situation too, but an attempt may be worthwhile as an alternative to amputation. There are some specific situations where the role of thrombolysis has been clarified. For acute thrombosis of a popliteal aneurysm, thrombolysis should not be used to open the aneurysm as there is a significant risk of massive distal embolisation. It may, however, be used to open the run-off arteries by passing the catheter through the aneurysm, as this can open up distal vessels for a surgical bypass. Alternatively, surgery can be undertaken as a primary procedure with the option to use intra-operative thrombolysis to open occluded distal vessels during the surgery [16].

Optimal results from thrombolysis

There is evidence that the results of thrombolysis for acute leg ischaemia can be optimised. Results from the patients treated by the Thrombolysis Study Group were returned to members annually as part of the process of comparative audit. The Group agreed to stop treating patients with acute onset claudication in 1998 [17]. The overall results on the NATALI database improved over the decade of enrolment, possibly as a result of surgeons and radiologists learning which patients to treat. In addition, selective series of patients reported by enthusiasts tend to have better results, suggesting as in so many areas of treatment, that there is a case-volume effect.

Good patient selection is the cornerstone of good practice. The information described above should allow individual guidance of risk intervention. It is clearly inappropriate to perform lysis on a high-risk patient when an alternative treatment exists. Using lysis in a high-risk situation can be justified, but only as a positive decision where a surgical option is lacking or equally high-risk (Figure 4). There are considerable issues around informed consent in these patients.

The actual technique of thrombolysis does not seem to be as important to outcome as good case selection. Early analysis of the Thrombolysis Surgical Group database showed no correlation between method of thrombolysis and outcome [18]. There are two main methods of intra-arterial thrombolysis: continuous low-dose infusion or accelerated

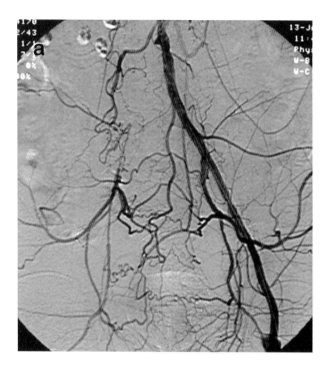

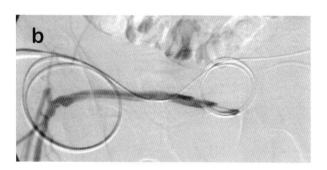

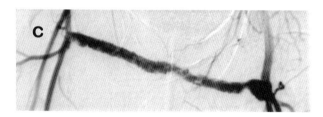

Figure 4. a) **Acute occlusion of a redo femoral cross-over graft after an acute attack of atrial fibrillation. The surgical alternative was aortobifemoral grafting. b) Low-dose thrombolysis with tPA given by direct graft puncture reopened the graft. c) Patent graft after thrombolysis with no obvious stenoses on duplex imaging.**

thrombolysis. Accelerated methods with pulse spray [19] or high-dose bolus tPA lysis [20] can reduce the time required to open an artery, but have never been shown to improve the overall results. Patients who present with acute critical ischaemia including a neurosensory deficit are at risk of early muscle necrosis and are therefore candidates for an accelerated technique. There is a significant risk that low-dose lysis will be too slow in these patients and that a limb may be lost despite successful recanalisation. A good interventional team will be flexible enough to use either technique and have the clinical judgement to decide which is appropriate. Good teamwork between surgeon and radiologist, and experience with the various techniques is vital.

When accelerated lysis is successful in a patient with critical ischaemia including a neurological deficit, a reperfusion syndrome can occur. Acute compartment syndrome is well recognised after surgical embolectomy, but rare after thrombolysis. A fasciotomy is occasionally required if there is swelling and tenderness in the anterior compartment muscles after successful lysis. This does pose problems in a patient who has just finished thrombolysis and who is probably anticoagulated with heparin, but if a fasciotomy is not done the benefits of thrombolysis are lost and amputation will follow.

The way ahead

It was only to be expected that new technology would offer alternatives in the management of acute leg ischaemia. Percutaneous removal of fresh clot either by aspiration embolectomy or percutaneous thrombectomy can be achieved with several modern devices. The aim of using these new devices is to reduce the risk of bleeding (and stroke) that exists with lytic therapy. There are two main problems: first, the cost of the device may be prohibitive; second, lysis is often required in addition, as the clot burden is simply reduced by the device and small distal vessels are not reopened. A variety of ingenious devices are now available and good results have been reported in individual case series [21]. None of the devices has ever been subjected to randomised comparison with surgery or primary thrombolysis. Some radiologists perform manual aspiration embolectomy before lysis and this could certainly be a cost-effective method of speeding up recanalisation and reducing the risks of bleeding. The problem is that larger arterial punctures are necessary with some of the interventional devices.

Other potential areas of advancement include new thrombolytic drugs and regimens. It is unlikely new agents will make much impact as the more effective the drug, in general, the higher the risk of bleeding complications. Fibrin specificity is probably an optimistic dream expounded by haematologists.

Minimising the risks

The main risk of intra-arterial thrombolysis is bleeding. Major haemorrhage occurred in 8% of episodes on the NATALI database, although minor but troublesome groin haematoma was much more frequent. Stroke is the most feared complication. In the NATALI database that included 1147 episodes, there were 26 strokes (2.3%), 20 of which were fatal [3]. Many of the strokes occurred after thrombolysis had finished, during therapeutic anticoagulation with heparin [22]. Approximately half the strokes associated with lysis are thrombotic rather than haemorrhagic, presumably because acute leg ischaemia is common in high-risk elderly arteriopaths. The stroke rate when intravenous thrombolysis is used for acute deep vein thrombosis is less than 1%, but these patients tend to be younger and fitter [23]. There is no known way to prevent stroke, but this complication has to be seen in the context of trying to prevent limb loss in elderly unfit patients, where surgery often has similar risks.

Likewise, it is difficult to prevent major bleeding complications. Monitoring the systemic fibrinolytic state with blood tests can be used to predict the risk of bleeding, but cannot be shown to be clinically valuable. Clinicians seldom stop lysis that seems to be working, even when coagulation tests suggest there is a systemic fibrinolytic state. Careful patient monitoring and good clinical care are more important. Some clinicians recommend that patients should be treated in Intensive Care, but pressure on beds means that most hospitals in the UK do not have that luxury. Local guidelines and protocols have been developed that can inform and educate the individual health care teams [24]. Contemporary pathways of care have been created for thrombolytic treatment of acute leg ischaemia that enable early diagnosis of complications during lysis at a stage when treatment can be instituted successfully [25]. Other catheter-related complications such as peri-catheter thrombosis and distal embolisation that were a problem in the 1980s are now uncommon, due mainly to advances in interventional equipment.

The future of thrombolysis is secure

A thrombolytic agent (usually tPA) is available on the shelf in all interventional radiology suites in the UK. Thrombolysis is now firmly instituted in mainstream vascular practice and is one of a number of options for treatment in patients with acute leg ischaemia. Owing to the great variation in patients with acute leg ischaemia, it is not surprising that global trials that compared surgery and lysis have not demonstrated the superiority of one particular technique. In good units, the management of acute leg ischaemia will be shared between vascular surgeons and radiologists, making joint decisions.

The first two decades of research into thrombolysis have produced information that can help clinicians make their choices. High-risk patients can be identified and in some of these, thrombolysis may still be justified. This information has at least improved the process of informed consent. New thrombolytic agents and techniques are unlikely to make much impact, but as in so many other areas of health care delivery, improved results come from standardising approaches to care. Informed case selection, teamwork in management and the institution of local care pathways should be employed by clinicians keen to provide an optimal service. Thrombolysis is here to stay. It remains an excellent alternative to surgery in selected patients with acute leg ischaemia.

Summary

◆ Twenty years of experience with intra-arterial thrombolysis for acute leg ischaemia has produced a wealth of clinical and research experience.

◆ The bleeding risks of thrombolytic therapy have made some clinicians circumspect about its routine use.

◆ Enthusiasts have learned the lessons from analysis of the randomised trials and the NATALI database to help identify patients likely to benefit from lysis.

◆ Best results are achieved by vascular surgeons and radiologists working together, using the breadth of available techniques, but with management tailored to the individual.

◆ Thrombolysis has now assumed a stable and important role as an alternative to surgery in the management of selected patients with acute leg ischaemia.

References

1. Braithwaite BD, Earnshaw JJ. Arterial embolectomy: a century and out. *Br J Surg* 1994; 81: 1705-6.

2. Porter JM. Thrombolysis for acute arterial occlusion of the legs. *N Engl J Med* 1998; 338: 1148-51.

3. Earnshaw JJ, Whitman B, Foy C on behalf of the Thrombolysis Study Group. National Audit of Thrombolysis for Acute Leg Ischemia (NATALI): clinical factors associated with early outcome. *J Vasc Surg* 2004 (in press).

4. Richards T, Pittathankal AA, Magee TR, *et al*. The current role of intra-arterial thrombolysis. *Eur J Vasc Endovasc Surg* 2003; 26: 166-9.

5. Eliason JL, Wainess RM, Proctor MC, *et al*. A national and single institutional experience of acute lower extremity ischaemia. *Ann Surg* 2003; 238: 382-9.

6. Dotter CT, Rosch J, Seaman AJ. Selective clot lysis with low-dose streptokinase. *Radiology* 1974; 111: 31-7.

7. Ouriel K. Current status of thrombolysis for peripheral arterial occlusive disease. *Ann Vasc Surg* 2002; 16: 797-804.

8. Ouriel K, Shortell CK, DeWeese, JA, *et al*. A comparison of thrombolytic therapy with operative revascularization in the initial treatment of acute peripheral arterial ischaemia. *J Vasc Surg* 1994; 19: 1021-30.

9. The STILE Investigators. Results of a prospective randomized trial evaluating surgery versus thrombolysis for ischaemia of the lower extremity. *Ann Surg* 1994; 220: 251-68.

10. Ouriel K, Veith FJ, Sasahara AA for the Thrombolysis Or Peripheral Arterial Surgery (TOPAS) Investigators. A comparison of recombinant urokinase with vascular surgery as initial treatment for acute arterial occlusion of the legs. *N Engl J Med* 1998; 338: 1105-11.

11. Palfreyman SJ, Booth A, Michaels JA. A systematic review of intra-arterial thrombolytic therapy for lower limb ischaemia. *Eur J Vasc Endovasc Surg* 2000; 19: 143-57.

12. Berridge DC, Kessel D, Robertson I. Surgery versus thrombolysis for acute limb ischaemia: initial management (Cochrane Review). In: *The Cochrane Library*, Issue 3, 2003. Update Software, Oxford.

13. Comerota A, Weaver FA, Hosking JD, *et al*. Results of a prospective randomized trial of surgery versus thrombolysis for occluded lower extremity bypass grafts. *Am J Surg* 1996; 172: 105-112.

14. Neary B, Whitman B, Foy C, *et al*. Value of POSSUM physiology scoring to assess outcome after intra-arterial thrombolysis for acute leg ischaemia. *Br J Surg* 2001; 88: 1344-5.

15. Braithwaite BD, Davies B, Birch PA, *et al*. Management of acute leg ischaemia in the elderly. *Br J Surg* 1998; 85: 217-20.

16. Beard JD, Earnshaw JJ. Intra-operative use of thrombolytic agents. *BMJ* 1993; 307: 638-9.

17. Braithwaite BD, Tomlinson MA, Walker SR, *et al*. Peripheral thrombolysis for acute-onset claudication. *Br J Surg* 1999; 86: 800-4.

18. Thomas SM, Gaines PA on behalf of the Thrombolysis Study Group. Avoiding the complications of thrombolysis. *Br J Surg* 1999; 86: A710.

19. Armon MP, Yusuf SW, Whitaker SC, *et al*. Results of 100 cases of pulse spray thrombolysis for acute and subacute leg ischaemia. *Br J Surg* 1997; 84: 47-50.

20. Braithwaite BD, Buckenham TM, Galland RB, *et al* on behalf of the Thrombolysis Study Group. Prospective randomized trial of high-dose bolus versus low-dose tissue plasminogen activator infusion in the management of acute limb ischaemia. *Br J Surg* 1997; 84: 646-50.

21. Haskal ZJ. Mechanical thrombectomy devices for the treatment of peripheral arterial occlusions. *Cardiovasc Med* 2002; 3 (suppl 2): S45-S52.

22. Dawson K, Armon M, Braithwaite BD, *et al*. Stroke during intra-arterial thrombolysis: a survey of experience in the UK. *Br J Surg* 1996; 83: A568.

23. Meissner MH. Thrombolytic therapy for acute deep vein thrombosis and the Venous Registry. *Rev Cardiovasc Med* 2002; 3 suppl 2: S53-S60.

24. Working Party on Thrombolysis in the Management of Limb Ischemia. Thrombolysis in the Management of the lower limb peripheral arterial occlusion - a consensus document. *Am J Cardiol* 1998; 81: 207-18.

25. Whitman B, Parkin D, Earnshaw JJ. Management of acute leg ischaemia. In: *Pathways of care in vascular surgery*. Beard JD, Murray S, Eds. tfm publishing Ltd, Shrewsbury, 2002; 12: 99-106.

Chapter 21

Mechanical thrombectomy: is it worthwhile?

Derek A Gould, FRCP FRCR, Consultant Radiologist

Royal Liverpool and Broadgreen University Hospitals Trust, Liverpool, UK

Avoidance of the potentially devastating sequelae of vascular, thromboembolic occlusion requires expeditious diagnosis and intervention to re-establish blood flow and may involve any, or a combination, of the following.

Conservative management

This involves anticoagulation, with correction of any risk factors. Nevertheless, the conservative management of acute limb ischaemia, can result in dismal limb salvage and survival, and invasive methods to re-establish flow are therefore frequently required.

Traditional surgery

Traditional surgery involves either, mechanical methods, such as balloon thrombectomy with an occlusion balloon [1], direct extraction of thrombus, or bypass grafting. In these procedures, access is achieved via an incision under local or general anaesthesia. The perioperative mortality and morbidity is generally high.

Percutaneous thrombolysis

The use of thrombolytic agents to chemically dissolve thrombus has become widespread practice within vascular intervention, with well documented technical success, although the procedures are prolonged, labour intensive and require multiple reinterventions. Side-effects include haemorrhage and stroke, which may be embolic or haemorrhagic (see Chapter 20).

Mechanical thrombectomy

There is now a range of mechanical thrombectomy (MT) methods, designed specifically for percutaneous use and ranging from simple aspiration thrombectomy, to novel devices which perform mechanical fragmentation, mechanical extraction, and hydrodynamic disruption and extraction. In common with thrombolysis, MT may reveal a culprit, underlying lesion, amenable to secondary interventions. Risks of these devices include haemolysis, endothelial damage, embolisation and mechanical failure.

Which therapeutic modality?

In the process of determining therapeutic options, the clinical background is of great importance. In lower limb ischaemia, the presence of arrhythmia, previous claudication or previous surgery may suggest embolisation, native stenosis or intimal hyperplasia. An occluded aortobifemoral graft may be rapidly managed by surgery with simultaneous correction of an underlying outflow stenosis. Thrombolysis may be more prolonged in occlusion by organised embolus and may therefore be unsuitable where limb ischaemia is critical, with paralysis and muscle tenderness. The duration of occlusion will influence the choice of MT devices, as these are generally less effective in thrombus older than 14 days.

Given the morbidity of surgery, and the complications and prolonged nature of re-canalisation using thrombolysis, percutaneous MT seems to offer an attractive and rapid alternative. There are, however, few registries and fewer randomised studies of these devices. This short review will examine the rationale and some applications of MT devices used either in isolation or in combination with other interventional techniques including chemical thrombolysis.

Mechanical thrombectomy: mode of action

Most MT devices act through generation of focused energy using mechanical or hydraulic means to fragment thrombus, with some simultaneously extracting the resulting debris. They do not totally eliminate thrombus and the particles produced may be quite large: in one *in vitro* study, 2-7% of embolic particles were in excess of 24 microns [2]. The risk of particulate emboli in an already ischaemic limb cannot be ignored and it follows that there is a potential advantage in devices which extract any particles generated.

The amount of thrombotic material remaining following mechanical and thrombolytic methods of recanalisation of haemodialysis grafts in 35 patients was examined using angioscopy by Vesely [3]. The Cragg brush and the Treratola Percutaneous

Thrombectomy Device left the smallest residue and there were increasing amounts of thrombus with the Endovac, Hydrolyser, Amplatz Thrombectomy device, Angiojet and Oasis: the greatest thrombus residue was with the lyse and wait technique. The role of such residual thrombus, however, and the relative implications at different anatomical sites, particularly with regard to long-term patency, remains unclear. An attempt to assess vessel wall damage in the same study was unsuccessful owing to poor correlation amongst the observers.

MT devices restore blood flow by various combinations of redistribution, fragmentation, dispersal and extraction of thrombus. These mechanisms are described below.

Redistribution of occlusive thrombus without extraction

Conventional PTA will often be acting in this way. Certainly the majority of the volume of chronic occlusive material traversed and subjected to balloon dilation or stenting in conventional percutaneous transluminal angioplasty may be organised thrombus. This material is redistributed away from the vascular lumen, allowing distal reperfusion, but without intentional fragmentation, although embolisation can occur as a complication. Balloon dilation can also be used to macerate and redistribute thrombus during thrombolysis, with the objective of increasing the available surface area and accelerating lysis.

Fragmention and dispersal of thrombus

Very fresh acute thrombus, such as may occur during an interventional procedure, may be fragmented and dispersed by simple physical methods such as injection of heparinised saline [4], or by agitation using a guidewire or balloon dilation. Alternatively, and in older (up to 14 days), more organised thrombus, the application of greater levels of energy using specific MT devices which fragment without removal, produces particulate material which, theoretically, is microscopic and disperses harmlessly. In practice, such emboli are of variable size.

Small pulmonary emboli are created intentionally during some methods of elimination of thrombus from dialysis fistulae, (eg. balloon extraction methods), though these have generally not been shown of clinical significance. Many of these devices have been used in combination with chemical thrombolysis, when fragmentation accelerates recanalisation by exposing a greater surface area of thrombus to the lytic agents used.

Amplatz thrombectomy device (ATD)

The Amplatz thrombectomy device (Microvena, White Bear Lake, MN, USA) creates a vortex which draws thrombus into a fragmenting impeller. Fragments are not removed, but are intended to be small and dispersable. While effective in up to 78% of cases, it is prone to drive shaft fracture when used around acute angles, can cause haemolysis and the embolic fragments may be up to 1000 microns in diameter. Comparison of hydrodynamic methods (Oasis, Angiojet, Hydroliser) against the Amplatz thrombectomy device has shown a greater amount of emboli larger than 10 microns with the latter [5]. Cooper et al [6] used ATD in 18 vascular access grafts and noted the withdrawal of fragments of fibrotic myointima in the impeller housing, thus raising concerns over its use in native vessels.

Arrow-Treratola percutaneous thrombectomy device (PTD)

The Arrow-Treratola percutaneous thrombectomy device (Arrow International, Reading, PA, USA) is essentially a wall contact device which can be used over a guidewire with a rotating nitinol basket. It produces fragmentation, with embolic particles up to 3mm diameter. Vesely et al [3] showed particularly low volumes of residual thrombus in haemodialysis grafts using angioscopy. Its use in native vessels is, however, associated with endothelial disruption and the device is recommended principally for graft thrombectomy.

Brush techniques

The Cragg, and Castaneda 'over the wire', brushes are wall contact devices, designed as an adjunct to thrombolysis. They are effective in fragmenting and removing thrombus from occluded grafts, but can produce vessel wall damage in native vessel segments and there is a high incidence of distal embolisation. Castaneda et al investigated the wall effect of the PTD, the Fogarty catheter and the Castaneda brush and vascular damage was found to extend to the media with all devices [7]. Minimal wall injury must clearly be an objective of device development and might suggest an advantage for hydrodynamic methods.

Catheter fragmentation

Catheter fragmentation of thrombus can be performed with conventional catheters (eg. Grollman). A rotating mini pigtail device has been developed specifically for fragmentation of thrombus: it has an exit sidehole at the base of the pigtail to allow a guidewire to be passed up to, and exit alongside, the terminal pigtail section. The pigtail can then be manually rotated within the thrombus, producing fragmentation of thrombus / embolus and restoring antegrade flow. This simple MT device has been used in declotting of dialysis access, and also in the recanalisation of pulmonary embolic occlusion where there is life threatening haemodynamic disturbance, hypotension and hypoxia.

Percutaneous balloon thrombectomy

Conventional balloon embolectomy is difficult to perform percutaneously though the use of percutaneous balloons has a role in detaching the arterial plug during dialysis fistula recanalisation. The large capacity venous circulation can tolerate such emboli far more readily than would be the case in an arterial occlusion in an ischaemic limb.

Ultrasound thrombolysis

Ultrasound thrombolysis utilises the cavitation effect of sound frequencies of 20 to 45 KHz. Kruger evaluated intravascular ultrasound thrombolysis in vitro, finding it significantly less effective at reducing thrombus weight than the Amplatz thrombectomy device [8]. Use of the ultrasound device in four patients with iliac or femoropopliteal occlusion of up to one

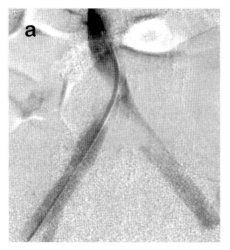

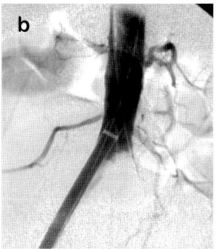

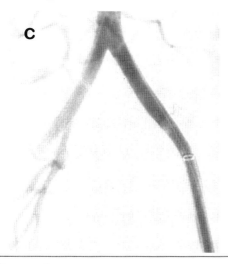

Figure 1. Aspiration of large aortic bifurcation embolus using a 16 French sheath. a) Large aortic bifurcation embolus. b) Aspiration from right arteriotomy using a 16 French sheath. c) After aspiration from left (distal flow defect on right is due to control at arteriotomy site).

year duration resulted in technical success in just one case. Ultrasound thrombolysis alone was considered insufficient to treat peripheral arteries *in vivo*. Silva *et al* however, suggested this method was highly effective for removing coronary thrombi prior to coronary intervention [9].

Extraction of thrombus

Surgical balloon thrombectomy

Surgical balloon thrombectomy was a landmark development in the management of acute ischaemia. Difficulty in removing adherent clot led to the development of latex corkscrew catheters [1], and conceptually, the MT catheter was born. Balloon embolectomy remains a mainstay of surgical methods today and has also been used percutaneously, in dialysis grafts (see above).

Percutaneous aspiration thrombectomy (PAT)

Percutaneous aspiration thrombectomy (PAT) was pioneered by Sniderman [10] and Starck [11]. Using a large syringe to produce suction via a catheter of modest lumen diameter such as a guide catheter (eg. Brite Tip, Cordis, Johnson and Johnson), removal of small to moderate amounts of thrombus or embolus can be performed, for example from the popliteal trifurcation following embolisation during angioplasty. Zehnder *et al* performed thromboaspiration in 93 infrainguinal occlusions with 90% technical success and 78% 12-month amputation-free survival. While aspiration was sufficient in 31%, lysis was required in 22% and PTA in 60%. Further secondary interventions were required in 30% within 12 months [12].

6-8 French catheters are suited to the femoropopliteal segment and 4-6 French, below the popliteal. Using large sheath diameters, larger (eg. pulmonary) emboli can be aspirated: the author has been successful in aspiration of a large aortic embolus in an acute Leriche syndrome, using a 16 French sheath (Cook, Copenhagen) via bilateral arteriotomy (Figure 1).

Fragmentation and extraction of thrombus

Mechanical impeller extraction devices use mechanical means to fragment thrombus and, often assisted by vacuum, extract the fragments.

Rotarex (Straub)

This mechanical, rotational device performs fragmentation and simultaneous extraction of thrombotic material. Zana *et al* [13] performed *in vitro* studies and found suitability to tubes of diameter 6-8mm, though with some distal embolisation.

Thrombex PMT

Thrombex PMT (Edwards Lifesciences LLC, Irvine, California, USA) uses a pre-evacuated, alarm protected, vacuum chamber for motorised cutting / extraction of thrombus. The device is passed over an .018" guidewire.

Hydrodynamic devices induce a local pressure gradient through rapid injection of saline through an accessory lumen in the catheter. A combined fragmentation effect with forced extraction of the fragmented material has been shown to produce varying degrees of technical success. However, there is variable ability to maintain an iso-volumetric fluid exchange. Only the Angiojet device has been shown to approach a ratio of applied saline to aspirated fluid of 1 (0.92) [5].

Oasis

Oasis (Boston Scientific, Galway, Ireland) uses the Venturi effect and consists of a three-lumen, 6 to 10 French over-the-wire, thrombectomy catheter: an inflow lumen is connected to an angiographic injector and an outflow lumen, to the collection bag. A three-way stopcock between the catheter connection and the injector allows quick refilling of the injector from a reservoir of heparinised saline solution. The device has a ratio of applied to aspirated fluid of 0.6, with consequent risk of anaemia. Haemolysis is minimal

though endothelial disruption has been reported after use of the Oasis device in dogs.

Hydrolyser

Hydrolyser (Cordis, Johnson and Johnson, Miami, Florida, USA) is an over-the-wire double lumen, 6 / 7 French device which also uses the Venturi principle, fragmenting thrombus and extracting the ensuing particles. Fluid overload and haemolysis are attendant risks in all such devices. In a randomised study, Barth [14] showed 89% clinical success using Hydrolyser in dialysis access fistulae, compared with 81% for thrombolysis. Baba *et al* [15] obtained technical success in five of seven males with arterial (6) and dialysis shunt (1) occlusion, concluding that Hydrolyser was more rapid than Fogarty embolectomy, with fewer complications, though clearly limited by the small size of the study.

Angiojet device (AJ)

The Angiojet device (AJ) (Possis Medical, Minneapolis, MN, USA) is a rheolytic thrombectomy device using the Bernoulli principle: a high pressure retrograde jet of normal saline creates a low pressure zone, drawing clot into the jet stream where it is fragmented and ejected via an exhaust lumen into a collection bag. The device is passed over an .035" or .014" guidewire and operated using a foot pedal with slow advancement through the obstruction. Operation is limited to 1 litre of saline infusate and (owing to haemolytic red cell damage) a total activation time of five to ten minutes. In the author's experience, frank haemoglobinuria can occur with prolonged (i.e. up to ten minutes) activation and there is therefore a potential for renal dysfunction. Potassium may be released by the process of haemolysis and may account for bradycardia and a sensation of breathlessness, which have been seen with use of AJ in central veins. A further disadvantage is the cost of the drive mechanism. The risk of fluid overload is low.

Various strategies for adjunct thrombolysis have been described with AJ, usually as formal infusion following suboptimal outcomes, though it is possible to administer lytics in place of heparin in the AJ infusate. In the 'power pulse spray' method, a small volume of high concentration lytics is administered on a few inflow strokes of the device.

Target areas for thrombectomy

Arterio-venous dialysis fistulae and dialysis grafts

This was an early application to be approved by the FDA and accounts for a moderate number of studies.

A multicentre randomised comparison of hydrodynamic thrombectomy using the Oasis device against pulse spray thrombolysis showed comparable technical success (95% for thrombectomy, 90% for thrombolysis) and clinical success of 89% and 81% respectively [14]. The cohort size was small (p=0.24 for clinical outcomes) but hydrodynamic thrombectomy was considered at least as effective as thrombolysis with treatment times significantly different at 16.8 and 23.4 minutes respectively (p<0.1).

The use of percutaneous balloon embolectomy, particularly for the resistant arterial plug, carries fewer of the concerns over embolisation that are present in peripheral arterial occlusion. Such emboli are readily dispersed in the large capacity venous circulation and symptomatic pulmonary embolism is rare, as is embolisation into the afferent artery (usually amenable to PAT). Gorriz et al performed vascular access recanalisation using balloon thrombectomy in 81 and Hydrolyser in 42 [16]. There was technical success in 97% with 14% early reocclusions (at <72 hrs) and 30% reocclusion on follow-up. There were segmental or subsegmental perfusion defects in 23% of perfusion lung scans following thrombecomy, but no related clinical sequelae.

In 22 patients with thrombosed dialysis grafts and fistulas, Schmitz-Rode et al, used a rotating mini pigtail to produce declotting in 100% cases with primary patency of 65% at three months [17].

Rocek et al used the PTD in ten native fistula occlusions, with PTA in all cases [18]. There was initial clinical success in nine with assisted primary patency in eight at six months.

Vogel et al randomised 40 patients with clotted dialysis grafts to the PTD Arrow-Trerotola device or the lyse and wait technique using 4mg of tPA [19]. Both groups had 95% angiographic success and similar overall procedure times, though there were bleeding complications in six of 20 in the thrombolysis group; none in the MT group.

Randomised studies of vascular access recanalisation using the Hydrolyser (Barth et al [14]) and ATD (Sofecleous [20]) have shown technical success equivalent to thrombolysis, while eliminating the bleeding complications of lytics. In a prospective, randomised trial of the AJ device against surgery in 153 cases with vascular access graft thrombosis, Vesely et al showed 73% technical success for AJ and 79% for surgery (p=0.41); three month primary patency was 15% and 26% respectively [21]. This difference approached significance, and indeed, in a meta-analysis, Green showed superiority of surgery over percutaneous methods [22].

Peripheral arteries, grafts and stent grafts

Acute limb ischaemia presents a major risk for limb loss and death. MT devices have been used to rapidly recanalise acute vascular occlusion in the upper [23] and lower limbs, in native vessels, stents and grafts. Ouriel considered that a reduction in the incidence of rheumatic heart disease has accounted for a change in the prevalence of acute arterial occlusion, from embolic to thrombotic [24]. In addition, increasing popularity of lower extremity arterial bypass grafts has led to a parallel increase in the incidence of graft occlusion as a cause of critical limb ischaemia.

In limb ischaemia, embolisation during recanalisation by MT devices has the potential for significant sequelae, in comparison with their use in the venous circulation. In practice, most arterial emboli can be removed using simple MT methodology such as transcatheter aspiration, possibly with adjunct thrombolysis.

The efficacy of MT devices has been defined by the amount of thrombus removed, with <50% lumen restoration generally regarded as technical failure.

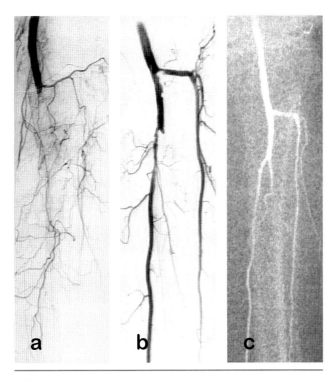

Figure 2. Pre and post-intervention: critical lower limb ischaemia treated by rheolytic thrombectomy with adjunct thrombolysis. a) Popliteal occlusion. b) Following rheolytic thrombectomy. c) Appearance following adjunct lytic infusion.

Canova *et al* reviewed 88 percutaneous thromboembolectomy procedures for acute infrainguinal embolic occlusion (claudication in 45, limb threat in 43). Using PAT with adjunct lysis and PTA as required, there was technical success in 97% with two major and two minor complications and one death within 30 days [25]. At eight years, primary clinical success was 76.5% and mortality 29.5%; ten of 16 interval failures were recurrent ipsilateral embolism.

Desgranges *et al* performed thromboaspiration in 33 cases of acute ischaemia due to popliteal or tibial occlusion, with additional PTA in seven; surgery was required for six failures [26]. 12-month limb salvage overall was 91% with primary patency of 88% at one month, 66% at 12 months. Similar results were obtained by Zehnder [27] in 89 cases of acute and subacute lower limb arterial occlusion; 31 were treated by thromboaspiration alone, with additional PTA in 69% and urokinase in 22%. Amputation-free

12-month survival was 78% though secondary interventions were required in 30%.

In a retrospective, multicentre review, 99 patients with native artery or graft, thrombotic occlusion (79% under 14 days duration) were managed using the AJ device. There was substantial or complete thrombus removal in 71%, partial in 22%, no change in 7% [28]. Adjunctive lysis was used in 37 cases and underlying stenoses were managed in 81 limbs. 30-day mortality was 7% and amputation rate, 4%.

Kasirajan *et al* [29] evaluated the AJ device in 65 acute and 21 subacute cases of limb threatening, arterial occlusion. Successful (61%) and partially successful (23%) cases overall stratified into 90% success in *in situ*, thrombotic occlusion and 60% in embolic occlusion. AJ was augmented with lytics in 50 (58%) cases but this was uniformly unsuccessful where MT had failed and indeed, produced angiographic improvement in only seven of the 50 cases.

Beyer-Enke *et al* [30] reported 80% primary clinical success with Hydrolyser, though 23% of patients died in the 3-year follow-up period. Silva *et al* have reported 95% one-month limb salvage using AJ, in the absence of any adjunctive thrombolysis [31]. In the author's experience, six of 18 cases of thrombotic occlusion at various anatomical sites required adjunct thrombolysis following AJ thrombectomy for significant, residual thrombus (Figure 2).

A report by Krajcer *et al* confirms the safe, effective applicability of rheolytic thrombectomy in aortic endograft thrombosis with success in restoring patency in all of six occluded endografts [32]: five of these cases were caused by graft kinking and adjunct stenting procedures were performed to maintain flow.

The case for adjunctive thrombolysis

While MT devices may not totally eliminate thrombus [3], it is unlikely that total removal of thrombus is universally necessary to obtain a lasting clinical outcome. There is, however, little evidence as to the amount of thrombus that can be left without adverse sequelae such as rethrombosis or embolisation. In view of this, many workers 'play safe' by administering adjunct lytics, though the precise indications are ill-defined. Perhaps because of this, there is considerable variation in the incidence and methods of adjunct thrombolysis, the latter ranging from bolus administration, to pulse and power pulse methods, to formal institution of lytic infusions.

Given the potential for significant complication with thrombolytic agents, a potential advantage of MT would seem to be rapid, low-risk recanalisation, with at least a reduced amount of any subsequent lysis, and at best, complete avoidance. Whether mechanical thrombectomy devices can achieve this 'holy grail' of complete, stand alone functionality, or whether adjunctive thrombolytic agents will continue to be needed [33] to a greater or lesser degree, is yet to be determined. While some randomised studies have been performed in the coronary arteries (lysis versus AJ: the VeGAS trial, Kuntz et al [34]) and in vascular access (see above), level I evidence has yet to be obtained for the use of MT devices in the lower limb.

Coronary arteries

While this review sets out to examine the role of MT in the territory of the interventional radiologist, much work has been performed in the coronary arteries, including one of the few, completed randomised studies of MT devices (VeGAS 2 study, Kuntz [34]) which showed similar technical outcomes after AJ (86%) and Urokinase (72%). AJ was also shown to be successful in 94% of coronary stent thromboses by Silva [35] who strongly recommended this as a treatment option. Rinfret et al [36] obtained 76% technical success with AJ in saphenous vein grafts and 66% in native coronary arteries. There is also limited experience with the Hydrolyser in the coronary vessels [37].

Cervico-cerebral vessels

There is limited documentation of MT devices applied to the intracranial circulation. Thrombolysis can be time-consuming and risks haemorrhage. Use of a nitinol basket has been shown to retrieve clot from the basilar artery in three of five patients, with

assistance by induced flow reversal by vertebral or subclavian balloon occlusion. Three of the cases required thrombolysis as adjunct or for failure; there was residual disability in two [38].

Lutsep et al performed catheter aspiration thrombectomy in two patients with internal carotid occlusion with a good clinical outcome in both [39]. Another small series of three cases of internal carotid occlusion was described by Bellon et al who achieved a measure of technical success in all three, with adjunct lysis, PTA and stent placement [40].

Chow et al used the AJ device in four procedures, in two patients with dural sinus thrombosis [41]. There were no significant neurological deficits at six months, apart from mild short-term memory loss in one. In a 54-year-old female with dural sinus thrombosis, Dowd et al reported an excellent outcome following hydrodynamic thrombectomy [42].

Pulmonary arteries

Massive pulmonary embolism with haemodynamic instability is generally an indication for rapid recanalisation of the obstructed pulmonary arteries, using surgical or thrombolytic techniques to lower pulmonary artery pressure and improve pulmonary blood flow and oxygenation. There is a role for PAT and devices such as Hydrolyser, Oasis and ATD. Both the AJ device and the rotating mini pigtail have been shown to reduce mortality and procedure time as compared with chemical thrombolysis [43].

Schmitz-Rode et al concluded the mini pigtail was useful in 20 high-risk patients with right ventricular failure to accelerate thrombolysis and as an alternative to surgical embolectomy; mortality in the treated group was 20% [44]. Fava et al used the Hydrolyser in 11 patents with additional thrombolysis in four; ten of these patients recovered and were discharged by the 11th day [43]. In the author's experience of the AJ in two cases of massive pulmonary embolism with haemodynamic instability, there was immediate technical success in two, one death within 24 hrs and one survival (Figure 3). On a cautionary note, Biederer et al reported fatal haemoptysis following use of the AJ device in massive PE in a 76-year-old female, possibly due to activation of the 6 French catheter in a vessel under 6mm diameter [45].

Using MT devices in this way, it appears that lifesaving haemodynamic improvement can be obtained by recanalisation of occluded central pulmonary arteries, with additional thrombolysis and where indicated, caval filtration.

Peripheral veins

Debilitating long-term sequelae can follow untreated lower limb deep vein thrombosis (DVT). Mechanical thrombectomy and chemical thrombolysis may act synergistically, within a week of onset, to rapidly reduce clot burden and complications [46] and a number of sources suggest this can be performed without routine use of IVC filtration [47].

Using MT to augment chemical thrombolysis, Vedantham et al achieved 82% procedural success in 28 symptomatic limbs with lower extremity DVT, placing stents in 18 limbs. MT removed significantly more thrombus when used after, than before, pharmacological thrombolysis, though there were significant bleeding complications in three cases and a mean infusion time of 23.1 hours was required. It was concluded that MT alone was unlikely to be effective for the complete treatment of such cases [47]. Nonetheless, the degree of severity of symptoms was not recorded in this study and the clinical indications and applicability of these techniques in preventing post-phlebitic syndrome remain unclear.

Central veins

MT devices can be applied to other central venous structures, for example Ries et al reported thrombus aspiration combined with thrombolysis in superior vena cava obstruction in an infant. Debulking of thrombus using MT can also be performed prior to SVC stenting in obstruction by invading neoplasm [48].

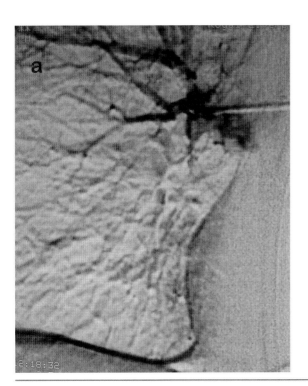
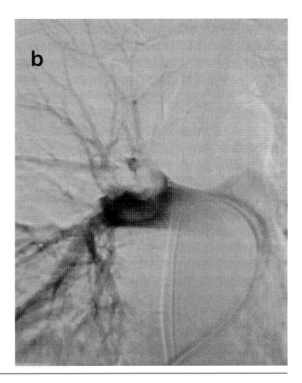

Figure 3. Pre and post-Angiojet thrombectomy in a 41-year-old male with massive pulmonary embolus and good clinical outcome. a) Massive PE. b) Following 6 French rheolytic thrombectomy.

Gu *et al* used the steerable Amplatz thrombectomy catheter to restore venographic patency in 23 dogs with infrarenal IVC thrombosis, though with residual mural thrombus in nine; 80% had rethrombosed by one month. Histopathological examination of explanted lungs in 11 animals showed arteriolar microemboli in four [49].

Muller-Hulsbeck has described the use of the ATD in ten patients with occluded TIPS shunts at a mean of 2.8 months post TIPS procedures [50]. Technical success in all cases was achieved with adjunct PTA in four and stent placement in five; primary patency was 60% at 11 months. A potential hazard reported by Fontaine *et al* is type 3 heart block during recanalisation of a TIPS shunt with the AJ device [51].

In a report on two portal vein occlusions, Bilbao *et al* obtained only fair results with MT and thrombolysis, with partial rethrombosis [52]. This reflects similar experience at the author's institution with occlusion following two AJ procedures in a single patient with portal vein occlusion.

Extravascular applications

MT devices have also been used in the urinary tract. Morello *et al* reported use of the AJ to remove bilateral renal pelvis mycetomas [53]. Htaik *et al* also used rheolytic thrombectomy to remove obstructive clot from a transplant ureter [54].

Conclusions

A number of methods and devices exist for the percutaneous removal of clinically important thrombotic and embolic occlusions. These range from simple PAT, which has been shown to be highly effective in lower limb embolic occlusion, to sophisticated mechanical and hydrodynamic devices to fragment, and in some cases, remove thrombus.

In ideal circumstances, MT devices are able to virtually eliminate thrombus with little need for additional intervention. Frequently however, further interventions are required for underlying stenosis (PTA

/ stent) or residual thrombus (adjunct thrombolysis). The amount of residual thrombus that can be left without precipitating reocclusion is unclear, though total removal of clot does not appear universally necessary to achieve a satisfactory outcome. There is no significant evidence as to when adjunct thrombolysis should be initiated, though this may be required in around 40% cases. Significant embolic debris seems more likely to occur with non-extracting, fragmentation devices than in fragment-extract devices. Where this occurs in peripheral arteries, further thrombectomy, aspiration or adjunct lysis are required.

Surgical bail out will be necessary in a number of cases. Indeed, it may be that the long-term surgical outcomes after revascularising dialysis access grafts are superior to percutaneous methods, though clinical practice must take into account the risks and invasiveness of the respective procedures.

MT is clearly of value in the armamentarium of the interventionalist, offering the potential for rapid recanalisation of thrombus with low risk of complication. At the least, most of these devices will debulk thrombus to a greater or lesser degree, facilitating the role of adjunctive thrombolysis. There is a need for carefully controlled randomised studies to compare MT devices with 'gold standards': thrombolysis and conventional surgery. Such studies should provide data to indicate when MT devices might act as a stand alone method, and when levels of residual thrombus are such as to require adjunct lysis. The short and long-term vessel wall effects of the various devices also require quantification. In dialysis access, firmer definition of the roles of MT devices and surgery is required.

As existing devices evolve, and new ones become available, these too will require evaluation, though devices which fragment and extract, rather than just fragment, are likely to be of greater clinical value in limb ischaemia. Randomised controlled trials are needed, to deliver the evidence for a more complete understanding of the role of these fascinating devices.

Summary

◆ Mechanical thrombectomy (MT) devices, alone or in various combinations, have wide ranging applications throughout the vascular tree.

◆ In acute lower limb arterial occlusion:-
  • MT devices may be highly effective but level I evidence for their use has yet to be obtained;
  • the indications and role of adjunct thrombolysis requires clarification;
  • embolic fragments which are well tolerated in the venous circulation may produce critical obstruction in the arterial circulation.

◆ Further, randomised studies are required to determine outcomes in acute limb ischaemia, thrombosed dialysis access and lower limb DVT.

References

1. Hill B, Fogarty TJ. The use of the Fogarty catheter in 1998. *Cardiovasc Surg* 1999; 7 (3): 273-278.

2. Stahr P, Rupprecht HJ, Voigtlander T, *et al.* A new thrombectomy catheter device (angiojet) for the disruption of thrombi: an *in vitro* study. *Catheter Cardiovasc Interv* 1999; 47(3): 381-9.

3. Vesely TM, Hovespian DM, Darcy MD, *et al.* Angioscopic observations after percutaneous thrombectomy of thrombosed haemodialysis grafts. *J Vasc Interv Radiol* 2000; 11: 971-977.

4. Greenberg RK, Ouriel K, Srivastava S, *et al.* Mechanical versus chemical thrombolysis: an *in vitro* differentiation of thrombolytic mechanisms. *J Vasc Intervent Radiol* 2000; 11(2 Pt I): 199-205.

5. Muller-Hulsbeck S, Grimm J, Leidt J, *et al.* In vitro effectiveness of mechanical thrombectomy devices for large vessel diameter and low pressure fluid dynamic applications. *J Vasc Intervent Radiol* 2002; 13: 831-839.

6. Cooper SG, Gaetz H, Sofocleous CT, Schur I, Patel RI. Hemodialysis graft mechanical thrombolysis with use of the Amplatz Thrombectomy Device: histopathologic evaluation of extracted myointimal tissue. *J Vasc Intervent Radiol* 1999; 0(3): 285-8.

7. Castaneda F, Li R, Patel J, DeBord JR, Swischuk JL. Comparison of three mechanical thrombus removal devices in thrombosed canine iliac arteries. *Radiol* 2001; 219(1): 153-6.

8. Kruger K, Deissler P, Zahringer M, *et al.* Intravascular ultrasound thrombolysis for recanalisation of peripheral arteries: evaluation of an *in vitro* model and results of a pilot study. *ROFO-Forschritte auf dem Gebiet der Rontgenstrahlen und der Bilderbenden V* 2002; 174(10): 1261-8.

9. Silva JA, Ramee SR. The emergence of mechanical thrombectomy; a clot burden reduction approach. [Review] [64 refs]. *Sem Intervent Cardiol* 2000; 5(3):137-47.

10. Sniderman AD. Salvage of a severely ischemic limb by arteriovenous revascularization: a case report. *Can J Surg* 1984; 27(3): 274-7.

11. Starck EE, McDermott JC, Crummy AB, Turnipseed WD, Acher CW, Burgess JH. Percutaneous aspiration thromboembolectomy. *Radiol* 1985; 156(1): 61-6.

12. Zehnder T, Birrer M, Do DD, *et al.* Percutaneous catheter thrombus aspiration for acute or subacute arterial occlusion of the legs: how much thrombolysis is needed? *Eur J Vasc Endovasc Surg* 2000; 20(1):41-6.

13. Zana K, Otal P, Fornet B, *et al. In vitro* evaluation of a new rotational thrombectomy device: the Straub Rotarex catheter. [Evaluation Studies. Journal Article] *Cardiovasc Intervent Radiol* 2001; 24(5): 319-23.

14. Barth KH, Gosnell MR, Aubrey M, *et al.* Hydrodynamic thrombectomy system versus pulse spray thrombolysis for thrombosed haemodialysis grafts: a multicentre prospective randomized comparison. *Radiol* 2000; 217: 678-684.

15. Baba Y, Inoue H, Sasaki M, *et al.* Percutaneous mechanical thrombectomy for thrombosed vessels with a hydrolyser (hydrodynamic thrombectomy catheter): clinical experience. [Japanese] *Nippon Igaku Hoshasen Gakkai Zasshi - Nippon Acta Radiologica* 2000; 60(1): 23-7.

16. Gorriz JL, Martinez-Rodrigo J, Sancho A, *et al.* [Endoluminal percutaneous thrombectomy as a treatment for acute vascular access thrombosis: long-term results of 123 procedures]. [Spanish] *Nefrologia* 2001; 21(2):182-90.

17. Schmitz-Rode T, Janssens U, Duda SH, Erley CM, Gunther RW. Massive pulmonary embolism: percutaneous emergency treatment by pigtail rotation catheter. *J Amer Coll Cardiol* 2000; 36(2): 375-80.

18. Rocek M, Peregrin JH, Lasovickova J, Krajickova D, Slaviokova M. Mechanical thrombolysis of thrombosed hemodialysis native fistulas with use of the Arrow-Trerotola percutaneous thrombolytic device: our preliminary experience. *J Vasc Intervent Radiol* 2000; 11(9): 1153-8.

19. Vogel PM, Bansal V, Marshall MW. Thrombosed hemodialysis grafts: lyse and wait with tissue plasminogen activator or urokinase compared to mechanical thrombolysis with the Arrow-Trerotola Percutaneous Thrombolytic Device. *J Vasc Intervent Radiol* 2001; 12(10): 1157-65.

20. Sofocleous CT, Cooper SG, Schur I, Patel RI, Iqbal A, Walker S. Retrospective comparison of the Amplatz thrombectomy device with modified pulse-spray pharmacomechanical thrombolysis in the treatment of thrombosed hemodialysis access grafts. *Radiol* 1999; 213(2): 561-7.

21. Vesely TM, Williams D, Weiss M, *et al.* Comparison of the angiojet rheolytic catheter to surgical thrombectomy for the

treatment of thrombosed hemodialysis grafts. Peripheral AngioJet Clinical Trial. *J Vasc Intervent Radiol* 1999; 10: 1195-1205.

22. Green LD, Lee DS, Kucey DS. Institute for Clinical Evaluative Sciences, Toronto, Ontario, Canada. A metaanalysis comparing surgical thrombectomy, mechanical thrombectomy, and pharmacomechanical thrombolysis for thrombosed dialysis grafts. *J Vasc Surg* 2002; 36(5): 939-45.

23. Zeller T, Frank U, Burgelin K, *et al*. Acute thrombotic subclavian artery occlusion treated with a new rotational thrombectomy device. *J Endovasc Ther* 2002; 9(6): 917-21.

24. Ouriel K. Current status of thrombolysis for peripheral arterial occlusive disease. *Ann Vasc Surg* 2002; 16(6): 797-804.

25. Canova CR, Schneider E, Fischer L, *et al*. Long-term results of percutaneous thrombo-embolectomy in patients with infrainguinal embolic occlusions. *Int Angiol* 2001; 20(1): 66-73.

26. Desgranges P, Kobeiter K, d'Audiffret A, Melliere D, Mathieu D, Becquemin JP. Acute occlusion of popliteal and/or tibial arteries: the value of percutaneous treatment. *Eur J Vasc Endovasc Surg* 2000; 20(2): 138-45.

27. Zehnder T, Birrer M, Do DD, *et al*. Percutaneous catheter thrombus aspiration for acute or subacute arterial occlusion of the legs: how much thrombolysis is needed? *Eur J Vasc Endovasc Surg* 2000; 20(1): 41-6.

28. Ansel GM, George BS, Botti CF, *et al*. Rheolytic thrombectomy in the management of limb ischaemia: 30-day results from a multicentre registry. *J Endovasc Ther* 2002; 9(4): 395-402.

29. Kasirajan K, Gray B, Beavers FP, *et al*. Rheolytic thrombectomy in the management of acute and subacute limb-threatening ischemia. *J Vasc Intervent Radiol* 2001; 12(4): 413-21.

30. Beyer-Enke SA, Deichen J, Zeitler E. [The long-term results after Hydrolyser-supported angioplasty - a prospective study]. [German] *ROFO-Fortschritte auf dem Gebiet der Rontgenstrahlen und der Bildgebenden V* 1999; 171(2):126-9.

31. Silva JA, Ramee SR, Collins TJ, *et al*. Rheolytic thrombectomy in the treatment of acute limb-threatening ischaemia: immediate results and six-month follow-up of the multicenter Angiojet registry. *Cathet Cardiovasc Diagn* 1998; 45: 386-393.

32. Krajcer Z, Gilbert JH, Dougherty K, *et al*. Successful treatment of aortic endograft thrombosis with rheolytic thrombectomy. *J Endovasc Ther* 2002; 9(6): 756-64.

33. Sharafuddin MJ, Sun S, Hoballah JJ, *et al*. Endovascular management of venous thrombotic and occlusive disease of the lower extremities. *J Vasc Interv Radiol* 2003; 14: 405-423.

34. Kuntz RE, Baim DS, Cohen DJ, *et al*. A trial comparing rheolytic thrombectomy with intracoronary urokinase for coronary and vein graft thrombus (the Vein Graft AngioJet Study [VeGAS 2]). *Amer J Cardiol* 2002; 89(3): 326-30.

35. Silva JA, White CJ, Ramee SR, *et al*. Treatment of coronary stent thrombosis with rheolytic thrombectomy: results from a multicenter experience. *Catheterization & Cardiovascular Interventions* 2003; 58(1): 11-7.

36. Rinfret S, Katsiyiannis PT, Ho KK, *et al*. Effectiveness of rheolytic coronary thrombectomy with the AngioJet catheter. *Amer J Cardiol* 2002; 90(5): 470-6.

37. Yingfeng L, Nakamura S, Tanigawa J, *et al*. Successful thrombus removal using 6Fr hydrolyser thrombectomy catheter in acute myocardial infarction via radial artery. *J Intervent Cardiol* 2001; 14(4): 443-9.

38. Mayer TE, Hamann GF, Brueckmann HJ. Treatment of basilar artery embolism with a mechanical extraction device: necessity of flow reversal. *Stroke* 2002; 33(9): 2232-5.

39. Lutsep HL, Clark WM, Nesbit GM, Kuether TA, Barnwell SL. Intraarterial suction thrombectomy in acute stroke. *Am J Neuroradiol* 2002; 23(5): 783-6.

40. Bellon RJ, Putman CM, Budzik RF, Pergolizzi RS, Reinking GF, Norbash AM. Rheolytic thrombectomy of the occluded internal carotid artery in the setting of acute ischemic stroke. *Am J Neuroradiol* 2001; 22(3): 526-30.

41. Chow K, Gobin YP, Saver J, Kidwell C, Dong P, Vinuela F. Endovascular treatment of dural sinus thrombosis with rheolytic thrombectomy and intra-arterial thrombolysis. *Stroke* 2000; 31(6): 1420-5.

42. Dowd CF, Malek AM, Phatouros CC, Hemphill JC 3rd. Application of a rheolytic thrombectomy device in the treatment of dural sinus thrombosis: a new technique. *Am J Neuroradiol* 1999; 20(4): 568-70.

43. Fava M, Loyola S. Applications of percutaneous mechanical thrombectomy in pulmonary embolism. *Techniques in vascular and interventional radiology* 2003; 6(1): 53-8.

44. Schmitz-Rode T, Janssens U, Duda SH, *et al*. Massive Pulmonary Embolism: percutaneous emergency treatment by pigtail rotation catheter. *J Am Coll Cardiol* 2000; 36(2): 375-80.

45. Biederer J, Schoene A, Reuter M, Heller M, Muller-Hulsbeck S. Suspected pulmonary artery disruption after transvenous pulmonary embolectomy using a hydrodynamic thrombectomy device: clinical case and experimental study on porcine lung explants. *J Endovasc Ther* 2003; 10: 99-110.

46. Frisoli JK, Sze D. Mechanical thrombectomy for the treatment of lower extremity deep venous thrombosis. *Techniques in vascular and interventional radiology* 2003; 6(1): 49-52.

47. Vedantham S, Vesely TM, Parti N, *et al*. Lower extremity venous thrombolysis with adjunctive mechanical thrombectomy. *J Vasc Intervent Radiol* 2002; 13: 1001-1008.

48. Ries M, Zenker M, Girisch M, Klinge J, Singer H. Percutaneous endovascular catheter aspiration thrombectomy of severe superior vena cava syndrome. *Archives of Disease in Childhood Fetal & Neonatal Edition* 2002; 87(1): F64-6.

49. Gu X, Sharafuddin MJ, Titus JL, *et al*. Acute and delayed outcomes of mechanical thrombectomy with use of the steerable Amplatz thrombectomy device in a model of subacute inferior vena cava thrombosis. *J Vasc Intervent Radiol* 1997; 8: 947-956.

50. Muller-Hulsbeck S, Hopfner M, Hilbert C, Kramer-Hansen H, Heller M. Mechanical thrombectomy of acute thrombosis in transjugular intrahepatic portosystemic shunts. *Investigative Radiology* 2000; 35(6): 385-91.

51. Fontaine AB, Borsa JJ, Hoffer EK, Bloch RD, So CR. Newton M. Type III heart block with peripheral use of the Angiojet thrombectomy system. *J Vasc Intervent Radiol* 2001; 12(10): 1223-5.

52. Bilbao JI, Vivas I, Elduayen B, *et al*. Limitations of percutaneous techniques in the treatment of portal vein thrombosis. *Cardiovasc Intervent Radiol* 1999; 22(5): 417-22.

53. Morello FA, Jr., Mansilla AV, Michael J. Wallace Removal of Renal Fungus Balls Using a Mechanical Thrombectomy Device. *AJR* 2002; 178: 1191-1193.

54. Htaik TT, Santaniello NA, Markmann JF, Shaked A, Clark TW. Treatment of obstructive nephroureteral clot with a rheolytic mechanical thrombectomy device. *J Vasc Intervent Radiol* 2003; 14(7): 933-6.

Chapter 22

Bypass or angioplasty for severe ischaemia of the leg: the BASIL trial

Jocelyn Bell, BSc MSc PhD, BASIL Trial Co-ordinator

Donald J Adam, MD FRCSEd, Senior Lecturer in Vascular Surgery and Consultant Vascular Surgeon

Andrew W Bradbury, BSc MD FRCSEd, Professor of Vascular Surgery and Consultant Vascular Surgeon

Research Institute (Lincoln House), Birmingham Heartlands Hospital, Birmingham, UK

Introduction

In the UK, at least 20,000 patients are treated for severe limb ischaemia (SLI) each year at an estimated cost to the NHS of £1 billion [1]. The relative indications for bypass surgery and angioplasty (PTA) remain controversial with strongly held and diametrically opposed views being expressed by surgical and radiological experts [2-4]. Two randomised controlled trials have suggested that surgery and PTA may achieve similar survival and limb salvage rates in certain patients [5,6]. However, both trials were small, included mainly patients with intermittent claudication and provide little or no evidence on which to base current treatment of patients with SLI. Clinicians' views are therefore almost entirely based on prejudices acquired during their training and the results of uncontrolled observational studies.

Many vascular surgeons still believe that surgery is the treatment of choice for virtually all patients affected by SLI. However, PTA is increasingly used as a first-line treatment and has a number of theoretical advantages: it may be safer, quicker and less expensive than surgery, suitable vein is not required, it is easily repeated and it may not prejudice subsequent surgical bypass if required [7,8]. In Leicester Royal Infirmary, for example, PTA accounts for over 85% of primary revascularisation procedures in patients with SLI [9]. Complex lesions are treated with a high primary technical success rate (over 80%), low major complication rate (less than 5%) and a short hospital stay. Furthermore, over 50% of patients with recurrent SLI can be successfully treated by means of further PTA [9-11]. Although surgery may well provide a better long-term anatomic patency, this may not translate into a superior clinical outcome overall because of the initial high morbidity and mortality; patients may not live long enough to reap the potential long-term patency benefits and, even if a PTA site does re-occlude, the limb may remain viable due to the development of collaterals.

The BASIL trial

The Bypass versus Angioplasty in Severe Ischaemia of the Leg (BASIL) trial is a multicentre randomised controlled trial funded by the Health Technology Assessment arm of the UK National Health Service (NHS) (Figure 1). The specific aim of the trial is to determine whether, in patients with SLI amenable to PTA or bypass surgery, adopting a 'PTA

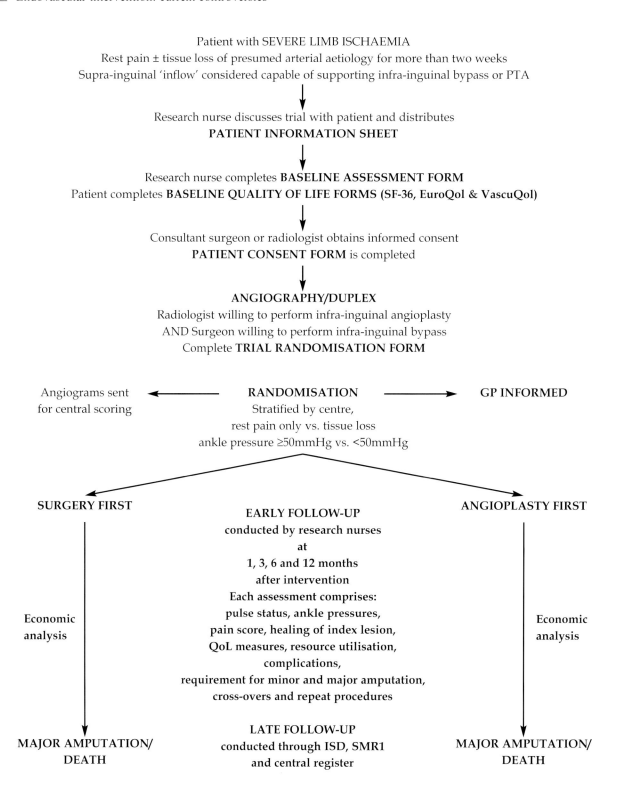

Figure 1. Outline of Bypass versus Angioplasty in Severe Ischaemia of the Leg (BASIL) Trial.

first' strategy rather than the traditional 'surgery first' strategy is associated with a better outcome in terms of:-

◆ amputation-free survival (primary end-point);
◆ abolition of symptoms, procedure complications, secondary and cross-over interventions, minor amputations, quality of life and cost-effective utilisation of NHS resources (secondary end-points).

Suitability for surgery or angioplasty: the Delphi consensus

Prior to the start of the BASIL trial, it became apparent that many of the vascular surgeons and radiologists who had indicated a willingness to participate had strong and fixed views as to the relative merits of surgery and PTA when it came to treatment of individual patients. These fixed ideas were largely a product of the particular institution in which they had trained, intuition and the relative availability of surgical and radiological resources, rather than a critical appraisal of a sound evidence base, which does not exist. It was considered that these fixed ideas were likely to hamper recruitment into the BASIL trial and that a Delphi consensus study could be used to:-

◆ define and quantify the level of agreement / disagreement amongst surgeons and radiologists regarding the preferred surgical and / or endovascular management of SLI;
◆ examine angiographic and clinical factors that impact upon these treatment preferences;
◆ establish a 'grey area of clinical equipoise' where patients could be randomised within BASIL.

A two-round Delphi consensus study was therefore conducted with the help of a panel of 20 consultant surgeons and 17 consultant interventional radiologists who had initially expressed a willingness to participate in the BASIL trial. Each panellist was presented with 149 angiographic representations of the lower limb ranging from minimal to severe disease. For each scenario panellists were asked to score their preferences for PTA, bypass surgery or primary amputation on an eight-point scale. Further, they were

asked to score each angiographic representation four separate times, on the basis of whether the patients had rest pain only or tissue loss, and whether a suitable vein was available for bypass. This meant that each panellist scored 596 scenarios. The median and range of these first-round responses for each scenario were then fed back to panellists so that each could see where their responses lay in relation to those of their peers. Panellists were given the opportunity to amend their responses in the second round by completing the questionnaire again.

Details of the BASIL trial Delphi consensus methods and the main findings have now been published [12,13]. The results of the consensus indicate substantial levels of disagreement between and among surgeons and radiologists with regard to the appropriateness of PTA, bypass surgery or primary amputation to treat SLI over a wide range of clinical and angiographic severities of disease. The panellists disagreed about the appropriateness of treatment in 81% of the scenarios in round one and 67% in round two. Disagreement was greater among surgeons compared with radiologists in both round one (83% vs. 65%) and round two (69% vs. 42%). Surgeons also demonstrated less convergence between rounds. This lack of consensus stems from an absence of an evidence base and means that the same patient may receive entirely different treatment depending on which hospital and consultant they attend. Although the Delphi study clearly demonstrated a large collective 'grey area of clinical equipoise', there is much less equipoise on the part of individual clinicians. Most clinicians have strong preferences as to how individual patients should be treated despite a complete lack of level I evidence to guide them. It was hoped that the results of this study, together with the recognition that current practice is not evidence-based, would encourage the randomisation of patients into the BASIL trial.

BASIL trial methodology

Patient recruitment into the BASIL trial commenced August 1999. Recruitment is due to finish in the spring or early summer of 2004 by which time it is hoped that a total of 450 patients will have been entered from 27 participating centres in England and Scotland. The

Table 1. Patient stratification into four groups at randomisation.

Clinical presentation	Ankle pressure ≥50mmHg	Ankle pressure <50mmHg
Rest/night pain only	A	B
Tissue loss ± rest/night pain	C	D

trial is due to finish in summer 2005 once all patients have been followed-up for a minimum of 12 months.

Patients with both critical (CLI) [14] and sub-critical limb ischaemia (SCLI) [15] are randomised within BASIL provided they have:-

◆ ischaemic rest pain requiring strong (opiate) analgesia for more than two weeks, or ulceration or gangrene of the foot or toes;
◆ no significant supra-inguinal disease, although aorto-iliac disease could be treated by surgery or PTA (± stent) prior to randomisation;
◆ given fully informed written consent;
◆ not got a degree of limb ischaemia, or a co-existing medical or surgical condition, that makes revascularisation inappropriate;
◆ an angiographic pattern of infra-inguinal disease that, in the opinion of the responsible consultant surgeon and radiologist, could be reasonably managed either by surgery or PTA in the first instance. In centres where treatment decisions for patients with SLI were routinely made on the basis of duplex findings, patient entry into BASIL could be decided from duplex results.

At randomisation, patients are stratified on the basis of their ankle pressure and clinical presentation into four groups as shown in Table 1.

Assessment of pre-intervention angiograms

In order to establish that both treatment groups are matched in terms of pattern and severity of arterial disease, copies of pre-intervention angiograms for all randomised patients are being scored. Two independent observers are scoring each angiogram blind to the treatment that the patient went on to receive using a modified Bollinger scoring system [16,17]. Each limb is being assessed from the common femoral bifurcation to the plantar arch with each vessel segment divided into two halves.

Clinical assessment

Prior to randomisation, relevant baseline information is collected including demographic data, risk factors, relevant past medical history, current medications, ankle pressures and ABPI and presenting symptoms, i.e. the presence of rest pain, ulceration and/or gangrene. Patients are randomised to either PTA or bypass surgery according to centre and stratification group on a 50:50 basis. Interventions are performed using the normal procedures of the participating centre and relevant details documented.

Patients are followed up at one, three, six, and 12 months after primary intervention, or until they meet a primary end-point of major amputation or death, either in a hospital-based clinic or by home visit. Ankle pressure measurements and changes in presenting symptoms (rest pain, ulceration and/or gangrene) are recorded at each follow-up. Details of any further or cross-over interventions during this follow-up period are recorded but the patients continue to be followed-up from the time of primary intervention. From 12 months onwards, patients return to normal clinical care but are followed-up through the Information and Statistics Division of the NHS in Scotland or regional Trusts in England.

Quality of life assessment

Patients are being asked to complete three quality of life questionnaires, the SF-36, EuroQol and the recently developed disease-specific instrument for lower limb ischaemia, VascuQol at Baseline and three, six and 12 months after primary intervention. The three questionnaires are also being posted to patients annually after 12-month follow-up.

Economic evaluation

Detailed information about length of stay in hospital and utilisation of equipment, drugs, time and personnel during interventions is being collected for each patient both at the time of the primary intervention and for any further interventions to the trial leg. At each follow-up visit self-reported data on primary care consultations, receipt of community health services and any further hospital out-patient visits and in-patient episodes are being collected. These data will be used to investigate the relative use of NHS resources and thereby the costs of treatments for the two patient groups.

Survey of non-randomised patients

In accordance with the CONSORT document, at the start of the BASIL trial an attempt was made to collect data on all patients presenting at participating centres with SLI who were deemed unsuitable for recruitment into BASIL. Data were collected from 491 patients who presented at eight different centres over periods between six and 15 months. However, as time progressed it was recognised that collecting data on all patients unsuitable for entry into BASIL at all participating centres was impossible for a number of reasons:-

◆ Patient care pathways differed between centres and, for example, in centres where patients were not admitted onto specialised vascular wards, ensuring that information was collected on all patients proved difficult.
◆ As more centres became involved in BASIL, manpower became stretched and it became difficult to ensure that data were collected on all patients.

◆ The relative enthusiasm of different consultants in the same centre to recruit patients into BASIL meant that patients suitable for the trial were not always randomised making data analysis difficult.
◆ It was frequently difficult, if not impossible, to determine why an individual patient was not deemed suitable for randomisation.

Because of the difficulties of obtaining meaningful information on all patients presenting with SLI at all centres, the first survey was abandoned and a more structured audit was undertaken. This survey was carried out in six of the major recruitment centres where manpower was available to complete the paperwork. The survey was limited to a six-month period between October 2001 and April 2002. Detailed data, equivalent to that collected for randomised patients at Baseline, were collected from all patients with SLI who underwent angiographic imaging during this period. Information was also collected on the type and location of arterial disease, the reason why the patient was deemed unsuitable for recruitment into BASIL and the treatment that they went on to receive. Although every attempt was made to collect the relevant data prospectively, this was not always possible and data had to be obtained retrospectively by interrogation of patient case notes. Full analysis of the data collected is still in progress. The results of the survey will be published in the near future.

Conclusions

The results of the BASIL trial will be presented in early 2006. The aim of treatment of patients with SLI is to guarantee a clinically optimal solution with long-term benefit within an acceptable economic frame. The results of the BASIL trial will provide the first level I evidence regarding the relative clinical and economic merits of PTA and bypass surgery in the treatment of patients with SLI. Furthermore, leaving aside the randomisation, it will be the largest most clinically and economically detailed cohort of treated patients with SLI ever described.

Summary

♦ Patients suffering from SLI are currently treated on the basis of personal experience and training of individual physicians, intuition and the results of uncontrolled observational studies often reported in single centre or even single operator series.

♦ The UK BASIL trial is a multicentre randomised controlled trial comparing the clinical and cost-effectiveness of PTA and bypass surgery as the first-line treatment of patients with SLI due to infra-inguinal arterial disease.

♦ The BASIL trial Delphi consensus confirmed that a substantial level of disagreement exists both between and among surgeons and radiologists with regard to the appropriateness of PTA, bypass surgery or primary amputation as first-line treatment for SLI.

♦ The high level of disagreement identified in the Delphi consensus reflects a large collective 'grey area of clinical equipoise' within which it was ethical to randomise patients into the BASIL trial.

♦ 450 patients with SLI will be randomised into the BASIL trial and have received first-line treatment by either PTA or bypass surgery. The outcomes of the BASIL trial will be presented in early 2006.

References

1. Vascular Surgical Society of Great Britain and Ireland. Critical limb ischaemia: management and outcome. Report of a national survey. *Eur J Vasc Endovasc Surg* 1995; 10: 108-113.

2. Parsons RE, Suggs WD, Lee JJ, *et al*. Percutaneous transluminal angioplasty for the treatment of limb threatening ischaemia: do the results justify an attempt before bypass grafting? *J Vasc Surg* 1998; 28: 1066-1071.

3. Varty K, Nydahl S, Nasim A, *et al*. Results of surgery and angioplasty for the treatment of chronic severe lower limb ischaemia. *Eur J Vasc Endovasc Surg* 1998; 16: 159-163.

4. Bolia A. Percutaneous intentional extraluminal (subintimal) recanalization of crural arteries. *Eur J Radiol* 1998; 28: 119-204.

5. Wolf GL, Wilson SE, Cross AP. Percutaneous transluminal angioplasty versus operation for peripheral arteriosclerosis. *J Vasc Surg* 1989; 9: 1-9.

6. Holm J, Arfridsson B. Chronic lower limb ischaemia. A prospective randomised controlled trial comparing 1-year results of vascular surgery and percutaneous transluminal angioplasty (PTA). *Eur J Vasc Surg* 1991; 5: 517-522.

7. Vraux H, Hammer F, Verhelst R, *et al*. Subintimal angioplasty of tibial vessel occlusions in the treatment of critical limb ischaemia: mid-term results. *Eur J Vasc Endovasc Surg* 2000; 20: 441-446.

8. Ray SA, Monty I, Buckenham T, *et al*. Clinical outcome and restenosis following percutaneous transluminal angioplasty for ischaemic rest pain or ulceration. *Br J Surg* 1995; 82: 1217-1221.

9. Molloy KJ, Nasim A, London NJM, *et al*. Percutaneous transluminal angioplasty in the treatment of critical limb ischaemia. *J Endovasc Ther* 2003; 10: 298-303.

10. Papavassiliou VG, Walker SR, Bolia A, Fishwick G, London N. Techniques for the endovascular management of complications following lower limb percutaneous transluminal angioplasty. *Eur J Vasc Endovasc Surg* 2003; 25: 125-30.

11. Salas CA, Adam DJ, Papavassiliou VG, London NJM. Percutaneous transluminal angioplasty for critical limb ischaemia in octogenarians and nonagenarians. *Eur J Vasc Endovasc Surg* 2004 (in press).

12. Bradbury AW, Bell J, Lee AJ, *et al*. Bypass or angioplasty for severe limb ischaemia? A Delphi consensus study. *Eur J Vasc Endovasc Surg* 2002; 24: 411-416.

13. Bradbury AW, Wilmink T, Lee AJ, *et al* on behalf of the BASIL Trial Delphi Consensus Group. Bypass versus angioplasty to treat severe limb ischaemia: factors that affect treatment preferences of UK surgeons and interventional radiologists. *J Vasc Surg* 2004 (in press).

14. Second European Consensus Document on Critical Limb Ischaemia. *Eur J Vasc Surg* 1992; 6(Suppl A): 1-32.

15. Wolfe JHN, Wyatt MG. Critical and sub-critical limb ischaemia. *Eur J Vasc Endovasc Surg* 1997; 13: 578-582.

16. Bollinger A, Breddin K, Hess H, *et al*. Semiquantitative assessment of lower limb atherosclerosis from routine angiographic images. *Atherosclerosis* 1981; 38: 339-346.

17. Smith FB, Lee AJ, Fowkes FGR, *et al*. Classification of site of peripheral atherosclerosis and observer variation using the Bollinger angiographic scoring system. *J Vasc Invest* 1995; 1: 79-85.

Chapter 23

Closure devices: indications and results

Stephen D'Souza, MRCP FRCR, Consultant Vascular Radiologist
Royal Preston Hospital, Lancashire Teaching Hospitals NHS Trust, Preston, UK

Introduction

Annually between 7.5 and 8 million percutaneous catheter-based procedures are performed worldwide [1]. Over the last decade there has been increasing interest in methods of achieving more rapid, predictable arterial puncture-site haemostasis. The demand for this new technology has been driven by the need for increased patient safety following the publication of guidelines, by the Royal College of Radiologists, UK [2] (Table 1), and the Society of Cardiovascular and Interventional Radiology, for maximum complication rates for diagnostic and interventional radiology procedures. A second factor has been the desire to perform more procedures on a day-case basis.

There are few publications regarding the usage of closure devices in patients with peripheral vascular disease [3,4], the majority of the literature relating to coronary diagnostic and interventional procedures.

With the advent of more complicated interventional procedures requiring:-

◆ peri-procedural anticoagulation;
◆ more complex procedures; and

◆ the use of antiplatelet agents, eg. aspirin and clopidogrel bisulphate or GP IIb/IIIa platelet inhibitors,

the incidence of puncture site complications is increasing [5,6,7]. Larger delivery systems in themselves may not adversely affect complication rates, however, their association with more complex, protracted procedures may [7].

Complication rates for diagnostic angiograms range from 0% to 1.1%, whereas in therapeutic procedures requiring anticoagulation and/or larger sheath sizes (6-8 French), the complication rates can rise to 1.3-3.4%. In cardiac series, with complex procedures and multiple antiplatelet therapies, local complication rates as high as 9% have been reported [6,7].

Any method or device that can significantly reduce time-to-ambulation, whilst reducing complication rates, or at least keeping them within acceptable limits, would be highly desirable. There are several arterial closure devices currently available that use different methods to address this problem. Whilst these devices appear to reduce the time required to achieve haemostasis and the time-to-ambulation [8,9,10], they have not significantly reduced the complication rates and in certain situations, they have introduced

Table 1. Royal College of Radiologists' recommended upper limit of complications.

Complication	Diagnostic angiography (%)	Interventional procedures (%)
Puncture site		
Haematoma (requiring transfusion, surgery, or delayed discharge)	3.0	4.0
Occlusion	0.5	0.5
Pseudoaneurysm	0.5	NS
A-V fistula	0.1	NS
Non-puncture site		
Distal embolisation causing tissue damage	0.5	0.5
Unintended occlusion of selected vessel	2.0	3.0
Vessel rupture/perforation requiring surgery	NS	0.5
Emergency surgery	NS	3.0

A-V: arteriovenous

NS: not specified.

Reproduced with permission from the Royal College of Radiologists [2].

new complications [8,11]. One study even identified an increase in overall complication rates with closure devices as compared to manual compression [12].

As a result of the immediate cost, availability and potential complications, currently only 10% to 15% of all catheter-based procedures performed worldwide utilise a vascular closure device for access site haemostasis [1].

This review looks at the way closure devices work, the evidence for their use, and suggests patients for whom they may confer most benefit.

The various methods of achieving haemostasis can be categorised as follows:-

◆ Manual compression.
◆ Mechanical compression.
◆ Collagen plug device.
◆ Suture mediated device.
◆ Patch technology.

Manual compression

This method is considered as the gold standard and was described by Seldinger *et al* [13] in 1953. It involves manual compression over the puncture site, for 20 to 30 minutes, followed by overnight bed rest. Haemostasis is achieved as a result of the formation of a fibrin and platelet plug following exposure of the blood to the collagen in the arterial wall at the puncture site.

In a study of early mobilisation following manual compression of arteriotomies, up to 6 French, following angioplasty, 90% of 128 patients were ambulant at four hours following gradual mobilisation after two hours of supine bed rest. This was achieved with no major puncture site complications and no delayed complications (beyond four hours) [14].

It should be remembered that manual compression is not without risk. Reported major complications, from femoral artery puncture, associated with manual compression include active or late puncture site bleeding requiring surgery, pseudoaneurysm, A-V fistula, retroperitoneal haematoma, large (>5.0cm) haematoma, requirement of two units blood transfusion, secondarily infected haematoma, and femoral artery and femoral vein thrombosis [15,16].

Reported minor complications include small (<5.0cm) non-surgical haematoma, less than two units blood transfusion, periprocedural and prolonged leg pain, leg weakness and numbness, prolonged oozing, ecchymosis, bruit, acute and prolonged painful mass, back pain, prolonged immobilisation, increased length of stay, increased resource utilisation, and increased costs [15,16].

Manual compression has certain other less obvious clinical limitations which include the need to omit anticoagulants and/or antiplatelet therapy prior to the procedure or administer protamine following the procedure and the potential risk of repuncture.

Mechanical compression

There are a number of devices designed to aid manual compression. These include the Femstop (RADI Medical Systems, Uppsala, Sweden), the Clamp-ease (Pressure Products, Rancho Palos Verdes, CA, USA), sandbags and pressure dressings.

Whilst these may free up the primary operator without significant detriment to the patient, each device is dependent on patient compliance and close supervision, and the length of hospital stay is unaltered when compared to manual compression.

The potential problems associated with the existing mechanical compression devices are similar in nature to those associated with traditional manual compression. However, mechanical compression significantly reduces the incidence of these complications [5].

More recently, Safeguard (Datascope Corp., NJ, USA), a pressurised assisted dressing, has been introduced which may overcome some of the problems of older mechanical devices. At present there is limited clinical information available on its use.

Collagen plug devices

These were the first commercially available devices to address the problem of achieving rapid haemostasis and early ambulation.

Angio-Seal ™ (Figure 1)

The Angio-Seal device (St Jude Medical, Stratford-upon-Avon, UK) creates a mechanical seal by sandwiching the arteriotomy between a bioabsorbable intravascular foot plate and a bovine collagen sponge. Haemostasis is achieved primarily through mechanical means and is supplemented by the platelet inducing properties of the collagen.

The millennium platform and millennium EV device uses a suture and tension spring to maintain tension between the two other elements. The device is designed for sealing punctures up to 8 French and is available in 6 and 8 French forms with subtle differences in the method of placement. Both devices have been used for diagnostic and therapeutic procedures. One problem with this device is that the tension spring has to be left in place for 20 minutes before true haemostasis is established. Often the patient remains in the department for this period.

A newer version, the Angio-Seal STS and STS PLUS platform, features a self-tightening suture, allowing procedures to be completed on the catheter lab table. Deployment is simpler than the earlier device and 6 and 8 French sizes are available. Both sizes are suitable for use in therapeutic procedures.

With both versions of the device, the anchor is resorbed in a process that is physically complete at approximately 30 days and chemically complete at approximately 90 days post-procedure. As a result, arterial re-puncture within 90 days is not recommended, to prevent displacement of the anchor. It may be possible to identify and avoid the anchor using ultrasound if any re-intervention is required.

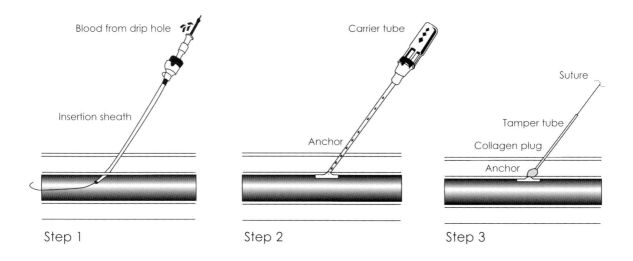

Step 1   Step 2   Step 3

Figure 1a. Angio-Seal STS deployment. The device is available in 6 French and 8 French versions. It consists of a delivery kit and three bioresorbable components: a flat 10mm X 2mm X 1mm anchor (footplate), a bovine collagen plug, and a suture that maintains tension between these two components. The delivery kit contains a guidewire, an insertion sheath, a dilator (arteriotomy locator), and a carrier tube. *Step 1* At the end of the procedure the insertion sheath/dilator is inserted over a guidewire. The 8 French device can be inserted over a standard 0.035″ wire but the 6 French version must be exchanged over the 0.032″ wire supplied. Correct placement is confirmed by blood exiting from the drip hole. Slowly pull back the whole system over the guidewire until blood stops and then reinsert 1.5cm. *Step 2* The guidewire and dilator are removed and the carrier tube containing the anchor, plug, and suture is inserted into the sheath. The anchor is deployed into the arterial lumen and pulled back to abut against the arteriotomy. *Step 3* The carrier tube and sheath are withdrawn to reveal a tamper tube that is used to tamp the collagen plug against the outer arterial wall and locks into place. The suture is cut below the skin. It is essential to cut the suture below the compaction marker, which is not bioresorbable.

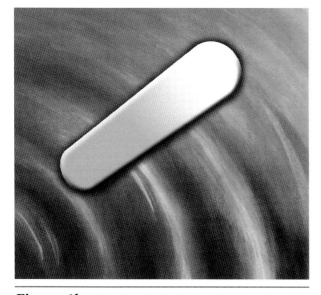

Figure 1b. The Angio-Seal STS device showing the flat 10mm X 2mm X 1mm anchor (footplate).

Vasoseal ™

The Vasoseal ES device (Datascope Corp, Montvale, New Jersey, USA) contains a purified bovine collagen plug delivered to the external surface of the artery. Collagen interacts with platelets in order to create a haemostatic seal directly over the arterial puncture site. This process is unaffected by aspirin or heparin. The device may be deployed after use of a 5-8 French sheath.

Duett™

The Duett device (Vascular Solutions Inc., Minneapolis, USA) comprises an ultra-fine (approximately 3 French) balloon catheter, which is passed through the arterial sheath (up to 9 French) and inflated in the lumen of the vessel. The balloon is elliptical in shape to reduce the likelihood of blocking the artery. The balloon is withdrawn to the arteriotomy site, which creates a temporary vascular seal, and 5-10mls of an extravascular procoagulant mixture is injected through the side arm of the sheath. The procoagulant consists of 50-60mg/ml of bovine microfibrillar collagen and 1000-2000 units/ml of bovine thrombin in isotonic saline. The procoagulant is mixed just prior to deployment.

Compression of the artery proximal to the puncture site is required for 2-5 minutes. Recommended ambulation times vary depending on sheath size, anticoagulation and/or antiplatelet agents and the angiographer's discretion.

Suture mediated devices

Perclose™ (Figure 2)

The Perclose (Abbott Vascular Devices, Redwood City, CA, USA) arterial closure device is designed to perform a percutaneous surgical closure of an arterial puncture using braided polyester sutures. Its primary healing is not dependent upon clot formation and can be used with patients who are anticoagulated or have undergone thrombolysis.

The original devices, Techstar 6F and Prostar 8F and 10F, contained one or two pairs of needles attached to one or two sutures. The device has an oversized hub and is passed over a guidewire. The needles are already attached to the suture and located in the intra-arterial shaft of the device. Once in place the needles pass from the lumen of the vessel, through the artery wall into the hub, taking the suture ends with them. A slipknot is tied to close the arteriotomy. The majority of published studies relate to these devices as opposed to the more recently introduced devices. The Prostar (8F and 10F) device, with two sutures and four needles, is still available.

More recently, the Closer S, a 6 French device, has replaced the Techstar 6F device. It can be used to close puncture sites up to 8 French. Larger sheath sizes can be accommodated if the device is deployed prior to arteriotomy dilation.

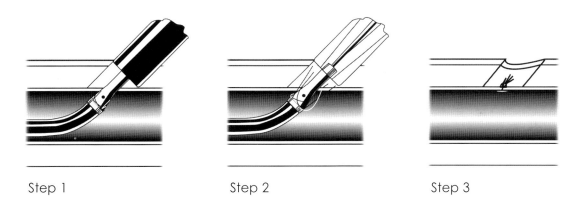

Step 1   Step 2   Step 3

Figure 2. Perclose Prostar deployment. The device is available in 8 French and 10 French versions. It consists of a shaft holding two pairs of needles connected by two braided polyester suture loops, and a rotating barrel used to facilitate the positioning of the device before needle deployment and to guide the needles during their travel through the subcutaneous tract. *Step 1* At the end of the procedure the sheath is removed and the device is inserted over a standard guidewire. Dilatation of the subcutaneous tract is needed to accept the oversize barrel. Correct positioning of the device with the barrel against the arterial wall is confirmed when pulsatile blood exits the marker lumen having entered the marker port within the artery. *Step 2* The needles are then deployed, passing from within the device in the arterial lumen, through the arterial wall and into the barrel. They take the suture ends with them and exit from the top of the device. *Step 3* The needles are cut from the sutures that are then freed from the device. The surgical knots are tied and slipped down onto the arterial wall whilst the device is removed. The knots are tightened with a knot pusher, achieving haemostasis, and the suture ends cut short.

As previously, the Closer S is inserted through the arteriotomy site, over a guidewire (Figure 3). Two needles pass from the hub of the device, through the artery wall into the lumen of the vessel where they attach to a plate that holds either end of the suture. As the needles are withdrawn, the stitch passes back through the arterial walls and a slipknot is tied to close the arteriotomy.

A newer version, the Perclose A-T (auto-tie), is now available (Figure 4). As the name suggests, the slipknot is created within the device, thus allowing quicker, easier and single-handed operation. Although there is some similarity in operation to the Closer device, there are significant changes. A structured training programme has been introduced to ensure correct operation.

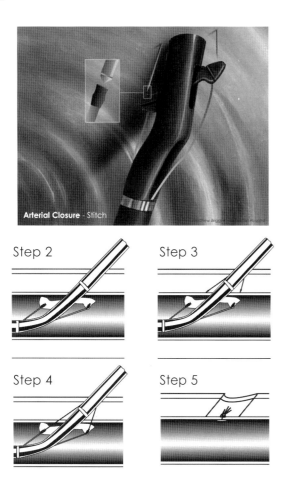

Figure 3. Closer S deployment. The device consists of a shaft containing a suture loop and separate needles, and a hub with a marker lumen, foot deployment lever, and needle plunger. It is supplied with a knot-tying device and knot pusher. *Step 1* At the end of the procedure, the sheath is removed and the device inserted over a standard guidewire. Correct positioning is confirmed by pulsatile blood from the marker lumen. *Step 2* Extension of the lever deploys the footplates, which carry the suture ends within the arterial lumen. *Step 3* Depressing the needle plunger deploys the needles from the shaft of the device within the subcutaneous tract. *Step 4* The needles then pass through the arterial wall and plug into the ends of the sutures in the footplates. Withdrawing the needle plunger from the device pulls the needles and suture ends through the arterial wall and up through the shaft of the device. The footplates are lowered again. *Step 5* The needles are cut from the suture, which is then freed from the device. The surgical knot is tied then slipped down onto the arterial wall whilst the device is removed. The knot is tightened with the knot pusher, achieving haemostasis, and the suture ends are cut short.

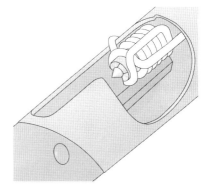

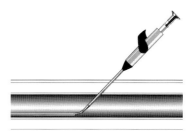

Figure 4. Perclose A-T deployment. The deployment procedure is very similar to that of the Closer S device. There are two significant differences. First, when the plunger is withdrawn, only one end of the suture appears, i.e one needle does not have a suture end attached to it. Second, the knot is already formed within the device and so this step is eliminated.

*X-Press*TM

The X-Press device (X-SITE Medical, Blue Bell, Pennsylvania, USA) is a suture-based vascular closure device designed to deliver single or multiple suture loops across the arteriotomy as the final step of a catheterisation procedure.

One small study (51 consecutive patients: 36 diagnostic angiography, 15 therapeutic interventions) demonstrated a 94% success rate in achieving haemostasis with the X-Press device. Patients in the study were successfully ambulated within approximately one hour following their catheterisation procedures. No major complications occurred. In a multicentre trial, results were not affected by the use of IIb/IIIa glycoprotein inhibitors [19].

*Sutura superstitch device*TM

This device is similar to the Closer S. However, it does not extend into the proximal portion of the artery. Needles pass from the shaft of the device, through the artery walls and attach to either end of a suture held on a footplate. The stitch is then pulled through the wall of the artery into the shaft of the device and a slipknot tied.

Deployment of collagen plug and suture mediated devices

Deployment success rates vary from 86% to 100%, with several authors reporting increased failure early in the learning curve. Warren experienced 14% non-deployment with Angio-Seal in the first 50 cases and 3.5% in the next 200 cases [20]. O'Sullivan quotes a 12% non-deployment rate for Angio-Seal in patients with peripheral vascular disease with the majority of failures early in their experience [3].

Deployment failure in 3.8% to 5.8% of cases is reported for the Duett device [10, 21].

Perclose (Prostar/Techstar) deployment failure rates vary from 3.6% to 12% [9,22]. However, some authors include in this figure residual oozing post-procedure requiring a short period of manual compression. This is often due to the dilatation of the

subcutaneous track to accept the oversize hub of the Prostar/Techstar device and therefore, does not represent arterial bleeding. In our experience, it does not occur with the Closer device because of its normal profile hub. Perclose devices have also been successfully deployed in the brachial and popliteal artery puncture sites, and to close inadvertent subclavian artery punctures created during central venous catheter insertion [23,24,25].

Time-to-ambulation

There is evidence that arterial closure devices are effective in achieving and reducing time to haemostasis [8,9,10]. A review of the literature of over 6000 patients managed with collagen plug devices revealed successful haemostasis in 50-98% for Vasoseal and 54-98% for Angio-Seal [21]. Variability in figures is partly accounted for by differences in use of antiplatelet and anticoagulant agents, and variation in time to removal of the sheath from the end of the procedure. Haemostasis has been achieved in one minute in 75% of patients in one study using Angio-Seal, and within two to five minutes in 95% of patients with the Duett device [15,26]. It should be noted that the Angio-Seal figure is slightly misleading, as the patient will require the suture and tension spring to remain in place for at least 20 minutes. The STS version has eliminated the need for this delay.

In a study of 80 patients with antegrade femoral punctures, a mean time to haemostasis of 5.2 minutes was achieved in 96% using the Prostar/Techstar Perclose devices [4]. With the Closer S device (Perclose) and now the Perclose A-T, the simplification of design and operation has reduced time to haemostasis as compared to the Prostar/Techstar device. In the author's experience with the Perclose A-T device, the time to haemostasis averaged less than a minute. This is in line with the manufacturer's claims.

Using Vasoseal, an ambulation time of one hour has been achieved with no increase in complication rate [27]. With the Perclose devices, short distance ambulation, except following thrombolysis, is possible immediately after depolyment. Our practice is to mobilise patients gently on return to the ward. If they have just undergone thrombolysis, mobilisation is delayed until the activated partial thromboplastin time (APTT) is below 140 seconds.

It must be remembered that traditional bed rest times for manual compression are arbitrarily set. One study showed no advantage of six hours bed rest over two hours post-manual compression following diagnostic cardiac catheterisation [28]. Furthermore, in a study of early mobilisation following manual compression of arteriotomies up to 6 French post-angioplasty, 90% of 128 patients were ambulant at four hours following gradual mobilisation after two hours of supine bed rest [14]. This was achieved with no major puncture site complications (Royal College of Radiologists' definitions - see Table 1) and no delayed complications (beyond four hours). These results support the view that for some therapeutic procedures outpatient angioplasty is possible without the use of closure devices.

Particular care and consideration should be exercised when using closure devices following angioplasty or stenting of an ipsilateral iliac artery, as any disturbance of flow at the puncture site may raise the possibility of post-intervention vessel thrombosis. The various devices have different effects in this respect. During Vasoseal deployment, occlusive pressure is required but once haemostasis is achieved, there is no flow disturbance. Similarly, with Duett, the balloon will cause considerable reduction in flow during deployment but once deflated, normal flow is restored. Flow disturbance from the Angio-Seal footplate is minimal in a normal calibre vessel but persists post-deployment. Insertion of the catheter of the Perclose devices over a wire should be atraumatic and any flow disturbance caused ceases post-deployment.

With the collagen plug devices, adequate haemostasis during device deployment is essential to prevent haematoma formation, this being particularly important in the use of Vasoseal due to its entirely extravascular nature. Any haematoma forming during Vasoseal deployment separates the collagen plug from the arterial wall making rapid haemostasis unlikely. In obese patients, this is a distinct possibility as proximal occlusive arterial compression may not be possible.

Complications

Unfortunately, but perhaps rather unsurprisingly, the use of arterial vascular closure devices has not eliminated the occurrence of puncture-site complications. Most of the published data on closure devices relates to cardiology patients and, in many of these studies, evidence of peripheral vascular disease was used as an exclusion criterion. However, complication rates are broadly similar in the few published series of patients with peripheral vascular disease [3, 4].

In a review of the world literature, Silber quotes minor complication rates of 8%, 5.9%, 5.3% and 2.1%, and major complication rates of 5.3%, 1.3%, 4% and 2.6% for Vasoseal, Angio-Seal, Perclose and Duett respectively [29]. In contrast, in a prospective study of 1605 cardiology patients, Shrake et al quote major complication rates of 0.6%, 3.2%, 2.3% and 1% for Vasoseal, Angio-Seal, Perclose and manual compression respectively [30]. A review of published data on over 6000 patients managed with Vasoseal or Angio-Seal showed no clinically relevant difference in minor complications compared with manual compression and no reduction in major complications [21].

Differences in the mechanism of action and methods of deployment of the devices can result in the potential for some specific individual complications:-

◆ Detachment and distal embolisation of the footplate of the Angio-Seal device has been reported by several authors [3, 8, 11].
◆ Intravascular placement of the collagen plug with Vasoseal has been reported with an incidence of between 0.3 and 2% [21].
◆ Arterial occlusion can occur with any device or manual compression, but stenosis of the punctured artery is again a reported complication of Angio-Seal, presumably due to the presence of the intravascular footplate [8, 11]. The other devices have a temporary effect on arterial flow, which returns to normal once haemostasis is achieved. Particular care and consideration should be exercised when using closure devices following angioplasty or stenting of an ipsilateral

iliac artery, as any disturbance of flow at the puncture site may raise the possibility of post-intervention vessel thrombosis.

◆ Adequate haemostasis during device deployment is essential to prevent haematoma formation, this being particularly important in the use of Vasoseal due to its entirely extravascular nature. Any haematoma forming during Vasoseal deployment separates the collagen plug from the arterial wall making rapid haemostasis unlikely. In obese patients, this is a distinct possibility as proximal occlusive arterial compression may not be possible.

◆ Delayed puncture site closure is not recommended, with the collagen plug devices, because of the increased risk of infection [18].

◆ A late soft tissue response caused by collagen can lead to scar formation and make future open surgical access difficult.

◆ The retrograde movement of the needles of the Prostar/Techstar, Perclose devices has resulted in device entrapment in the heavily scarred groins of patients with prosthetic grafts, requiring surgical removal (personal experience).

◆ Problems can occur with the needles attaching to the suture when using the Closer S device. The incidence of this has been reduced with the Perclose A-T.

◆ As all the collagen plug and suture mediated closure devices involve leaving a foreign body at the puncture site there is an increased risk of local infection, especially in the presence of a haematoma, and therefore, scrupulous aseptic technique should be observed [8, 26, 31].

It should be noted that the majority of recent studies still relate to older versions of the various devices. The Angio-Seal STS and Perclose A-T are significantly better than their predecessors and it is likely deployment failures and complication rates will decrease.

Patch technology

Recently, there has been increasing interest and availability of so called 'patch technologies' which encompass a group of products that augment manual compression. They consist of celluloid polymer patches coated with agents that are applied externally and accelerate the coagulation process when blood comes into contact with the patch, along the puncture tract. Manual compression is still required. However, they have a number of advantages:-

◆ Easy to use.
◆ Can be used in anticoagulated patients.
◆ Can be used in patients on antiplatelet therapy.
◆ No foreign body left in situ.
◆ No arterial or groin changes that preclude re-intervention or surgery.
◆ One size fits all.

At present, there is no clinical evidence that the time to ambulation is reduced with these devices.

Currently available patch products are the Syvec NT patch (Marine Polymer Technologies, Danvers, MA, USA), the D-Stat (Vascular Solutions, Inc, Minnesota, USA), the Chito-Seal (Abbott Vascular, Redwood City, CA, USA) and the Clo-Sur PAD (Scion Cardio-vascular, Miami, Florida, USA).

SyvecPatch™

The SyvecPatch consists of a celluloid polymer patch coated with poly-N-acetyl glucosamine (pGlcNAc). Where it comes into contact with blood, it invokes both clot formation and local vasoconstriction as part of its overall haemostatic effect [17]. Following the procedure the sheath is removed and the saline moistened SyvecPatch applied and held in place with manual compression for four minutes. Manual compression is maintained if oozing of blood occurs. Once haemostasis is achieved, the patch is left in place with a non-occlusive dressing for 24 hours.

In a study of 1000 consecutive patients (364 interventional procedures, 636 diagnostic procedures) only one serious complication (0.1%; pseudoaneurysm) occurred. Minor complications (small haematoma or slight ooze) occurred in 13 patients. Sheath sizes ranged from 4-12 French and 12% of patients were on anticoagulant and/or antiplatelet therapy. Neither factor affected outcome [17].

D-Stat™

D-Stat uses an adhesive dressing containing thrombin and is available for use in the UK. However, clinical information is limited. Application is the same as with the other two devices, although the company recommends an initial check after five minutes. Once haemostasis is achieved, the patch is left in place with a non-occlusive dressing for 12-24 hours. The patch can be used with puncture sites up to 8 French and in patients on anticoagulation and/or antiplatelet therapy.

Chito-seal™

As with the other devices the Chito-seal is a topical haemostasis pad. In this case, the active ingredient is Chitosan gel. Application is the same as with the other two devices, although the company recommends an initial check after 2-3 minutes. Once haemostasis is established, a dressing is applied and removed within 24hrs.

Future developments

Matrix VSG™

Matrix VSG (Vascular Sealing Gel) (Access Closure Inc., Palo Alto, CA, USA), is comprised of a synthetic polymer and delivery catheter. It is a tissue-adherent, flexible sealant, consisting of two fully synthetic, non-thrombogenic liquids that, when mixed together, rapidly crosslink to form a biocompatible absorbable poly(ethyleneglycol)-based hydrogel. The gel solidifies within seconds of injection and provides secure haemostasis within one minute.

To achieve haemostasis, Matrix VSG is injected through a standard introducer sheath while the delivery catheter provides temporary haemostasis. After injection of the polymer, the delivery catheter is removed and non-occlusive pressure is maintained for one to three minutes.

SoundSeal Noninvasive Haemostasis System™

SoundSeal Noninvasive Haemostasis System® Pending (Therus Corp., Seattle, WA, USA) is an ultrasound-based device that noninvasively targets and delivers to the puncture site, ultrasound energy that induces puncture site sealing in seconds. The approach is independent of the puncture size and the patient's coagulation status because the mechanism of sealing is not dependent on clotting. The device is noninvasive, and no foreign materials are introduced into the catheter track, thereby reducing the risk of complication.

Angiolink EVS™

Angiolink EVS is a staple mediated device that provides a mechanical closure of the arteriotomy site. The device deploys a titanium staple, which expands to 13 French before closure to ensure adequate tissue capture. At present, it is awaiting approval and, at the time of writing, the company was unable to provide any clinical research data (personal communication with company).

Conclusions

As with any situation where there are a number of solutions to a problem, no single method of achieving haemostasis is perfect. Without doubt, the most important step in reducing puncture site complications is good technique and operator experience, both with regards to the initial puncture and the use of the favoured closure device.

In the UK, operator choice will be limited by product availability (not all devices described are available in the UK), available facilities (without a recovery bay and dedicated nursing staff, promoted cost saving may not be achievable) and financial constraints.

The data makes it difficult to recommend the use of closure devices in all patients, but there are certain circumstances and patient types for which their use may be particularly advantageous:-

◆ The earlier ambulation times achieved may facilitate day-case angioplasty and/or stenting, even when large sheaths are used and the patients are highly anticoagulated. The cost of the device should be offset by the savings in bed occupancy and nursing time.

- Patients with cardiorespiratory disease who are unable to lie flat for prolonged periods can sit up shortly after a procedure if a closure device is used.
- The risk of performing procedures in patients that are unable to lie still, (eg. confused patients, psychiatric patients, and patients with movement disorders) may be greatly reduced.
- The use of closure devices in patients who are unable to stop their anticoagulants, (eg. those with prosthetic heart valves) or who have undergone thrombolysis should greatly reduce the risk of bleeding and other puncture site complications.

Arterial closure devices have been shown to reduce the time-to-haemostasis and ambulation, but complication rates are similar when compared with manual compression. As a result of this and the additional costs of these devices, their widespread use is not the norm. It should be remembered that multiple patient-satisfaction surveys have consistently identified the importance of patient comfort, ease in ambulation, and the need to 'improve the overall interventional experience', but this remains a low priority in healthcare [32].

In our practice, manual compression is usually sufficient for diagnostic angiography and interventional procedures using small sheaths. For interventional procedures using larger sheaths, particularly in the context of a day-case service and the other specific applications discussed, the use of arterial closure devices has been greatly beneficial.

Acknowledgement

The author would like to thank Matthew Briggs, Department of Medical Illustration, Royal Preston Hospital, for his help with the illustrations.

Summary

- Avoid diagnostic angiography where possible. Consider magnetic resonance angiography or Doppler ultrasound.
- Common femoral artery punctures should be single wall, single pass over femoral head. If uncertain, use ultrasound guidance.
- Prolonged procedures increase the risk of puncture site complications.
- Manual compression should be used for small puncture sites.
- Closure devices have their place in the management of larger puncture sites especially in highly anticoagulated patients. However, the operator must be fully trained in their use.

References

1. Strategic growth opportunities in cardiovascular interventional treatment drives cardiology sector. American Health Consultants. BBI Newsletter. 2001; 5: 1-6.

2. The Royal College of Radiologists. The Royal College of Radiologists Standards in Vascular Radiology. London, BFCR, 1999.

3. O'Sullivan GJ, Buckenham TM, Belli AM. The use of the Angio-Seal hemostatic puncture closure device in high-risk patients. *Clin Radiol* 1999; 54: 51-5.

4. Duda SH, Wiskirchen J, Erb M, *et al*. Suture-mediated percutaneous closure of antegrade femoral arterial access sites in patients who have received full anticoagulation therapy. *Radiology* 1999; 210: 47-52.

5. Prayck JB, Wall TC, Longabaugh P, *et al*. A randomised trial of vascular hemostasis techniques to reduce femoral vascular complications after coronary intervention. *Am J Cardiol* 1998; 81: 970-6

6. Muller DW, Shamir KJ, Ellis SG, Topol EJ. Peripheral vascular complications after conventional and complex percutaneous coronary interventional procedures. *Am J Cardiol* 1992; 69: 63-68.

7. Waksman R, Spencer BK III, Douglas JS, *et al*. Predictors of groin complications after balloon and new device intervention. *Am J Cardiol* 1995; 75: 886-9

8. Eidt JF, Habibipour S, Saucedo JF, *et al*. Surgical complications from hemostatic puncture closure devices. *Am J Surg* 1999; 178: 511-6.

9. Gerckens U, Cattelaens N, Lampe EG, *et al*. Management of arterial puncture site after catheterization procedures: evaluating a suture-mediated closure device. *Am J Cardiol* 1999; 83: 1658-63.

10. Ellis S, *et al*. Duett femoral artery closure device versus manual compression after diagnostic or interventional catheterization: Results of the SEAL trial. *Circulation* 1999; 100 (Suppl 1): 2703.

11. Goyen M, Manz S, Kroger K, *et al*. Interventional therapy of vascular complications caused by the hemostatic puncture closure device Angio-seal. *Catheter Cardiovasc Interv* 2000; 49: 142-7.

12. Dangas G, Mehran R, Kokolis S, *et al*. Vascular complications after percutaneous coronary interventions following hemostasis with manual compression versus arteriotomy closure devices. *J Am Coll Cardiol* 2001; 38: 638-641.

13. Seldinger SI. Catheter replacement of the needle in percutaneous arteriography. *Acta Radiol* 1953; 39: 366-376

14. Butterfield JS, Fitzgerald JB, Razzaq R, *et al*. Early mobilization following angioplasty. *Clin Radiol* 2000; 55: 874-7.

15. Kussmaul WG, Buchbinder M, Whitlow PL, *et al*. Rapid arterial hemostasis and decreased access site complications after cardiac catheterization and angioplasty: results of a randomized trial of a novel hemostatic device. *J Am Coll Cardiol* 1995; 25: 1685-1692.

16. Duffin DC, Muhlestein JB, Allison SB, *et al*. Femoral arterial puncture management after percutaneous coronary procedures: a comparison of clinical outcomes and patient satisfaction between manual compression and two different vascular closure devices. *J Invas Cardiol* 2001; 13: 354-362.

17. Nader RG, Garcia JC, Drushal T, *et al*. Clinical evaluation of Syvek patch in patients undergoing interventional, EPS and diagnostic cardiac catheterisation procedures. *J Invas Cardiol* 2002; 14: 305-7

18. Carere RG, Webb JG, Miyagishima R, *et al*. Groin complications associated with collagen plug closure of femoral arterial puncture sites in anticoagulated patients. *Cathet Cardiovasc Diagn* 1998; 43: 124-9

19. Mehta H, Chatterjee T, Windecker S, *et al*. Novel femoral artery puncture closure device in patients undergoing interventional and diagnostic cardiac procedures. *J Invas Cardiol* 2002; 14: 9-12.

20. Warren BS, Warren SG, Miller SD. Predictors of complications and learning curve using the Angio-Seal closure device following interventional and diagnostic catheterization. *Catheter Cardiovasc Interv* 1999; 48: 162-6.

21. Silber S. Hemostasis success rates and local complications with collagen after femoral access for cardiac catheterization: Analysis of 6007 published patients. *Am Heart J* 1998; 135: 152-6.

22. Baim DS, Knopf WD, Hinohara T, *et al*. Suture-mediated closure of the femoral access site after cardiac catheterization: results of the suture to ambulate and discharge (STAND I and STAND II) trials. *Am J Cardiol* 2000; 85: 864-9.

23. Kulick DL, Rediker DE. Use of the Perclose device in the brachial artery after coronary intervention. *Catheter Cardiovasc Interv* 1999; 46: 111-2.

24. Hoffmann K, Schott U, Erb M, *et al*. Remote suturing for percutaneous closure of popliteal artery access. *Cathet Cardiovasc Diagn* 1998; 43: 477-82.

25. Berlet MH, Steffen D, Shaughness G, *et al*. Closure using a surgical closure device of inadvertent subclavian artery punctures during central venous catheter placement. *Cardiovasc Intervent Radiol* 2001; 24: 122-4.

26. Silber S, Tofte AJ, Kjellevand TO, *et al*. Final report of the European multi-center registry using the Duett vascular sealing device. *Herz* 1999; 24: 620-3.

27. Schickel SI, Adkisson P, Miracle V, *et al*. Achieving femoral artery hemostasis after cardiac catheterization: a comparison of methods. *Am J Crit Care* 1999; 8: 406-9.

28. Logemann T, Luetmer P, Kaliebe J, *et al*. Two versus six hours bed rest following left-sided cardiac catheterization and a meta-analysis of early ambulation trials. *Am J Cardiol* 1999; 84: 486-8.

29. Silber S. 10 years of arterial closure devices: a critical analysis of their use after PTCA. *Z Kardiol* 2000; 89: 383-9.

30. Shrake KL. Comparison of major complication rates associated with four methods of arterial closure. *Am J Cardiol* 2000; 85: 1024-5.

31. Cooper CL, Miller A. Infectious complications related to the use of the Angio-Seal hemostatic puncture closure device. *Cathet Cardiovasc Interv* 1999; 48: 301-3.

32. Rickli H, Unterweger M, Sutsch G, *et al*. Comparison of costs and safety of a suture-mediated closure device with conventional manual compression after coronary artery interventions. *Cathet Cardiovasc Interv* 2002; 57: 297-302.

PART V. Renal and mesenteric disease

Chapter 24

Renal angioplasty and stenting: indications and results

Jon G Moss, FRCS FRCR, Consultant Interventional Radiologist

Interventional Radiology Unit, North Glasgow Hospitals University NHS Trust

Gartnavel Hospital, Glasgow, UK

Introduction

In 1978, Andreas Gruentzig published a short communication in the *Lancet* describing the world's first renal angioplasty (PTRA). It was reported as a triumph '...blood pressure fell to normal and renal plasma flow increased' [1]. It was proposed that PTRA would be an alternative to surgical revascularisation. It is interesting to reflect upon these words 25 years later. There is little doubt that with the advent of stents, endovascular methods have largely replaced surgical techniques as the primary method of renal revascularisation in the majority of patients. However, (and this is the crux of the problem), the encouraging clinical response that Gruentzig reported in this single patient has not been reproduced in larger series and indeed, randomised controlled trials (RCTs). Considerable sceptism and controversy persists after all these years and we still have much to learn about the role of renal revascularisation in patients with atherosclerotic renal artery stenosis.

Incidence and pathophysiology

Renal artery stenosis (RAS) is an anatomical description of a lesion, which may lead to a variety of pathophysiological disease processes or simply exist as a silent lesion throughout life. By far the commonest aetiology is atherosclerosis, although in some parts of the world the less common arteridites are more prevalent. The mechanism whereby RAS can lead to hypertension through the renin-angiotensin pathway is well described and will not be repeated here. The process whereby atherosclerotic renovascular disease (ARVD) can lead to impaired renal function is much less well understood. The notion that reduced blood flow is the answer is naïve in the extreme and other processes such as cholesterol embolisation, small vessel atherosclerosis and hypertensive glomerulosclerosis, frequently coexist. Although we know that complete renal artery occlusion usually leads to loss of renal function there is no clear relationship between the degree of RAS and renal function [2]. Indeed, the group from Guy's hospital in London have shown that in patients with unilateral RAS, the glomerular filtration rate (GFR) is often higher in the stenotic kidney that the normal contralateral side [3]!

Arteridites

The arteridites make up a rare group of disparate disorders of which the most common is fibromuscular disease. There is little controversy regarding their management and, therefore, will not be discussed in this chapter.

Atherosclerosis

Atherosclerotic renovascular disease (ARVD) is very prevalent in the West, and is a disease of ageing. A post-mortem study from over three decades ago showed the incidental finding of significant ARVD (defined as >50% RAS) in over 40% of patients aged over 75 years [4], irrespective of their cause of death. This high prevalence should be of no surprise, as a similar proportion of aged patients are likely to have significant coronary, cerebrovascular and peripheral vascular disease (PVD). ARVD has been shown to be frequently associated with these conditions. As so many patients are likely to have 'clinically silent' ARVD, it is not possible to estimate the true prevalence of the condition in the general population. However, using a definition of >60% RAS as determined by Doppler ultrasound, Hansen *et al* did show that 6.8% of 834 community-based people aged over 65 years had significant (and incidental) ARVD [5]. ARVD can present with hypertension, acute or chronic renal failure, cardiac failure or with one of the extra-renal vascular pathologies alluded to above.

Although much of the original research involved renovascular hypertension, there has been a renewed interest focusing on renal impairment. ARVD is now the commonest cause of end-stage renal failure in patients aged over 60 years on renal replacement therapy, accounting for at least 25% of this group [6]. Renal revascularisation by either an endovascular or open surgical method has the potential to alter this process and prevent progression to end-stage renal failure. Two randomised trials, one in the UK (ASTRAL) and the other in Holland (STAR), are comparing renal stenting with best medical treatment to test this hypothesis and should report in five years.

Natural history

ARVD is a progressive disorder. Prospective sequential doppler studies have indicated that stenoses <60% have a 42% of progressing to >60%

and those >60% have an 11% chance of progressing to occlusion over a two-year period with consequent loss of functioning renal mass [7-8]. This is probably the strongest (and maybe the only), argument for renal revascularisation. However, a more recent study has suggested a lower rate of RAS progression and that other factors, such as hypertension, may be more important than RAS in determining progression to renal atrophy [9].

Clinical presentation

ARVD is often a silent symptomless disease and indeed, when it does manifest with symptoms - hypertension, renal insufficiency and pulmonary oedema - there may be other more prevalent causes for these very same symptoms. So, it is often impossible to determine the role of ARVD and it is not uncommon for renal revascularisation to be used almost as a diagnostic test.

ARVD should always be considered in patients presenting with hypertension and/or renal failure who have evidence of atheromatous disease. Specific clinical features include ACE-inhibitor related renal dysfunction, or unexplained pulmonary oedema, but the presence of femoral, renal or aortic bruits and the co-existence of severe extra-renal vascular disease are the main clinical pointers [10]. In patients with severe (often systolic) hypertension, especially when unresponsive to three or more antihypertensive agents, increased vigilance for RAS is advised [11].

Clinical features suggestive of ARVD are:-

◆ Hypertension.
◆ Renal insufficiency.
◆ Other vascular disease.
◆ ACE-inhibitor induced renal insufficiency.
◆ Unexplained pulmonary oedema.
◆ Vascular bruits.

Indications for revascularisation

It is not clear at present which patients with ARVD benefit from renal revascularisation. Each patient has to be considered on their own merits and the potential

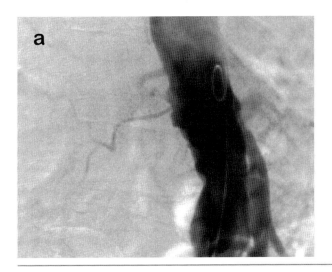
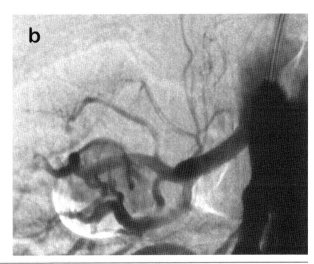

Figure 1. The patient presented with acute renal failure. (a) An angiogram shows bilateral renal artery occlusion. An ultrasound scan indicated the right kidney to be 10cm in length. (b) A right renal stent restored blood flow to the kidney, and renal function was re-established.

benefits of treatment weighed against the complications. The following is a reasonable list of indications and in some of these there is no other alternative active treatment. Patients should be adequately informed regarding the uncertain therapeutic response and the potential complications (see results and complications):-

◆ Severe hypertension resistant to full medical therapy.
◆ ACE-inhibitor induced uraemia.
◆ Deteriorating renal function.
◆ Flash pulmonary oedema.
◆ Acute renal failure with a good sized kidney (Figure 1).
◆ Severe stenosis in a single functioning kidney?

Treatment

It has been recognised for many years that PTRA had a high technical failure rate in ostial ARVD which resulted from the elastic recoil of the aortic cushions of atheroma which were simply temporarily displaced by the inflated balloon. It was not until stents were developed in the early '90s that this problem was addressed.

A single RCT compared PTRA with stenting in 85 patients with ostial lesions [6]. The technical success rates of stents was superior to PTRA (88% versus 55%) and primary 6-month patency, likewise superior (75% versus 29%). The trial was stopped prematurely following an interim analysis of the data. The results of this trial came as no surprise to many radiologists who recognised the poor technical results that PTRA gave when dealing with ostial disease. Consequently, stents have become the treatment of choice for ostial disease. Advances in cross-sectional imaging have also revealed that the vast majority of atherosclerotic lesions are ostial even when a conventional angiogram suggests otherwise [13]. This is due to the aortic wall becoming elongated out towards the diseased artery giving the impression of a non-ostial lesion on angiography. Therefore, PTRA has been largely surpassed by stenting for ARVD.

Although not all and possibly the majority of patients with ARVD are unlikely to benefit from renal stenting, optimal medical therapy is appropriate for all:-

◆ Cessation of smoking.
◆ Antiplatelet agents (eg. aspirin).
◆ Statins: the target total cholesterol should be <5 mmol/l. If cholesterol is already lower than this at

Table 1. Randomised controlled trials in renovascular disease.

Trial	Year	Number	Arms	Result
Malmo [14]	1993	58	Surgery vs PTRA	Technical and primary patency better with surgery Secondary patency equal. PTRA first choice
Scottish & Newcastle [15]	1998	55	Medical vs PTRA for blood pressure	Modest systolic BP improvement only in bilateral disease with PTRA
EMMA [16]	1998	49	Medical vs PTRA for blood pressure	Reduction in drug requirement with PTRA
Van de ven [12]	1999	85	Stent vs PTRA for patency	Primary stent better technical success and patency
DRASTIC [17]	2000	106	Medical vs PTRA for blood pressure	No significant differences

presentation, then current evidence would suggest that the patient should still receive statin therapy.

◆ Antihypertensive therapy: patients may require combinations of several antihypertensive drugs to effect blood pressure control (target <140/80, or 125/75 in those with significant proteinuria). Surprising as it might initially seem, both ACE-inhibitors and A-II receptor blockers are optimal antihypertensive choices for patients with ARVD, especially if patients have evidence of chronic parenchymal disease, with proteinuria. Clearly, careful monitoring of renal function is indicated, especially in patients with significant bilateral RAS, or RAS affecting a solitary kidney.

◆ Optimise anti-diabetic therapy where appropriate.

Results of renal endovascular revascularisation

This is a complicated area, which has been divided into several sections. The problems partly stem from the different outcome measures, eg. blood pressure, renal function, technical success and patency, the evolution of technology, i.e. PTRA, stents and surgical reconstruction. More recently, several RCTs [12,14-17] (Table 1) have been published and several others are underway. The final picture is therefore far from complete.

Angioplasty or surgical revascularisation?

Only one RCT has compared PTRA with surgical (mainly endarterectomy) revascularisation [14]. This small study (n=58) found that the technical success rate was higher in the surgical group (97% versus 83%) and the primary 2-year patency superior (96% versus 75%). However, the secondary patency rates were similar and the authors suggested that PTRA should be the first treatment provided adequate surveillance and reintervention was available. This trial (1993) predated the stent era.

Angioplasty or stents?

A single RCT compared PTRA with stenting in 85 patients with ostial lesions [12]. The technical success rate in the stent arm was superior to PTRA (88%

versus 55%) as was primary 6-month patency (75% versus 29%). The trial was stopped prematurely following an interim analysis of the data. The clinical outcomes in the two groups were similar although the study was not powered to detect differences in blood pressure or renal function.

Stents or surgery?

There are no trials to answer this question and it seems unlikely there ever will be. The two treatments are so different in nature that patient recruitment would be very difficult. Although it is unlikely that the patency rates of any endovascular technique will match those of surgical reconstruction, the increased morbidity and mortality of surgery will restrict its use to the young and fit with a long life expectancy. These patients are rare in the atherosclerotic renovascular field. A rare indication for surgery is a failed attempt at stenting, which most commonly occurs with complete occlusions. It has been suggested that complications such as cholesterol embolisation may be less common with surgical revascularisation as there is usually no instrumentation of the lesion prior to clamping. The perceived advantages of an endovascular approach seem obvious to many, particularly in the aging high-risk vasculopath.

Clinical results

The clinical results of renal revascularisation are the most crucial and the least well understood. There are very many publications usually emanating from individual centres of excellence that have been published over the last 25 years. A recent meta-analysis [18] compared the results of PTRA (10 articles, 644 patients) with stenting (14 articles, 678 patients). None were RCTs. Stent placement had a higher technical success rate and lower restenosis rate and the complication rate was similar for both techniques. The cure rate for hypertension was higher (20% vs 10%) and the improvement rate for renal function was lower (30% vs 38%) after stent placement than PTRA. Although these analyses should not be totally discredited there is a limited amount of information that can be gleaned from non-randomised studies of this nature.

Three RCTs have compared revascularisation (essentially PTRA) with best medical treatment [15-17] in patients with hypertension. None were designed or powered to assess renal function although some renal outcome data is available. The trials were all small; the largest recruited 106 patients. Many patients were excluded before randomisation and slow recruitment restricted patient numbers. Blood pressure is notoriously difficult to measure and reproduce, and the three trials used different measurement criteria. All reported only short-term results (3-54 months). Of the total 210 patients only two were treated with stents. Patient cross-over from one arm to the other was frequent and occurred in 44% in the largest trial. None of these trials produced any good evidence to support the routine use of angioplasty in the treatment of hypertension, although there was some reduction in the drug burden in the PTRA arm in all three studies. This limited benefit had to be tempered by the complications of PTRA, which included one nephrectomy. The confidence limits in all these trials was wide and consequently, they had little power to detect moderate but potentially worthwhile clinical benefits.

There are two published meta-analyses of the three trials [19-20]. Both come to the same conclusion, namely that the effect of PTRA on hypertension was at best modest and none of these small trials were powered to detect changes in renal function (Figure 2). A moderate, but clinically worthwhile benefit could not be excluded and further large scale randomised trials are required. Two such trials (ASTRAL and STAR) are currently recruiting patients.

Complications of endovascular treatment

Although often seen as a minor event in comparison to surgical revascularisation it would be naïve to assume that an endovascular procedure is risk-free. The literature quotes complications rates ranging from 0-66% for renal PTRA/stenting [21]. Most of the series are retrospective with no agreed reporting standards or definitions.

In the single RCT comparing surgery with PTRA [14], the major complication rate following PTRA was 17% versus 31% following surgery with minor

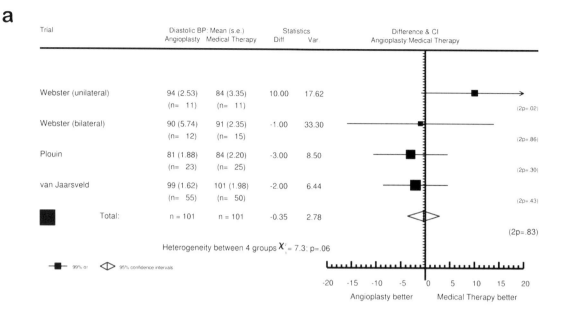

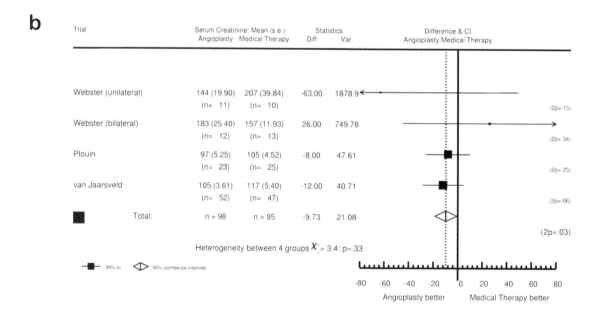

Figure 2. Forrest plots from a meta-analysis comparing the results of PTRA with medication alone in patients with hypertension (a) and impaired renal function (b).

complications in 48% of the PTRA group versus 7% in the surgical group. The Dutch RCT comparing PTRA with stenting reported a 39% complication rate following PTRA and 43% following stenting [12]; most of these complications were minor and groin-related.

With advances in technology and imaging, many complications can be avoided or at least minimised (Table 2). Temporary impairment of renal function due to contrast nephropathy is the most frequent complication. Efforts to minimise this are shown in Table 2, but once it does occur, supportive treatment usually suffices. Cholesterol embolisation is perhaps

Table 2. Prevention and management of endovascular complications.

Complication	Prevention	Treatment
Groin haematoma, pseuodaneurysm	Small platform systems Closure devices	Supportive Thrombin injection
Contrast nephropathy	Hydration Minimise contrast load Carbon dioxide Acetylcysteine	Supportive
Cholesterol embolisation	Minimise manipulations Small platform systems Protection devices	Supportive
Renal artery perforation	Correct balloon size	Balloon tamponade Covered stent
Retroperitoneal bleed (perirenal)	Avoid stiff tipped guidewire Avoid distal guidewire placement	Supportive

the most significant complication, which can be clinically silent and is often under appreciated. The onset is insidious (over 1-3 weeks) and may be associated with an elevated ESR, eosinophilia and the typical livedo reticularis skin rash. The prognosis is guarded and little can be done beyond general supportive measures. The future lies in the use of protection devices; preliminary results are encouraging although a dedicated system still needs to be developed to meet the special challenges of the renal artery anatomy [22-23]. Surgical salvage should be exceptional nowadays and often is too late to save a kidney due to the relatively short warm ischaemic time.

Recent imaging and technical advances

A detailed description of renal angioplasty and stenting is outside the remit of this chapter and suggested reading includes the following reference [24]. A brief description of some of the more recent advances is given below.

Imaging

3D gadolinium enhanced magnetic resonance imaging has rapidly evolved over recent years and has become the preferred imaging modality of choice for RAS in most centres where this technology is available [25]. There is potentially a wealth of additional information to be gleaned from MR imaging and we can look forward in the foreseeable future to a 'one-stop' investigation that will give individual renal function and prognostic indicators in addition to detailed anatomical images. There is some evidence that measurement of the resistive index using ultrasound may help predict the outcome of renal revascularisation; a RI of >70 indicating a poor result [26].

Drugs and devices

Research continues into drugs, which either prevent contrast nephropathy (acetylcysteine, fenoldopam) or replace conventional contrast with

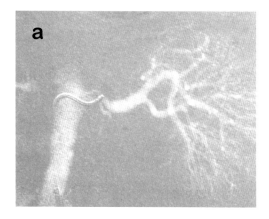

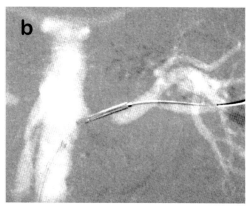

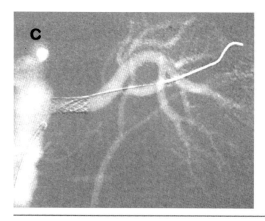

Figure 3. Renal stenting procedure undertaken using CO_2 alone as the imaging contrast media.

less nephrotoxic agents (iodixanol, carbon dioxide) (Figure 3). Dedicated imaging trains on the fluoroscopic angiographic units have improved the resolution of carbon dioxide acquired images.

Miniaturisation of balloons and stents have brought us into the 'small platform' era reducing the size of the puncture site and perhaps causing less trauma at the stent site. With the advent of groin closure devices outpatient stenting may become a reality.

It is hoped that with the evolution of effective protection devices that cholesterol embolisation becomes a thing of the past.

Finally, although restenosis is not a major issue with renal stents, it seems likely that drug eluting or other coated stent technology will further reduce the incidence of restenosis.

Conclusions

The last 25 years has seen PTRA being replaced by stenting for atheromatous disease of the renal arteries. The minimally invasive nature of stenting in the comorbid vascular patient has made it the revascularisation technique of choice in comparison to open surgical techniques. Clinical trials have failed to demonstrate a significant clinical gain for patients with hypertension. At the same time the pharmacological control of hypertension has improved considerably and renal revascularisation is unlikely to have a large role in the management of these patients in the future.

It remains to be seen whether renal stenting will have a useful effect on renal function. The hope is that it will and thereby reduce the need for renal replacement therapy in this group of patients. Research will continue in other clinical areas, for example the cardiac substudy looking at a possible cardiac benefit from renal revascularisation.

Summary

◆ Non-atheromatous RAS should be treated by PTRA.

◆ ARVD is common and associated with hypertension and impaired renal function. The pathophysiology is poorly understood.

◆ Technical success and primary patency following surgery is superior to PTRA.

◆ Meta-analysis of three RCTs shows no clear improvement in renal function or blood pressure following PTRA compared with best medical treatment.

◆ The above trials are underpowered and may have missed a worthwhile clinical benefit.

◆ Two large RCTs are underway to determine whether renal stenting improves renal functional outcomes.

References

1. Gruentzig A, Vetter W, Meier B, et al. Treatment of renovascular hypertension with percutaneous transluminal dilatation of a renal artery stenosis. Lancet 1978; April: 801-802.

2. Suresh M, Laboi P, Mamtora H, Kalra PA. Relationship of renal dysfunction to proximal arterial disease severity in atherosclerotic renovascular disease. Nephrol Dial Transplant 2000;15: 631-636.

3. Farmer CKT, Reidy J, Kalra PA, Cook GJR, Scoble JE. Individual kidney function before and after renal angioplasty. Lancet 1998; 352: 288-289.

4. Schwartz CJ, White TA. Stenosis of the renal artery: an unselected necropsy study. Br Med J 1964; 2: 1415-1421.

5. Hansen KJ, Edwards MS, Craven TE, et al. Prevalence of renovascular disease in the elderly: a population-based study. J Vasc Surg 2002; 36(3): 443-51.

6. Mailloux LU, Napolitano B, Belluci AG, et al. Renal vascular disease causing end-stage renal disease, incidence, clinical correlates and outcomes: a 20-year clinical experience. Am J Kidney Dis 1994; 24: 622-29.

7. Zierler RE, Bergelin RO, Isaacson JA, Strandness DE Jr. Natural history of atherosclerotic renal artery stenosis: a prospective study with duplex ultrasonography. J Vasc Surg 1994; 19: 250-258.

8. Caps MT, Zierler RE, Polissar NL, et al. Risk of atrophy in kidneys with atherosclerotic renal artery stenosis. Kidney Int 1998 Mar; V53(3): 735-42.

9. Crowley JJ, Santos RM, Peter RH, et al. Progression of renal artery stenosis in patients undergoing cardiac catheterisation. Am Heart J 1998; 136:913-918.

10. Shurrab AE, Mamtora H, O'Donoghue D, Waldek S, Kalra PA. Increasing the diagnostic yield of renal angiography for the diagnosis of atheromatous renovascular disease. Br J Radiol 2001; 74: 213-8.

11. Maxwell MH, Bleifer KH, Franklin SS, Varady PD. Cooperative study of renovascular hypertension: Demographic analysis of the study. JAMA 1972; 220: 1195-1204.

12. Van de ven PJG, Kaatee R, Beutler JJ, et al. Arterial stenting and balloon angioplasty in ostial atherosclerotic renovascular disease: a randomised trial. Lancet 1999; 353: 282-86.

13. Kaatee R, Beek FJA, Verschuyl EJ, et al. Atherosclerotic Renal Artery Stenosis: Ostial or Truncal. Radiology 1996; 199: 637.

14. Weibull H, Bergqvist D, Bergentz S-E, et al. Percutaneous transluminal renal angioplasty versus surgical reconstruction of atherosclerotic renal artery stenosis: a prospective randomised study. J Vasc Surg 1993; 18: 841-52.

15. Webster J, Marshall F, Abdalla M, et al. Randomised comparison of percutaneous angioplasty vs continued medical therapy for hypertensive patients with atheromatous renal artery stenosis. Journal of Human Hypertension 1998; 12: 329-335.

16. Plouin P-F, Chatellier G, Darne B, et al. Blood pressure outcome of Angioplasty in atherosclerotic renal artery stenosis. Hypertension 1998; 31: 823-829.

17. Van Jaarsveld BC, Krijnen P, Pieterman H, et al. The effects of balloon angioplasty on hypertension in atherosclerotic renal artery stenosis. N Engl J Med 2000; 342: 1007-14.

18. Leertouwer TC, Gussenhoven EJ, Bosch JL, et al. Stent placement for renal arterial stenosis: where do we stand ? A meta-analysis. Radiology 2000; 216: 78-85.

19. Ives N, Wheatley K, Stowe RL, et al. Continuing uncertainty about the value of percutaneous revascularisation in atherosclerotic renovascular disease: a meta-analysis of randomised trials. Nephrol Dial Transplant 2003; 18: 298-304.

20. Nordmann AJ, Woo K, Parkes R, et al. Balloon angioplasty or medical therapy for hypertensive patients with atherosclerotic renal artery stenosis? A meta-analysis of randomised controlled trials. Am J Med 2003; 114: 44-50.

21. Beek FJA, Kaatee R, Beutler JJ, et al. Complications During Renal Artery Stent Placement for Atherosclerotic Ostial Stenosis. Cardiovasc. Intervent Radiol 1997; 20: 184-190.

22. Henry M, Klonaris C, Henry I, et al. Protected renal stenting with the PercuSurge Guardwire device: a pilot study. J Endovasc Ther 2001; 8: 227-237.

23. Holden A, Hill A. Renal angioplasty and stenting with distal protection of the main renal artery in ischaemic nephropathy: early experience. *J Vasc Surg* 2003; 38: 962-8.

24. Moss JG. Renal and visceral artery intervention. In: *Textbook of endovascular procedures,* 1st edition. Dyet, Ettles, Nicholson and Wilson (Eds). Churchill Livingstone, Edinburgh, 2000: 151-173.

25. Tan KT, Van Beek EJR, Brown PWG, *et al.* Magnetic resonance aniography for the diagnosis of renal artery stenosis. A meta-analysis. *Clin Radiol* 2002; 57: 617-624.

26. Radermacher J, Chavan A, Bleck J, *et al.* Use of Doppler Ultrasonography to Predict the Outcome of Therapy for Renal-Artery Stenosis. *New Engl J Med* 2001; 6; 410-417.

Chapter 25

Mesenteric revascularisation: is it worthwhile?

Graham J Munneke, MRCP FRCR, Clinical Fellow, Interventional Radiology

Thomas M Loosemore, MS FRCS, Consultant Vascular Surgeon

Anna-Maria Belli, FRCR, Consultant Radiologist

St George's Hospital, London, UK

Introduction

Chronic mesenteric ischaemia presents as postprandial abdominal pain, significant weight loss and 'food fear' where patients avoid eating for fear of provoking pain. Clinically apparent mesenteric ischaemia is rare despite autopsy series quoting mesenteric vessel atherosclerosis in 35-70% of unselected patients [1]. This is because excellent collateral communication exists between the mesenteric vessels. At least two vessels must be significantly stenosed to provoke symptoms. When the blood flow is insufficient to meet the physiologic demands of the gastrointestinal tract, the patients become symptomatic. The natural history of these mainly atherosclerotic lesions is progression. Thrombotic occlusion of a pre-existing stenosis precipitates acute ischaemia and bowel infarction. Even with swift diagnosis and treatment this is associated with a very high mortality.

Mesenteric ischaemia was first described more than a century ago. The first reports of angioplasty as a therapeutic option in the visceral circulation were in 1980, shortly followed by a small series with encouraging results [2]. However, percutaneous transluminal angioplasty (PTA) and stenting have as yet not achieved widespread acceptance as first line treatment and many of the patients offered endovascular therapy are those deemed high risk for surgery. The disease usually presents in the over 60 age group and is three times more common in women. It is associated with the usual vascular risk factors and is frequently accompanied by atherosclerosis in other vascular territories. Non-atherosclerotic causes include fibromuscular dysplasia, Takayasu's disease, Sneddon's syndrome [3] and aortic dissection. The ultimate goal of revascularisation is to alleviate pain, improve nutritional status and most importantly, prevent bowel infarction.

Imaging

With advances in diagnostic imaging the mesenteric circulation can now be evaluated non-invasively by a variety of modalities with accurate results.

Stenoses of the coeliac axis and superior mesenteric artery (SMA) may be seen on colour Doppler ultrasound as a narrowing followed by post-stenotic dilatation and turbulent flow. Measuring an increase in peak systolic velocity within the vessel provides objective evidence of a haemodynamically

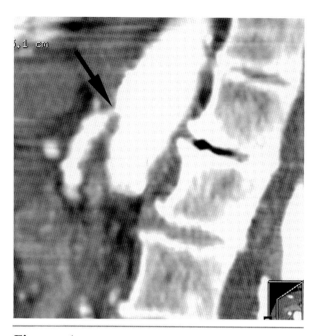

Figure 1. CT angiogram in a patient with a characteristic history of chronic mesenteric ischaemia. This demonstrates occlusion of the coeliac axis and tight stenosis of the SMA (arrow).

significant stenosis. A peak systolic velocity of greater than 275cm per second predicts a stenosis of at least 70%, with a sensitivity of 92% and a specificity of 96% [4]. Unfortunately, ultrasound is time-consuming and heavily operator-dependent. There is a high technical failure rate related to interposed bowel gas. Ultrasound contrast agents may reduce the failure rate by enhancing reflection of the ultrasound beam, improving vessel visibility and Doppler signal.

The advent of multi-channel Computed Tomography (CT) allows rapid scanning of the patient at very fine collimation. This isotropic data can then be reformatted in any plane avoiding the stair step reformatting artifacts of previous generation spiral scanners (Figure 1). Heavily calcified plaques are readily identified on CT prior to intervention. The main disadvantage of CT angiography is its use of a large volume of contrast medium in patients that may have associated renovascular disease.

Contrast-enhanced Magnetic Resonance Angiography (MRA) avoids irradiation and uses gadolinium which is not nephrotoxic in the doses required for the scan. Angiographic images can be generated from the 3D volume acquired during scanning. However, MRA tends to overestimate stenosis and only reliably images the proximal portions of the vessel.

These non-invasive imaging methods are likely to replace angiography in the initial diagnosis of mesenteric vascular disease. They also have application in the follow-up of patients after intervention.

Depending on the availability of non-invasive imaging methods, angiography may still be required. A lateral flush aortogram is the best way of assessing the origins of the mesenteric arteries and selective angiography is only performed when intervention is being performed.

Acute mesenteric ischaemia

Acute mesenteric ischaemia (AMI) is a common cause of an acute abdomen in the elderly. Patients classically present with severe pain and relatively unimpressive abdominal signs. AMI may be caused by arterial or venous occlusion. The diagnosis is often not made until laparotomy when extensive infarcted bowel is found. The surgical options are usually resection with a planned second look laparotomy at 24 hours postoperatively or the abdomen is simply closed if the extent of the infarcted bowel is thought to be too great to be compatible with survival. Occasionally at laparotomy the small bowel appears ischaemic but viable. If there is no arterial pulsation in the mesentery, surgical revascularisation should be considered.

The available evidence for endovascular therapy in AMI is limited to a few case reports and a small series of patients treated with local thrombolysis. A major difficulty with such series is the basis on which the diagnosis was made, particularly if there were no peritoneal signs. Brountzos et al [5] performed balloon angioplasty and stenting of the superior mesenteric artery (SMA) in a patient with acute worsening of chronic mesenteric ischaemia. The patient was said to have peritoneal signs but at exploratory laparotomy 24 hours after endovascular therapy, there was only some discolouration of the small bowel but no evidence for necrosis and no bowel resection was required. The patient apparently made a full recovery. The series [6] reported the results of local catheter directed thrombolysis for acute SMA embolus in ten patients with no peritoneal signs. Nine out of ten patients had a technically successful lysis and seven of the nine were clinical successes. The two patients with technical but not clinical success were found to have necrotic bowel at laparotomy. In another series of 12 patients reported by Sheeran et al [1], five presented as emergencies with acute deterioration of chronic abdominal symptoms. Two of these had peritoneal signs at presentation and had bowel resections followed by endovascular stenting. All three of the patients with no suggestion of necrotic bowel at presentation subsequently developed abdominal signs and had necrotic bowel at laparotomy.

Surgical series have shown that prompt diagnosis and resection of non-viable bowel are associated with an improved outcome [7,8]. The initial management of these patients should be resection of non-viable bowel. Other therapies which delay the removal of necrotic bowel are not in the patient's best interests. There may be a role for endovascular therapy followed by exploratory laparoscopy to assess bowel viability but currently there is not enough evidence to support this strategy.

Indications for treatment

The main criteria for therapy are stenosis or occlusion of at least two of the mesenteric vessels, in a patient with postprandial abdominal pain and significant weight loss. Treatment of asymptomatic patients with abnormal angiograms should be avoided. The only possible exception to this rule is where prophylactic revascularisation may be required in patients with occlusive disease of the SMA and coeliac axis who are due to have abdominal aortic aneurysm repair. The inferior mesenteric artery (IMA) may be sacrificed during surgery with obvious detrimental effect in these patients.

Before intervention, care should be taken to exclude other causes for abdominal pain and weight loss. Many of the treatment failures in the literature are due to undiagnosed intra-abdominal malignancy or

extrinsic compression of the coeliac axis from the median arcuate ligament (MALC) of the diaphragm. Typical appearances of MALC are a non-ostial, asymmetric narrowing on the superior aspect of the coeliac artery, which is accentuated on expiratory angiograms. Many patients with angiographic evidence of compression of the coeliac artery by the MALC are entirely asymptomatic. Indeed, there is debate as to whether symptoms related to the MALC are from intestinal ischaemia or compression of the adjacent sympathetic nerve plexuses. Irrespective of pathogenesis, symptomatic patients should be treated by surgical release of the ligament, not endovascular therapy.

Technique

Prior to intervention, findings from non-invasive imaging should be confirmed by angiography. A flush aortogram in the lateral projection will demonstrate the vessel origins. Anterioposterior projections allow the collateral supply to be appreciated. Selective catheterisation of the vessels should be avoided until the time of intervention to minimise the chance of spasm and inadvertent occlusion. A transfemoral approach is usually successful but if this fails, an upper limb approach such as via the brachial may be required [9]. Either a long sheath or a guiding catheter are desirable, as they provide a stable platform for PTA and stent deployment and facilitate repeated angiograms without catheter exchange. The vessel to be treated is catheterised with a pre-shaped catheter, the most widely used being the cobra and sidewinder (Figure 2). The stenosis or occlusion is then traversed with a guidewire and the catheter advanced across the lesion. 'Roadmapping' software which superimposes an angiographic image on live fluoroscopy may be helpful during this and subsequent angioplasty. After confirming that the catheter is intra-luminal, a bolus of 5000 units of heparin should be given and regular small doses of intra-arterial antispasmodic such as glyceryl trinitrate may be of use. Once the guidewire has been advanced as distally as possible into the target vessel, angioplasty may be performed with an appropriately sized balloon. The coeliac axis and SMA range from 6-8mm but the IMA is much smaller averaging 3mm. Following PTA a completion angiogram and paired

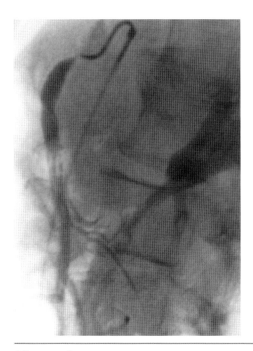

Figure 2. The same patient as in Figure 1. A long sheath is in place and the SMA has been selectively catheterised with a sidewinder 1 catheter. This confirms a significant ostial stenosis.

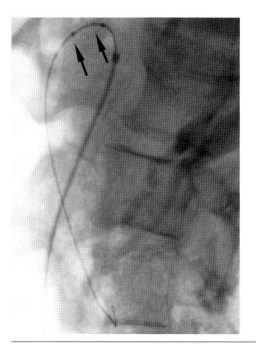

Figure 3. Once again the same patient. A Rosen wire is across the SMA stenosis and a balloon-expandable stent (arrows) has been deployed. Notice that the stent is not particularly radio-opaque.

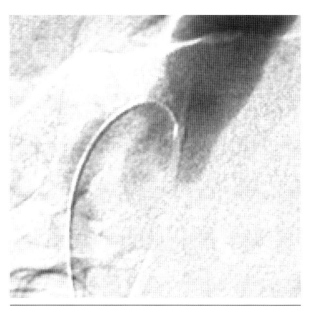

Figure 4. Post-stenting angiogram shows the SMA to be widely patent.

pressure measurements distal to the lesion and in the aorta should be taken. A residual stenosis of >30% or a pressure gradient of more than 10% of systolic blood pressure are indications for a stent. Primary stenting is indicated in ostial stenoses which is analagous to the renal territory and occlusions. Flow limiting dissection following PTA is another indication for stents. Stents may be of the balloon-expandable or self-expandable varieties. The former allows extremely precise deployment across ostial lesions with a small (2mm) amount protruding into the aortic lumen (Figures 3 and 4). Frequent check angiograms through the sheath or guiding catheter provide guidance for accurate stent placement.

Endovascular management of chronic mesenteric ischaemia

As a function of the rarity of the condition, the published results of intervention for chronic visceral ischaemia are limited to case reports and small series. Only two comparisons of surgical and endovascular therapy exist, neither of which is a randomised trial. The available data on angioplasty and stenting for chronic mesenteric ischaemia is presented in Table 1 on an intention to treat basis. Most studies show high

Table 1. The results of endovascular therapy.

	No. of patients	No. of arteries treated	Technical success	Clinical success	Long-term relief of symptoms	Primary assisted relief of symptoms	Patency	Mean follow-up (months)	Complication rate	30-day mortality
AbuRahma 2003 [9]	22	24	23/24 96%	21/22 95%	11/22 50%	12/22 55%	6/20 30%	26	0/22 0%	0/22 0%
Sharafuddin 2003 [10]	25	26	24/25 96%	22/25 88%	20/25 80%	22/25 88%	23/25 92%	15	3/25 12%	1/25 4%
Pietura 2002 [11]	6	9	6/6 100%	6/6 100%	4/6 66%	N/A	4/6 66%	18	0/6 0%	0/6 0%
Cognet 2002 [12]	16	23	16/16 100%	16/16 100%	14/16 88%	16/16 100%	N/A	26	2/16 12%	0/16 0%
Matsumoto 2002 [13]	33	47	32/33 97%	29/33 88%	24/33 73%	28/33 85%	N/A	38	5/33 13%	0/33 0%
Kasirajan 2001 [14]	28	32	28/28 100%	N/A	66 %	N/A	73%	36	5/28 18%	3/28 11%
Sheeran 1999 [1]	12	13	11/12 92%	11/12 92%	9/12 75%	10/12 83%	9/12 75%	16	0/12 0%	1/12 8%
Maspes 1998 [15]	23	41	22/23 96%	17/23 74%	15/23 65%	N/A	N/A	27	2/23 9%	0/23 0%
Nyman 1998 [16]	5	6	5/5 100%	5/5 100%	5/5 100%	5/5 100%	2/5 40%	21	2/5 40%	0/5 0%
Allen 1996 [17]	19	24	18/19 95%	15/19 79%	12/19 63%	14/19 74%	N/A	36	2/19 11%	1/19 5%
Rose 1995 [18]	8	9	3/9 30%	7/8 88%	5/8 63%	N/A	N/A	9	2/8 25%	1/8 13%
Hallisey 1995 [19]	16	25	14/16 88%	14/16 88%	9/16 56%	12/16 75%	N/A	28	1/16 6%	1/16 6%
Odurny 1988 [20]	10	19	8/10 80%	8/10 80%	3/10 30%	6/10 60%	N/A	11	1/10 10%	1/10 10%
Golden 1982 [2]	7	7	6/7 86%	6/7 86%	6/7 86%	N/A	3/3 100%	28	0/7 0%	0/7 0%

initial technical and clinical success but there is a tendency for restenosis and a need for re-treatment. The procedure is extremely well tolerated with average morbidity and mortality rates of 11.1% and 4.1% respectively.

An early series [17] on PTA in chronic mesenteric ischaemia consisted of 19 patients, all of whom were considered extremely poor surgical candidates. Angioplasty was technically successful in 18 out of 19 patients. The single failure resulted in dissection and then thrombosis of the SMA. The patient died despite emergency surgical revascularisation and bowel resection. This occurred prior to the availability of stents and nowadays the situation may have been salvaged by stenting. Complete symptomatic relief was achieved in 15 patients. This was sustained in 12 patients and two of the three patients with recurrence of symptoms, were successfully re-treated. Rose *et al* [18] showed that while only 30% of their procedures were technically successful by accepted angiographic criteria (<30% residual stenosis following PTA), patients derived symptomatic improvement as long as there was some increase in the vessel lumen diameter. Excluding a patient with pancreatitis who was misdiagnosed and one patient with arcuate ligament compression, all of their patients had initial pain relief despite the low technical success rate.

The results from early series mainly pertain to angioplasty alone but more recently, results with stenting have become available. As in the renal artery, the long-term patency of stenting may prove to be superior than with angioplasty alone.

Sharafuddin *et al* [10] have recently reported their experience of stenting in 22 consecutive patients with chronic mesenteric ischaemia and three liver transplant patients with coeliac axis stenosis. The only technical failure was in a patient with extrinsic compression of the coeliac axis by the median arcuate ligament. In addition to this there were two clinical failures. Of note, both of these patients only had moderate stenosis of a single artery and one of them subsequently failed to improve with bypass surgery. If these three patients are excluded, the primary assisted clinical benefit in this study is 100% at a mean of 15 months follow-up. The only peri-procedure death in this group was a patient with advanced intra-abdominal carcinoid.

In another series of angioplasty and stenting [9], once again the only technical failure was in a patient who ultimately had curative surgery for median arcuate ligament entrapment. Twenty-one patients were successfully treated, only two of whom had both the SMA and coeliac axis revascularised. The mean age of the patients was 69.2 and all were deemed to be high surgical risks. No perioperative mortality or major morbidity was reported and there were no late cases of mesenteric infarction over the study period. At a mean of 26 months, 61% of the 18 patients still available for follow-up were asymptomatic. However, patency as assessed by duplex ultrasound was only 30%. Approximately half of these patients with restenosis >70% were asymptomatic. The majority of the symptomatic restenoses were amenable to retreatment but required several interventions for in-stent restenosis. The authors comment, that the low patency rate may be due to their documentation with ultrasound rather than inferring patency from lack of symptoms.

In 2002, Matsumoto [13] published updated data on patients treated at his institution between 1981 and 1999. The patients treated at the start of his series, at a time when only angioplasty was performed, had been previously reported on in 1995. Latterly he performed both angioplasty and stenting. Stents were placed for residual stenosis of 30% or greater post PTA, a flow limiting dissection post PTA and recurrent stenosis within 12 months of PTA. PTA alone was performed in 21 patients and PTA and stenting in 12. There were four immediate clinical failures. Two of these patients had undiagnosed intra-abdominal malignancy as the cause of their symptoms. The authors now routinely obtain abdominal CT scans on all patients prior to intervention. The third failure was related to MALC. In the last patient there was only partial relief of symptoms following a technically favourable angioplasty. The patient was rendered pain-free following surgical revascularisation. All the procedure-related morbidity was from access site problems. There were no episodes of acute mesenteric ischaemia and no early deaths. Brachial arterial access resulted in more complications than femoral, 12% verses 4%. A higher long-term clinical success rate for stenting failed to reach statistical significance. The 5-year survival rate in this study of 76.1% compares favourably with recently published surgical series quoting figures of 54-79% [21,22,23,24,25].

The effect of stenting on outcome is still not entirely clear. Matsumoto [13] found that stenting resulted in a higher technical success of 100%, compared with 81.3% for PTA, but this did not confer a statistically greater long-term clinical success. Although some authors [10] have reported high patency rates following stenting, others have suffered significant in-stent restenosis [9]. In-stent restenosis may be treated by PTA, cutting balloon angioplasty [26] or further stenting. Other options such as drug eluting stents and brachytherapy have not been reported in the visceral circulation.

Surgical management of chronic mesenteric ischaemia

Surgical revascularisation of the mesenteric circulation can be achieved by endarterectomy, antegrade or retrograde bypass grafting and re-implantation of the artery. Inflow of bypass grafts may be from the supracoeliac aorta (antegrade) or from the infrarenal aorta or common iliac artery (retrograde). Outflow may be to just the coeliac or SMA or a bifurcated graft to both. Controversies remain over the relative benefit of antegrade as opposed to retrograde bypass. In common with the literature on endovascular treatment, most of the surgical series are small and the objective long-term follow-up of graft patency is poor, making meaningful comparison of the different techniques difficult. The antegrade method results in a straighter course to the SMA and coeliac axis, with less chance of graft kinking but requires a more extensive dissection and the risks from aortic cross-clamping are significantly higher. The supracoeliac aorta may be accessed without the need for thoracotomy and its associated morbidity by means of a medial visceral rotation. Retrograde grafting from the more familiar territory of the infrarenal aorta requires less exposure but it may be diseased and the grafts are more prone to kinking. Prosthetic grafts are considerably more resistant to kinking than vein grafts. Several series have shown that the method of reconstruction or the type of graft material have no influence on outcome or late clinical success [8,23,25].

The results of recent surgical series are presented in Table 2. They all report high technical success rates of between 97% and 100% and good long-term relief of symptoms of 76% to 93%. Comparison of results between endovascular and surgical studies is difficult because of differing follow-up and presentation of results. Nevertheless, the results of surgery appear to be more durable than angioplasty and stenting. Significantly, this is at the expense of greater mortality and morbidity, range 0-14.7% and 19-66% respectively. The largest series from the United States Nationwide Inpatient Sample [28] included 336 patients. In this group the in-hospital death rate was 14.7% and only 73.4% of patients were discharged home. The mean length of hospital stay was 18.3 days. Some of the recent series on stenting with modern devices, through low profile delivery systems have technical and clinical results comparable to surgery whilst maintaining low mortality and morbidity rates.

Single or multiple vessel revascularisation?

In surgical series, multivessel or complete revascularisation was performed on most patients. Proponents of complete revascularisation argue that it is associated with decreased symptomatic recurrence, improved graft patency and survival [23,29]. In Hollier's series [29] 5-year graft patency was 90% for three vessel reconstruction but 0% for single vessel. However, Foley et al [22] reported comparable results to multivessel reconstruction with single vessel retrograde grafting to the SMA. Their 5-year recurrence rate was only 6%. Other authors have found no significant difference in the results for single and multivessel reconstruction [8,25]. However, this may be related to the small numbers in the available series. Because of the catastrophic consequences of thrombosis of a single vessel graft, most authors recommend multivessel reconstruction when practical. The situation may be different in endovascular treatment where gradual restenosis occurs rather than acute thrombosis. The high immediate clinical success of the mainly single vessel endovascular revascularisation also suggests that treating more than one vessel is unnecessary.

Table 2. The results of surgery.

	No. of patients	No. of arteries treated	Technical success	Clinical success	Long-term relief of symptoms	Patency	Mean follow-up (months)	Complication rate	30-day mortality
Park 2002 [8]	98	179	95/98 97%	N/A	74/80 93%	43/54 79%	23	21/98 21%	3/98 3.1%
Jimenez 2002 [24]	47	92	100%	N/A	N/A	69%	31	31/47 66%	4/47 9.7%
Mateo 1999 [23]	85	130	100%	100%	76%	64/85 75%	36	28/85 33%	7/85 8%
Johnston 1995 [21]	21	43	100%	N/A	N/A	86%	120	19%	0%
Moawad 1997 [27]	24	38	100%	100%	78%	78%	60	45%	4%
Derrow 2001 [28]	336	N/A	N/A	N/A	N/A	N/A	N/A	44.6%	14.7%
Rose 1995 [18]	9	16	100%	7/9 78%	7/8 88%	N/A	34.5	3/9 33%	1/9 11%

However, some authors have proposed that endovascular treatment of single vessels is the reason for its lower durability; this has yet to be proven. Indeed, Matsumoto [13] found no difference in primary clinical success and survival in those who had multivessel as opposed to single vessel endovascular treatment. Sharafuddin *et al* [10] found that treatment of a coeliac axis stenosis in the presence of an SMA occlusion was associated with good clinical outcome without the need to tackle the SMA occlusion. In general, it would seem reasonable to attempt multivessel treatment if the lesions are technically favourable. This may in time provide more durable results.

Conclusions

Is mesenteric revascularisation worthwhile? Yes, the evidence is that it is an effective treatment in patients who otherwise suffer intractable symptoms and risk developing acute ischaemia.

Whilst AMI is best treated surgically, the improved results of recent endovascular series in treating chronic mesenteric ischaemia indicate that it is a viable treatment option in most patients, not just those who pose a high surgical risk. PTA and stenting can produce results comparable to surgery but with lower complication and mortality rates. In-stent restenosis can be safely retreated with low morbidity in the first instance. If there is repeated restenosis or if the endovascular option is technically impossible, open surgery is still an option.

Summary

◆ The mesenteric circulation can be imaged non-invasively.

◆ The treatment of acute mesenteric ischaemia should be surgical.

◆ Surgery produces durable results in chronic mesenteric ischaemia but morbidity and mortality are higher than with endovascular methods.

◆ The technical and clinical results of PTA and stenting are now approaching those of surgery, although this is based on small numbers.

◆ Recurrent stenosis is often amenable to repeat angioplasty.

◆ Intra-abdominal malignancy and MALC should be excluded prior to treatment.

References

1. Sheeran SR, Murphy TP, Khwaja A, *et al.* Stent placement for treatment of mesenteric artery stenoses or occlusions. *J Vasc Intervent Radiol* 1999; 10(7): 861-867.

2. Golden DA, Ring EJ, McLean GK, *et al.* Percutaneous transluminal angioplasty in the treatment of abdominal angina. *Am J Roentgen* 1982; 139: 247-249.

3. Khoo LA, Belli AM. Superior mesenteric artery stenting for mesenteric ischaemia in Sneddon's syndrome. *Br J Radiol* 1999 Jun; 72(858): 607-609.

4. Moneta GL. Screening for mesenteric vascular insufficiency and follow-up of mesenteric artery bypass procedures. *Semin Vasc Surg* 2001; 14(3): 186-192.

5. Brountzos EN, Critselis A, Magoulas, *et al.* Emergency endovascular treatment of a superior mesenteric artery occlusion. *Cardiovasc Intervent Radiol* 2001; 24: 57-71.

6. Simo G, Echenagusia AJ, Camunez F, *et al.* Superior mesenteric arterial embolism: local fibrinolytic treatment with urokinase. *Radiology* 1997; 204: 775-779.

7. Brandt LJ, Boley SJ. AGA technical review on intestinal ischaemia. *Gastroenterology* 2000; 118: 954-968.

8. Park WM, Cherry KJ, Chua HK, *et al.* Current results of open revascularization for chronic mesenteric ischaemia: a standard for comparison. *J Vasc Surg* 2002; 35: 853-859.

9. AbuRhama AF, Stone PA, Bates MC, *et al.* Angioplasty/stenting of the superior mesenteric artery and celiac trunk: early and late outcomes. *J Endovasc Ther* 2003; 10: 1046-1053.

10. Sharafuddin MJ, Olson CH, Sun S, *et al.* Endovascular treatment of celiac and mesenteric arteries stenoses: application and results. *J Vasc Surg* 2003; 38: 692-698.

11. Pietura R, Szymanska A, El Furah M, *et al.* Chronic mesenteric ischaemia: diagnosis and treatment with balloon angioplasty and stenting. *Med Sci Monit* 2002; 8(1): PR8-12.

12. Cognet F, Ben Salem D, Dranssart M, *et al.* Chronic mesenteric ischaemia: imaging and percutaneous treatment. *Radiographics* 2002; 22: 863-880.

13. Matsumoto AH, Angle JF, Spinosa DJ, *et al.* Percutaneous transluminal angioplasty and stenting in the treatment of chronic mesenteric ischaemia: results and long-term follow-up. *J Am Coll Surg* 2002; 194(1 Suppl): S22-31.

14. Kasirajan K, O'Hara PJ, Gray BH, *et al.* Chronic mesenteric ischaemia: open surgery versus percutaneous angioplasty and stenting. *J Vasc Surg* 2001; 33: 63-71.

15. Maspes F, Mazzetti di Pietralata G, Gandini R, *et al.* Percutaneous transluminal angioplasty in the treatment of chronic mesenteric ischaemia: results and 3 years of follow-up in 23 patients. *Abdom Imaging* 1998; 23(4): 358-363.

16. Nyman U, Ivancev K, Lindh M, *et al.* Endovascular treatment of chronic mesenteric ischaemia: report of five cases. *Cardiovasc Intervent Radiol* 1998; 21: 305-313.

17. Allen RC, Martin GH, Rees CH, *et al.* Mesenteric angioplasty in the treatment of chronic intestinal ischaemia. *J Vasc Surg* 1996; 24: 415-423.

18. Rose SC, Quigley TM, Raker EJ. Revascularization for chronic mesenteric ischaemia: comparison of operative arterial bypass grafting and percutneous transluminal angioplasty. *J Vasc Intervent Radiol* 1995; 6: 339-349.

19. Hallisey MJ, Deschaine J, Illescas FF, *et al.* Angioplasty for the treatment of visceral ischaemia. *J Vasc Intervent Radiol* 1995; 6: 785-791.

20. Odurny A, Sniderman KW, Colapinto RF. Intestinal angina: percutaneous transluminal angioplasty of the celiac and superior mesenteric arteries. *Radiology* 1988; 167: 59-62.

21. Johnstone KW, Lindsay TF, Walker PM, *et al.* Mesenteric arterial bypass grafts: early and late results and suggested surgical approach for chronic and acute mesenteric ischaemia. *Surgery* 1995; 118: 1-7.

22. Foley MI, Moneta GL, Abou-Zamzam AM, *et al.* Revascularization of the superior mesenteric artery alone for treatment of intestinal ischaemia. *J Vasc Surg* 2000; 32: 37-47.

23. Mateo RB, O'Hara PJ, Hertzer NR, *et al.* Elective surgical treatment of symptomatic chronic mesenteric occlusive disease: early results and late outcomes. *J Vasc Surg* 1999; 29: 821-832.

24. Jimenez JG, Huber TS, Ozaki CK, *et al*. Durability of antegrade synthetic aortomesenteric bypass for chronic mesenteric ischaemia. *J Vasc Surg* 2002; 35: 1078-1084.

25. Cho J, Carr JA, Jacobsen G, *et al*. Long-term outcome after mesenteric artery reconstruction: a 37-year experience. *J Vasc Surg* 2002; 35: 453-460.

26. Munneke GJ, Engelke C, Morgan RA, Belli AM. Cutting balloon angioplasty for resistant renal artery in-stent restenosis. *J Vasc Intervent Radiol* 2002; 13(3): 327-331.

27. Moawad J, McKinsey JF, Wyble CW, *et al*. Current results of surgical therapy for chronic mesenteric ischaemia. *Arch Surg* 1997; 132: 613-619.

28. Derrow AE, Seeger JM, Dame DA, *et al*. The outcome in the United States after thoracoabdominal aortic aneurysm repair, renal artery bypass, and mesenteric revascularization. *J Vasc Surg* 2001; 34: 54-61.

29. Hollier LH, Bernatz PE, Pairolero PC, *et al*. Surgical management of chronic intestinal ischaemia: a reappraisal. *Surgery* 1991; 90: 940-946.

PART VI. Imaging

Chapter 26

Imaging for endovascular aneurysm repair

Maarten J van der Laan, MD, Resident Surgery
St. Antonius Hospital, Nieuwegein, The Netherlands

Lambertus W Bartels, PhD, Physicist
Image Sciences Institute, University Medical Center, Utrecht, The Netherlands

Jan D Blankensteijn, MD, Professor and Chief Division of Vascular Surgery
University Medical Center Nijmegen, Nijmegen, The Netherlands

Introduction

In order to select appropriate candidates for endovascular aneurysm repair (EVAR), the radiologist or vascular surgeon must rely on accurate imaging. The limitations of the available endograft devices require the assessment of several anatomic features of an abdominal aortic aneurysm (AAA) prior to endoluminal repair. We will discuss the relevant anatomic features as well as the imaging techniques that are used in preoperative evaluation of an AAA patient. The specific techniques to be discussed are Digital Subtraction Angiography (DSA), Computed Tomography Angiography (CTA), Magnetic Resonance Imaging (MRI) and Magnetic Resonance Angiography (MRA). We will address the advantages and limitations of each of these techniques, and we will include a discussion of the post-imaging processing used for CTA and MRA highlighting their unique advantages for preoperative imaging.

In the postoperative follow-up, most centres use a CTA based follow-up program. A dedicated follow-up in combination with image post-processing is an accurate and sensitive tool for monitoring these patients. MRI and MRA techniques have developed a great deal over the last decade. MRI gives excellent soft tissue contrast, a high sensitivity for non-nephrotoxic contrast agents and does not utilise ionizing radiation. For postoperative imaging, MRI has already been demonstrated as an accurate and sensitive method of follow-up [1]. The exact role for MRI and MRA techniques in preoperative planning has not yet been clearly defined.

For the follow-up after EVAR, several imaging modalities have been suggested [2-11]. MRI has been demonstrated to be even more sensitive to endoleak detection [12]. MRI can also be used for other aspects of the EVAR follow-up, such as the determination of aneurysm sac size change and graft patency. Although MRI has not yet been accepted as a commonly used tool for the EVAR follow-up, it is a modality with great potential.

Pre-procedural imaging

Advances in CTA and MRA imaging techniques have substantially decreased DSA's role in pre-procedural imaging. In fact, many endovascular centres have eliminated DSA from their imaging protocol and use CTA alone. The main reasons for eliminating DSA stem from the combined risks and potential complications of arterial puncture and iodinated contrast, both of which are requirements of the procedure. In addition, DSA does not provide additional information when compared to a dedicated CTA.

Despite its potential usefulness, DSA does have significant limitations. DSA is unable to detect actual aneurysm dimensions, as it only reveals the true lumen and not the associated thrombus. Also, this imaging method does not accurately detect calcification at the aortic bifurcation and within the iliac vessels, a very important aspect of pre-procedure imaging. By contrast, CTA allows for the accurate assessment of all of these important issues in pre-procedure imaging. As we will discuss, the combination of MRI and MRA may provide accurate pre-procedural imaging as well as CTA in the near future.

Computed Tomography Angiography

Spiral CTA has taken DSA's place as the gold standard for pre-EVAR imaging [13]. As previously mentioned, high-quality pre-procedural imaging is essential for patient selection, endograft sizing, and procedure planning. Spiral CTA with post-imaging processing provides all of the necessary information and has made DSA relatively superfluous in most instances. Post-imaging processing of spiral CTA data has proven to be superior over the two-dimensional DSA projection for both patient selection and endograft sizing [14].

Our standardised CTA acquisition protocol utilises one un-enhanced scan and another using 140ml Ultravist (Berlex Laboratories, Montville, NJ). The raw data is sent to a post-imaging workstation for exact analysis.

Modern multislice helical CT scanners are able to image the entire abdomen a lot faster than the spiral single slice scanners, thus reducing motion artifacts. Multislice scanners can also produce thinner slices, leading to a more isometric voxel size. This technology will slightly increase the in-plane resolution, because of reduced partial-volume effect, but the resolution of reconstructed planes will improve significantly compared to normal spiral CTA.

In order to evaluate a patient's suitability for EVAR, it is essential to measure the diameter and length of the infrarenal aortic neck and both common iliac arteries. CTA provides tissue contrast that easily distinguishes between lumen mural thrombus and aortic wall. In combination with post-imaging processing, this provides the basis for exact measurements. Furthermore, it is important to depict the amount of thrombus and calcium in the infrarenal neck, common iliac arteries, and the external iliac arteries [15].

Aortic length and diameter measurements allow the choice of an endograft of the right anatomical configuration. Commercially available post-imaging processing software, or workstations, can be used to perform these measurements [16].

The last step in pre-procedure imaging is planning the intervention. In most AAAs, the aorta is elongated and tortuous. This anatomy may result in a more difficult introduction through one of the iliac systems or in a very angulated infrarenal neck, complicating graft delivery. Using a three-dimensional model of the aortic lumen, the correct angulation and rotation of the C-arm during the intervention can be assessed (Figure 1). The origin of the most distal renal artery is essential to the exact placement of the proximal attachment system. The hypogastric artery origin is important for proper placement of the distal attachment systems. In our experience, a rotation and angulation of the C-arm based upon pre-procedural measurements on the three-dimensional model results in precise placement of the endograft without losing precious millimeters in the proximal and distal seal zones [17].

CTA has drawbacks as well, but most involve the post-procedure follow-up. Patients require lifelong CTA scan surveillance after EVAR. This can not only result in a potentially high accumulated dose of radiation, but also a repeated load of iodine containing contrast agent, with a possible influence on renal function.

Magnetic Resonance Imaging and Magnetic Resonance Angiography

New developments in MR hardware have made faster scanning at a high resolution possible. MR

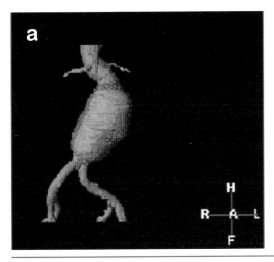
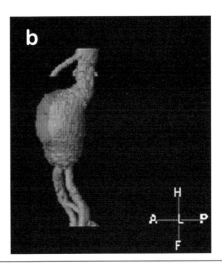

Figure 1. A 3D shaded surface model of a pre-operative AAA. a) The anterior posterior view and b) the lateral view. The model can be rotated in any way the observer thinks best.

angiography techniques make use of gadolinium-based contrast agents and allow fast three-dimensional imaging of the abdominal aorta and branches, as well as of the iliac arteries. Gadolinium is non-nephrotoxic so the risk of inducing further renal insufficiency is absent in MRA. MRI has some other theoretical advantages over CTA, including inherent three-dimensionality, excellent soft tissue contrast, and lack of ionizing radiation. Nevertheless, to extract all the necessary information from MR for patient selection, sizing, and procedure planning, several scans need to be obtained.

We use a standardized MR protocol. After the initial survey, we obtain the following scans: a T1-weighted spin echo, a T2-weighted turbo spin echo, a high-resolution three-dimensional contrast-enhanced (CE) MRA, and a post-contrast T1-weighted spin echo (as pre-contrast). For the three-dimensional CE-MRA, we administer 25ml of gadolinium contrast agent. However, a simple high-resolution three-dimensional CE-MRA is not enough. This scan can offer an excellent depiction of the aortic lumen and all patent side branches, but because of the pronounced T1-weighting of this scan, the intrinsic tissue contrast is minimal. Exact measurements of the aortic infrarenal neck cannot be done on this scan unless a part of the T1-weighting is given up. The vessel wall and thrombus are not clearly distinguishable and measuring the lumen alone is insufficient. Additional

non-contrast-enhanced, T2-weighted turbo spin echo and T1-weighted spin echo MRI scans are necessary. A T1-weighted post-contrast scan is particularly well suited for patient selection and sizing because it provides a good contrast between lumen, thrombus, and vessel wall.

The maximum intensity projection (MIP) images of the three-dimensional CE-MRA are comparable to a three-dimensional DSA. They allow the same assessment as DSA; the length and angulation of the aneurysm neck, any associated renal artery stenosis, iliac artery tortuosity or stenosis, patency of internal iliac arteries, and luminal diameter of the iliac vessels and the external iliac arteries. However, neither MRI nor MRA will depict calcium, which can be a problem in a tortuous iliac system or a short aortic neck. Raw MRI and MRA data can be sent to a post-imaging workstation for exact measurements and detailed analysis.

Image post-processing

Processing of the acquired images (whether they are gathered through CTA or MRI/MRA) is essential in the pre-procedural analysis of a patient. Taking measurements on the hard copies of a scan can be inaccurate. For instance, an angulated neck will look wider on an axial slice than when measurements are

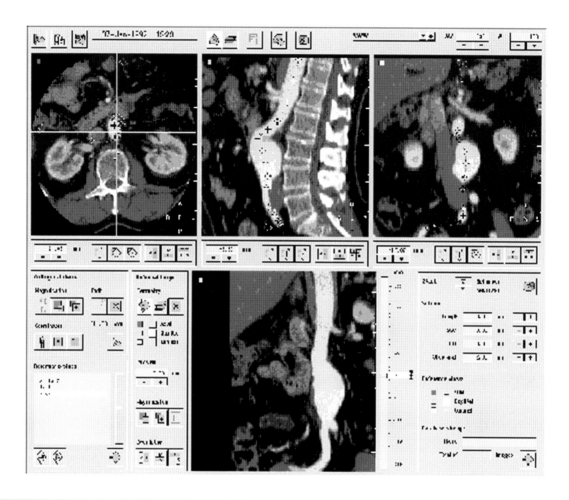

Figure 2. An example of the image post-processing. A central lumen line (CLL) is drawn and exact measurements are done in the curved linear reformat (CLR) and the multiplanar reconstruction (MPR).

taken perpendicular to the central lumen line (CLL) (Figure 2). Furthermore, the window level and width of an axial slice on a hard copy is fixed, making it difficult to distinguish lumen from calcium. Using a higher window width, the amount of calcium is easily assessed. Inaccurate measurements can lead to inappropriate graft placement, or use of the wrong size endograft. These mistakes can lead to an endoleak, or to the covering and possible occlusion of one of the renal or the hypogastric arteries.

Post-imaging processing can be done on several commercially available programs. We have been using Philips EasyVision workstation, release 4 (Philips Medical Systems, Best, The Netherlands). It is also possible to submit raw CTA data commercially

(Preview, Medical Media Systems, West Lebanon, NH), and obtain prefabricated, three-dimensional, shaded-surface reconstructions of lumen, thrombus, and calcium. With this system, the physician can select the most suitable endograft by simulating the endograft in the three-dimensional aneurysm image on the computer screen. A relatively new PC-based program called Vitrea (Vital Images, Plymouth, MN) is also available. This program can process raw data or Dicom III images. One of the major advantages of the Vitrea system is that fully automated, three-dimensional, shaded-surface reconstructions are incorporated into the program. The program is user-friendly, but the range of measurements that can be performed on the system is limited.

The following post-imaging processing options are useful in the assessment of an AAA: cine-mode, multiplanar reconstruction (MPR) formats, MIP, and three-dimensional shaded surface reconstructions.

Once a patient is accepted for endovascular grafting, these three-dimensional images are useful for determining the surgical plan. By viewing and rotating the virtual aneurysm in any direction, the tortuosity of the access arteries and angulation of the aortic lumen can be appreciated.

As discussed, imaging remains a crucial part of the preoperative planning for EVAR. We believe that CTA is the current standard of care, especially when combined with post-imaging processing.

Postoperative imaging

It has been shown that endoleaks can occur at any time and that aneurysm sac enlargement can start after a prolonged period of shrinkage [18]. Patients, therefore, need to be monitored for life following EVAR. The long-term durability and outcome following this treatment is still unknown [18-21].

Computed Tomography Angiography

Endoleak detection, aneurysm sac size change, size and type of endoleak, graft migration, and endograft patency are the most important aspects in the EVAR follow-up [22-26]. In order to have the highest sensitivity for endoleak detection, size change and the other parameters, a dedicated CTA scan protocol must be used. Our CTA scan protocol consists of a non-contrast enhanced scan, a CE-CTA using 140ml of Ultravist and delayed CT series two and four minutes after the CE scan.

Evaluation consists of a comparison of the non-contrast-enhanced scan to the subsequent scans. This is best done on a separate image processing workstation as described earlier. The use of delayed series has been shown to be an effective tool to trace small type II endoleaks.

An essential part of our follow-up is the tracking of size change by volume measurements of the non-

luminal aneurysm sac. Volume measurements have been shown to be more sensitive to size change than are diameter measurements [14]. These volume measurements are obtained by a process of manual segmentation of the lumen and total aneurysm volume on a separate graphical workstation.

Endoleak detection with CTA can be difficult because of the relative insensitivity of this technique to iodinated contrast agent. Even with the use of the most dedicated CTA protocols, endoleaks may be missed [19,27-30]. There are a significant number of patients with a growing aneurysm sac after EVAR, without a detectable endoleak on CTA or on conventional angiography [19,29]. In some of these patients, this might be due to a hygroma-like process [31]. In others, it is possible that CTA is not sensitive enough. The super-selective digital subtraction angiography technique is mainly reserved for specific cases and cannot be used routinely for surveillance because of its invasive nature [32].

In addition, the evaluation of sac size by using diameter or volume measurements can be difficult using CTA. The moderate amount of soft tissue contrast involved does not always allow an accurate demarcation of the aneurysm wall, especially in inflammatory aneurysms. Another limitation of CTA is the difficulty in detecting stenosis in the endograft. Maximum Intensity Projections (MIP) not only depict the endograft lumen but also calcium, bone, metal and other signal intense tissues, making appreciation of the lumen difficult.

Magnetic Resonance Imaging and Angiography

MRI might be more appropriate for follow-up after EVAR than CTA due to its excellent soft tissue contrast, its inherent three dimensionality, and its extreme sensitivity to gadolinium contrast agent. Moreover, the signal losses resulting from the metallic stent and calcium cannot be confused with contrast agent and are, therefore, less disturbing in low artifact metals, like nitinol or tantalum. The absence of ionizing radiation and the ability to use a non-nephrotoxic contrast agent give MRI an additional advantage over CTA in EVAR follow-up [1,33,34,35-37]. Furthermore,

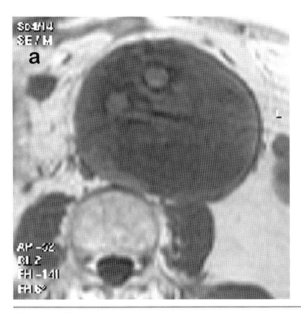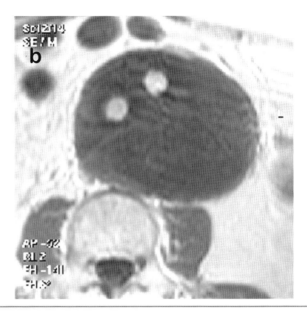

Figure 3. Geographically identical slices of an AAA patient. a) The pre-CE T1-weighted scan and b) the post-CE T1-weighted scan. The only difference between the scans is the CE.

recent developments in MR hardware, such as SENSE (parallel imaging) and ultra-fast gradient systems, have made fast dynamic scanning possible. These techniques have the potential to depict the contrast dynamics in and around the aneurysm sac and might, therefore, be of use for determining the origin of an endoleak and assessment of endograft patency.

The excellent soft tissue contrast of MRI can be used to detect local variations in thrombus consistency on T1- and T2-weighted images as described by Castrucci et al [38]. Hygroma-like processes as described by Risberg et al [31] could also be revealed in this way. The clear liquid-like material from the hygroma will have a high signal intensity on a T2-weighted image in contrast to older organised thrombus.

We have developed a postoperative MR scan protocol in order to evaluate all aspects of post-EVAR follow-up. For all MRI examinations a quadrature wrap-around synergy body coil was used as receive coil. All examinations started with localizer scans, after which the following diagnostic scans were acquired: a T1-weighted spin echo; a T2-weighted turbo spin echo; a dynamic 3D CE-MRA using SENSE factor 2

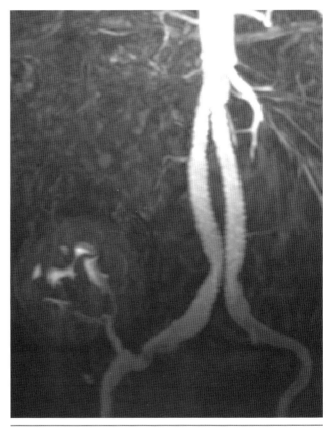

Figure 4. An MIP anterior-posterior view of a 3D MRA of a patient with a bifurcated endograft in place.

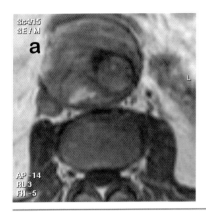
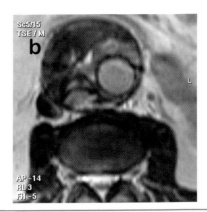
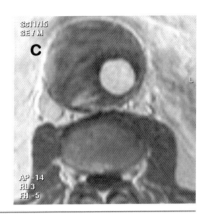

Figure 5. Geographically identical slices of an AAA patient. a) The pre-CE T1-weighted scan, b) the pre-CE T2-weighted scan and c) the post-CE T1-weighted scan.

(approximately 6.5s per volume) during which 20ml contrast agent was administered; a 3D CE-MRA during which 20ml contrast agent was administered with a pre-determined delay; a post-contrast T1-weighted spin echo (as pre-contrast); and a post-contrast T1-weighted spin echo.

The reconstructed source images are sent to a separate image post-processing workstation for accurate evaluation. The combination and especially the comparison of these scans results in high sensitivity for endoleaks. For this purpose, we mainly use the T1-weighted pre-contrast scan and the T1-weighted post-contrast scan (Figure 3), the only difference between the two scans being the 40ml contrast agent administered in scan three and four. For the exact determination of the type of endoleaks, the 3D CE-MRA in combination with the dynamic CE series can be very helpful (Figure 4). The dynamic CE scan results in 10 3D volumes, 4.5-6.5 seconds after each other, depending on the required coverage. The added temporal resolution can give the ultimate proof of site of inflow of an endoleak, negating the need for an additional diagnostic DSA.

Interpretation of the acquired images is, however, time-consuming and difficult. In order to have this temporal resolution, some of the spatial resolution has to be sacrificed compared to the static CE-MRA scan. The evaluation of size change can best be done on the second T1-weighted post-contrast scan. Because of the smaller voxel dimensions there is less partial volume effect and segmentation of the non-luminal volume is more accurate. The T1-weighted scans in

combination with the T2-weighted scan can provide information on thrombus organisation in the aneurysm sac and thereby the effectiveness of exclusion (Figure 5) [31].

Image post-processing after EVAR

The processing of the acquired images of patients after endovascular repair is similar to the pre-procedural image post-processing. CTA or MRI/MRA data is loaded onto a separate graphical workstation. Again, measurements from hardcopy scans is inaccurate and leads to decreased sensitivity for treatment failure.

Cine-mode, multiplanar reformats, segmentations of the lumen and the non-luminal aneurysm sac are useful image post-processing options in the assessment of an AAA after endovascular repair. For a more detailed analysis and for accurate diameter and length measurements the central lumen line is drawn in the MPR. Curved linear reformats allow accurate measurement of the aneurysm diameter in a plane perpendicular to the vessel axis. CLR allows accurate length measurements as well, used for the evaluation of graft migration and aneurysm deformation.

Manual segmentations of the non-luminal thrombus provide the most sensitive way to evaluate size change over time [14]. As stated earlier this is a labour-intensive method but is of great value in the follow-up program.

Conclusions

In the preoperative imaging for EVAR, CTA is the imaging modality of choice. All necessary assets of the patient selection, endograft sizing and planning can be done on these images provided a standardised, accurate image post-processing protocol is used. Accurate measurements and planning on an image post-processing workstation will decrease the risk of misplacement and inadequate seal.

Postoperatively, a dedicated CTA protocol will be able to detect most problems, provided it is combined with an adequate image post-processing protocol. There is accumulating evidence for the value of MRI and MRA techniques after EVAR and this modality seems to be much more sensitive to endoleak detection than CTA is. Furthermore, the combination of the high soft tissue contrast before and after contrast enhancement and the possibility of performing dynamic CE-MRA might very well make MRI the imaging modality of choice after EVAR in the future.

Summary

- MRI and MRA have some inherent disadvantages that make them inadequate for preoperative imaging.
- DSA has become obsolete in the preoperative evaluation.
- CTA in combination with a dedicated image post-processing protocol is the preoperative image modality of choice.
- Postoperatively, a dedicated CTA protocol combined with an adequate image post-processing protocol will be able to detect most problems.
- MRA and MRI techniques seem to be more sensitive to endoleak detection than CTA is.
- MRI might very well become the imaging modality of choice after EVAR in the future.

References

1. Haulon S, Lions C, McFadden EP, et al. Prospective evaluation of magnetic resonance imaging after endovascular treatment of infrarenal aortic aneurysms. Eur J Vasc Endovasc Surg 2001; 22(1): 62-69.
2. Beebe HG. Imaging modalities for aortic endografting. J Endovasc Surg 1997; 4(2): 111-123.
3. Broeders IA, Blankensteijn JD, Olree M, Mali W, Eikelboom BC. Preoperative sizing of grafts for transfemoral endovascular aneurysm management: a prospective comparative study of spiral CT angiography, arteriography, and conventional CT imaging. J Endovasc Surg 1997; 4(3): 252-261.
4. Isokangas JM, Hietala R, Perala J, Tervonen O. Accuracy of computer-aided measurements in endovascular stent-graft planning: an experimental study with two phantoms. Invest Radiol 2003; 38(3): 164-170.
5. Lutz AM, Willmann JK, Pfammatter T, et al. Evaluation of aortoiliac aneurysm before endovascular repair: comparison of contrast-enhanced magnetic resonance angiography with multidetector row computed tomographic angiography with an automated analysis software tool. J Vasc Surg 2003; 37(3): 619-627.
6. Rubin GD, Walker PJ, Dake MD, et al. Three-dimensional spiral computed tomographic angiography: an alternative imaging modality for the abdominal aorta and its branches. J Vasc Surg 1993; 18(4): 656-664.
7. Wyers MC, Fillinger MF, Schermerhorn ML, et al. Endovascular repair of abdominal aortic aneurysm without preoperative arteriography. J Vasc Surg 2003; 38(4): 730-738.
8. Fletcher J, Saker K, Batiste P, Dyer S. Colour Doppler diagnosis of perigraft flow following endovascular repair of abdominal aortic aneurysm. Int Angiol 2000; 19(4): 326-330.
9. Golzarian J, Murgo S, Dussaussois L, et al. Evaluation of abdominal aortic aneurysm after endoluminal treatment: comparison of color Doppler sonography with biphasic helical CT. Am J Roentgenol 2002; 178(3): 623-628.
10. Haulon S, Lions C, McFadden EP, et al. Prospective evaluation of magnetic resonance imaging after endovascular treatment of infrarenal aortic aneurysms. Eur J Vasc Endovasc Surg 2001; 22(1): 62-69.
11. White RA, Donayre CE, Walot I, Woody J, Kim N, Kopchok GE. Computed tomography assessment of abdominal aortic aneurysm morphology after endograft exclusion. J Vasc Surg 2001; 33(2 Suppl): S1-10.
12. Haulon S, Willoteaux S, Koussa M, Gaxotte V, Beregi JP, Warembourg H. Diagnosis and treatment of type II endoleak after stent placement for exclusion of an abdominal aortic aneurysm. Ann Vasc Surg 2001; 15(2): 148-154.
13. Beebe HG, Kritpracha B, Serres S, Pigott JP, Price CI, Williams DM. Endograft planning without preoperative arteriography: a clinical feasibility study. J Endovasc Ther 2000; 7(1): 8-15.
14. Wever JJ, Blankensteijn JD, Mali WP, Eikelboom BC. Maximal aneurysm diameter follow-up is inadequate after endovascular abdominal aortic aneurysm repair. Eur J Vasc Endovasc Surg 2000; 20(2): 177-182.
15. Broeders IA, Blankensteijn JD. Preoperative imaging of the aortoiliac anatomy in endovascular aneurysm surgery. Semin Vasc Surg 1999; 12(4): 306-314.
16. Yeung KK, van der Laan MJ, Wever JJ, van Waes PF, Blankensteijn JD. New post-imaging software provides fast and accurate volume data from CTA surveillance after endovascular aneurysm repair. J Endovasc Ther 2003; 10(5): 887-893.
17. Broeders IA, Blankensteijn JD. A simple technique to improve the accuracy of proximal AAA endograft deployment. J Endovasc Ther 2000; 7(5): 389-393.
18. Buth J, Harris PL, van Marrewijk C, Fransen G. The significance and management of different types of endoleaks. Semin Vasc Surg 2003; 16(2): 95-102.
19. Gilling-Smith GL, Martin J, Gould D, et al. Freedom from endoleak after endovascular aneurysm repair does not equal treatment success. Eur J Vasc Endovasc Surg 2000; 19: 421-425.
20. Harris P, Brennan J, Martin J, et al. Longitudinal aneurysm shrinkage following endovascular aortic aneurysm repair: a source of intermediate and late complications. J Endovasc Surg 1999; 6(1): 11-16.
21. Laheij RJ, Buth J, Harris PL, Moll FL, Stelter WJ, Verhoeven EL. Need for secondary interventions after endovascular repair of abdominal aortic aneurysms. Intermediate-term follow-up results of a European collaborative registry (EUROSTAR). Br J Surg 2000; 87(12): 1666-1673.
22. Blankensteijn JD. Regarding 'changes in aneurysm volume after endovascular repair of abdominal aortic aneurysm'. J Vasc Surg 2002; 36(2): 412-413.
23. Buth J, Laheij RJ. Early complications and endoleaks after endovascular abdominal aortic aneurysm repair: report of a multicenter study. J Vasc Surg 2000; 31(1 Pt 1): 134-146.
24. Gould DA, Edwards RD, McWilliams RG, et al. Graft distortion after endovascular repair of abdominal aortic aneurysm: association with sac morphology and mid-term complications. Cardiovasc Intervent Radiol 2000; 23(5): 358-363.
25. Harris PL, Vallabhaneni SR, Desgranges P, Becquemin JP, van Marrewijk C, Laheij RJ. Incidence and risk factors of late rupture, conversion, and death after endovascular repair of infrarenal aortic aneurysms: the EUROSTAR experience. European Collaborators on Stent/graft techniques for aortic aneurysm repair. J Vasc Surg 2000; 32(4): 739-749.
26. White GH, May J, Waugh RC, Chaufour X, Yu W. Type III and type IV endoleak: toward a complete definition of blood flow in the sac after endoluminal AAA repair. J Endovasc Surg 1998; 5(4): 305-309.
27. Gilling-Smith G, Brennan J, Harris P, Bakran A, Gould D, McWilliams R. Endotension after endovascular aneurysm repair: definition, classification, and strategies for surveillance and intervention. J Endovasc Surg 1999; 6(4): 305-307.

28. Veith FJ, Baum RA, Ohki T, *et al.* Nature and significance of endoleaks and endotension: summary of opinions expressed at an international conference. *J Vasc Surg* 2002; 35(5): 1029-1035.

29. Wever JJ, Blankensteijn-JD, Eikelboom-BC. Secondary endoleak or missed endoleak? *Eur J Vasc Endovasc Surg* 1999; 18: 458-460.

30. Schurink GW, Aarts NJ, Wilde J, *et al.* Endoleakage after stent-graft treatment of abdominal aneurysm: implications on pressure and imaging - an *in vitro* study. *J Vasc Surg* 1998; 28(2): 234-241.

31. Risberg B, Delle M, Eriksson E, Klingenstierna H, Lonn L. Aneurysm sac hygroma: a cause of endotension. *J Endovasc Ther* 2001; 8(5): 447-453.

32. Mita T, Arita T, Matsunaga N, *et al.* Complications of Endovascualr Repair for Thoracic and Abdominal Aortic Aneurysm: an Imaging Spectrum. *Radiographics* 2000; 20 (5): 1263-1278.

33. Engellau L, Larsson EM, Albbrechtsson U, *et al.* Magnetic Resonace Imaging and MR Angiography of Endoluminally Treated Abdominal Aortic Aneurysms. *Eur J Vasc Endovasc Surg* 1998; 15: 212-219.

34. Haulon S, Lions C, McFadden EP, *et al.* Prospective evaluation of magnetic resonance imaging after endovascular treatment of infrarenal aortic aneurysms. *Eur J Vasc Endovasc Surg* 2001; 22(1): 62-69.

35. Haulon S, Willoteaux S, Koussa M, Gaxotte V, Beregi JP, Warembourg H. Diagnosis and treatment of type II endoleak after stent placement for exclusion of an abdominal aortic aneurysm. *Ann Vasc Surg* 2001; 15(2): 148-154.

36. Runge VM. Safety of approved MR contrast media for intravenous injection. *J Magn Reson Imaging* 2000; 12(2): 205-213.

37. Neschis DG, Velazquez OC, Baum RA, *et al.* The role of magnetic resonance angiography for endoprosthetic design. *J Vasc Surg* 2001; 33(3): 488-494.

38. Castrucci M, Mellone R, Vanzulli A, *et al.* Mural thrombi in abdominal aortic aneurysms: MR imaging characterization - useful before endovascular treatment? *Radiology* 1995; 197(1): 135-139.

Chapter 27

Three-dimensional rotational angiography

Jos C van den Berg, MD PhD, Interventional Radiologist

St. Antonius Hospital, Nieuwegein, The Netherlands

Introduction

Over the last 30 years balloon angioplasty and stenting has become a well accepted treatment for peripheral stenotic and occlusive arterial disease. In addition, over the last decade the endovascular treatment of peripheral arterial aneurysms has evolved due to the development of covered stents.

The diagnostic tests used in the assessment of peripheral vascular disease are also rapidly evolving. Currently, helical CT, CT angiography (using multislice scanners), gadolinium-enhanced MR angiography, calibrated angiography or (intravascular) ultrasound and Duplex ultrasound have gained acceptance as screening tests to detect and demonstrate peripheral aneurysmal and stenotic vascular disease.

The purpose of this chapter is to describe the use of three-dimensional rotational angiography (3D-RA) in pre-interventional interpretation of anatomic morphology and measurement of target vessels, and in the monitoring of peripheral endovascular interventions.

Technique of 3D rotational angiography

Acquisition and reconstruction

The basis of 3D-RA is conventional rotational angiography. This is obtained by performing a constant speed motorized movement of the C-arm around the patient during continuous contrast injection.

There are several ways to obtain three-dimensional images from rotational angiographic runs. One method consists of an examination in two phases, where at first the C-arm makes a sweep acquiring images that act as a mask for the subsequent data acquisition. Subsequently, a return sweep is performed whilst contrast is injected throughout the entire period of data acquisition. Images are then transferred to a workstation, where they are converted into pseudo-computed tomography slices (the image intensifier being considered a multiline detector). Using specific algorithms, to correct for image intensifier and contrast distortion, the data set is reconstructed into a volume-rendered technique [1,2].

The other technique of obtaining three-dimensional rotational angiography (3D-RA) is used in our institution and is directly based on conventional rotational angiographic images (Integris Allura, Philips Medical Systems, Best, The Netherlands). The system allows for two different movements: a roll movement that covers 180 degrees of rotational range with 30 degrees/sec rotational speed acquired during six seconds and a propeller movement that covers 240 degrees of movement range with 55 degrees of rotational speed completed within four seconds. The propeller movement is the preferred technique used for carotid studies and the vessels above the diaphragm, as it requires a lower contrast volume due to faster arc movement. This reduces the radiation dose. A drawback of increasing the rotational speed is a decrease in resolution of the acquisition, yielding images with decreased sharpness [1].

During either movement, 100 cine-fluoroscopic images are obtained with a frame rate of 12.5 or 25 frames/sec respectively, and the area of interest is placed in the system's isocenter. The image-intensifier entrance radiation dose in this fluoromode is 15µR/image, resulting in a total image-intensifier dose of 1.5mR/run.

Contrast injection is required throughout the acquisition of the images (four and six seconds for the propeller and roll movement respectively). The images obtained during the rotational studies (Figures 1a and 2a) are transferred to a 3D-RA workstation, where a default reconstruction is completed without user interaction as a background process (Figures 1b and 1e). During this reconstruction process two different types of image correction are done: pincushion distortion correction that is used to diminish environmental influences caused by the earth's magnetic field; and an isocenter correction that corrects all movement imperfections introduced by the rotating C-arc. This results in a negligible degree of visual distortion [3]. Both the corrections are based on the parameters that are calculated during calibration of the system, performed during routine maintenance. As the system is intrinsically calibrated, no additional calibration to perform measurements is required. The reconstruction method is based on the Feldkamp back-projection algorithm [4]. The reconstructions can be displayed in three different reconstruction matrices: 128^3, 256^3 and 512^3. The latter is used only if the visualisation of sub-millimeter

(micro-size) vessels is required. The total time that accounts for the image transfer and the reconstruction process of the default reconstruction amounts to 75 seconds.

The obtained 3-D volume can then be rotated and viewed in any direction. A reconstructive zoom technique (Figures 1c, 1f and 2b) can be used to make extra reconstructions of the area of interest, thus saving time, radiation dose to the patient and reducing the volume of contrast medium. Cut planes can be made at any position in the volume and measurements can be made (Figure 1d).

The use of automated vessel analysis (AVA) software allows determination of vessel geometrical properties on the user defined vessel portions/segments, such as the length, diameter, and area of the vessel segment of interest. The analysis is divided into two successive steps: definition of the central vessel axis and any branching points along the vessel trajectory and secondly, the analysis of the cross-sections positioned perpendicular to the defined vessel axis. The software provides an endoscopic view (virtual angioscopy), used for evaluation of the vessel interior. Furthermore, any point of the analysed vessel segment along the traced trajectory can be viewed in a cross-sectional view, which provides maximum and minimum vessel diameter measured at that particular position. Finally, a plot of vessel diameter distribution between the start and the end point of the vessel analysis can be drawn. The area and diameter of the stenosis and the length of the stenotic segment are measured and indicated in a histogram. Interactive dragging of the analysis borders allows enhanced definition of stent location and desired stent length (Figures 2c-2e).

Recent developments in software also allow visualisation of calcifications. Assessment and visualisation of the vessel's hyperdense plaque extent and location is based on a new acquisition protocol, especially designed for this particular purpose. The protocol requires creation of two runs: the calcification run and the contrast run. The first run is based on lowered kV numbers that decrease the radiation penetration rate and enhance visualisation of the soft tissue. As the vessel calcifications have increased attenuation in comparison with the

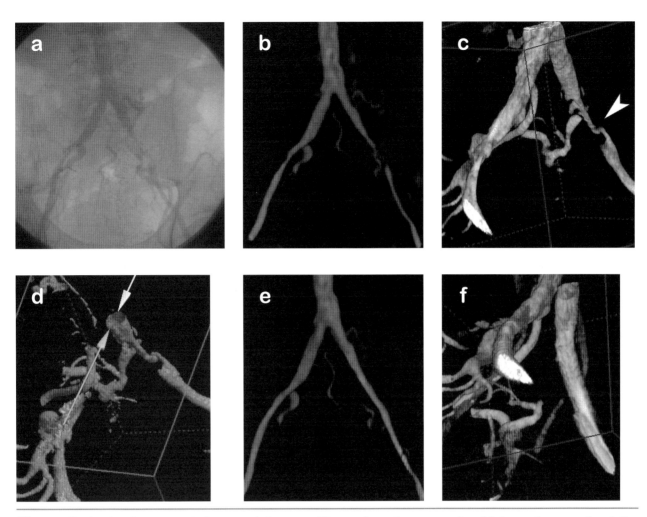

Figure 1. a) Cinefluoroscopic image of the aortoiliac region, demonstrating high-grade stenosis of the proximal right external iliac artery, and subtotal stenosis of left common and external iliac artery. b) 3D-RA of the same region: default reconstruction depicts stenoses in both iliac arteries. c) 3D-RA: reconstructive zoom of the left iliac artery, optimally depicting the subtotal stenosis (arrowhead) of the common and external iliac artery. d) 3D-RA: shaded-surface display with cutplane (pale grey lines) and measurement arrows allowing diameter measurement. e) 3D-RA: default reconstruction after bilateral stent placement; good angiographic result. f) 3D-RA: reconstructive zoom of the left iliac artery, showing complete resolution of the stenosis after stent placement.

surrounding soft tissue, the depiction of it is greatly enhanced. The second run is a standard contrast run, which is taken immediately after completion of the first run. After both the runs are acquired and reconstructed, the reconstruction superimposition is performed. In order to allow a perfect alignment of the reconstructions, a motion compensation technique is employed. The compensation diminishes consequences of possible patient movements introduced in the interval between the acquisitions of the runs and compensates for vessel pulsation. The

final reconstruction delineates the calcified masses and allows the assessment of the relation between the residual vessel lumen and the hyperdense plaque that is normally protruding into the lumen (Figure 2f).

The same method of superimposition of the two runs, taken with different acquisition settings, provides an improved depiction of stent location and its relation to the calcified plaque and vessel wall (Figures 2g and 2h).

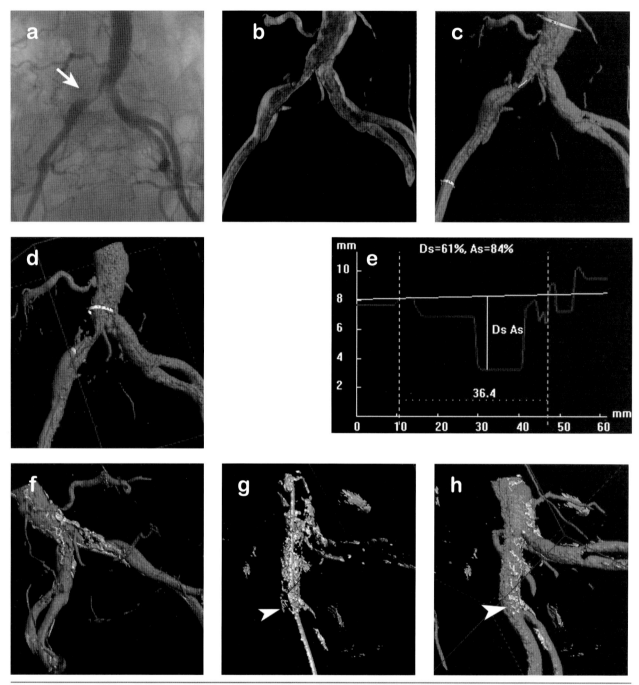

Figure 2. a) Cinefluoroscopic image of the aortoiliac region, demonstrating high-grade stenosis of the proximal right common iliac artery (arrow). b) 3D-RA: reconstructive zoom of the right common iliac artery and distal aorta demonstrating the stenosis in the right common iliac artery. c) 3D-RA: automated vessel analysis demonstrating the central lumen line running from the distal aorta (pale grey ring), to the right external iliac artery; along this line automatic diameter measurements can be displayed. d) 3D-RA: automated vessel analysis with rings placed just proximal and distal to a stenosis. e) Graph related to image depicted in figure 2d, demonstrating length of trajectory (36.4 mm), percentage of diameter and area stenosis (Ds, As); x-axis length, y-axis vessel diameter. f) 3D-RA: superimposition of shaded surface display and calcified plaque, demonstrating the heavily calcified nature of the common iliac lesion. g) 3D-RA: volume rendered image from calcification run after stent placement demonstrating plaque and stent struts (arrowhead). h) Volume rendered image obtained from a calcification run demonstrating plaque, catheter, as well as struts of the stent (arrowhead).

Radiation exposure and contrast medium dose

Although at first impression radiation exposure in an examination yielding 100 images seems to be an issue, the image-intensifier dose per image in the fluoromode of 15μR (leading to a total dose of 1.5mR) is much lower than with conventional angiography. Digital subtraction angiography using the same system can be performed at two dose levels: 200μR/image or 300μR/image. With a typical run of the iliac territory consisting of at least ten images, this will result in a total radiation exposure of 2mR and 3mR per run respectively. Since at least two oblique projections are required, this leads to an image-intensifier dose of 4-6mR. Other investigators found that the use of 3D-RA (even using the two-phase acquisition) does not lead to an increase of the dose delivered to the patient, and can even be reduced [1,5].

Although the amount of contrast for one rotational angiographic run exceeds the amount for a single, classic angiographic injection, the total amount of contrast is not significantly increased because one run will suffice [6]. For example, in our institution, standard projections of the aorto-iliac region include three views (AP, LAO and RAO), using a total contrast volume of 45ml (three times 15ml at a flowrate of 15ml/s). Using 3D-RA, visualising this region takes a total contrast volume of 48ml (injection rate 8ml/s). This is considerably lower than the amount needed for aortic imaging (requiring 120-150ml for a single acquisition) as advocated by others [1,7]. This might be caused by the difference in acquisition technique.

In order to keep the contrast volume to a minimum, catheter choice is very important. With flush catheter injections it is important to create a bolus of contrast running downstream, and upwards spill should be prevented. This feature of upstream contrast material dispersion is present to the greatest extent when using straight flush catheters, and to a lesser extent with pigtail catheters. Optimal contrast bolus injecting is achieved with so-called 'tennis-racket' and universal flush catheters [8]. In non-selective large vessel studies, a universal flush type catheter is used, while for selective studies (renal artery, carotid artery) the appropriate type of selective catheter is chosen on the basis of patient's anatomy. For an aorto-iliac study (from the infrarenal abdominal aorta to the distal external iliac arteries), a total amount of 48ml of contrast injected over six seconds (flow-rate 8ml/s), while for selective studies (renal arteries, visceral arteries and supra-aortic vessels), a flow-rate of 4-6ml/s is sufficient.

Because of the direct injection of contrast into the area of interest, timing of contrast-injection is not as difficult to optimise as in CT-angiography and MR-angiography [2].

Accuracy

Measurements on 3D-RA systems performed using well-defined test phantoms demonstrated that in all orientations of the phantom, the measured size deviated less than 2% from the actual size [9]. A comparison of IVUS and 3D-RA in an animal model demonstrated a high accuracy of the 3D-RA measurements [1]. *In vitro* comparison of CTA, MRA and 3D-RA in a cerebral aneurysm model, demonstrated the accuracy of measurements on 3D-RA to be as good as the other two modalities [10,11]. Others also found an excellent correlation between measurements obtained with MPR, 3D rotational angiography and intravascular ultrasound. Pitfalls remain when inappropriate window/level or threshold settings are being used, thus obscuring anatomic detail, leading to over- or underestimation of vessel size [1,11]. In order to avoid this, correlation of the volume rendered images and the original rotational angiographic images should always be made, or automated computer measurements (such as AVA), can be used to overcome this problem [11].

Because of precise calibration, accurate length and diameter measurements can be performed without the use of (costly) calibrated catheters [1,2,4,7].

Clinical aspects

The use of three-dimensional reconstructions is well known in MR-imaging and helical (multi-slice) CT. However, low spatial resolution, motion artifacts and limitations in visualisation of flow propagation are considered the most important disadvantages of CT and MRI [12]. 3D-RA is a relatively new technique that has initially been applied successfully in neuroradiological interventions, where it is a helpful

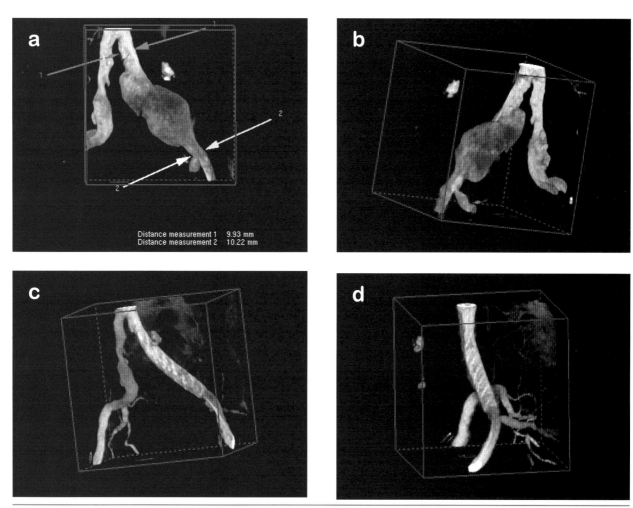

Figure 3. a) 3D-RA: volume rendered reconstructive zoom of left iliac region demonstrating a true aneurysm of the common iliac artery; arrows indicate the level where diameter measurements are performed. b) 3D-RA: volume rendered image; same region viewed with different angulation and skew; the relationship of the aneurysm to the hypogastric artery is clearly demonstrated; this tube position was used to monitor stent placement. c) 3D-RA: volume rendered image after covered stent placement showing exclusion of the aneurysm. d) 3D-RA: volume rendered image after covered stent placement demonstrating good patency of left hypogastric artery.

tool in the assessment of intracranial aneurysms and arteriovenous malformations [13-16]. One of the most critical issues in dealing with vascular diseases of the brain such as aneurysms or arterio-venous malformations is the accurate delineation of the pertinent anatomy. Rotational angiography (without three-dimensional reconstruction) has been demonstrated as a reliable technique for the multidirectional depiction of the internal carotid artery. In general, it demonstrates a more severe maximum internal carotid artery stenosis than does conventional two- or three-directional digital subtraction

angiography (DSA) [6,12,17,18]. Conventional rotational angiography has been demonstrated to show lesion morphology (eg. dissection/ulcers) to advantage [19].

Furthermore, 3D-RA offers the possibility to view the volume from different angles, which allows the physician to determine the optimal projection (angulation and skew) of the x-ray tube needed to facilitate the endovascular intervention (Figures 3 and 4), and assist the interventionalist in navigating through tortuous vasculature [5,20]. In addition, 3D reconstructions may give a better description of stenoses [7], and the

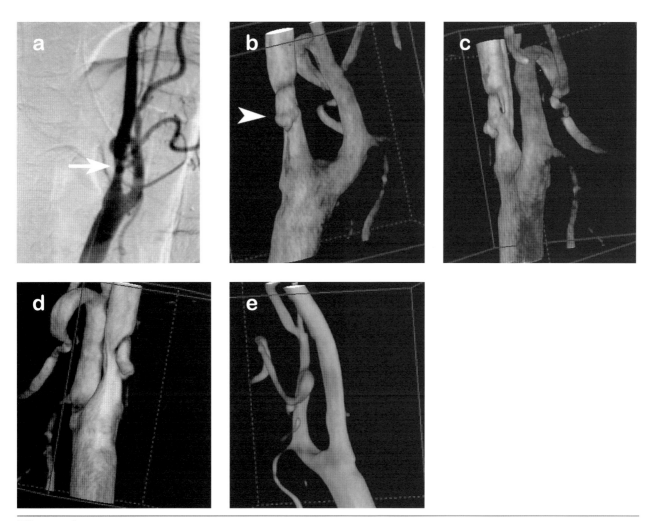

Figure 4. a) Digital subtraction angiography: carotid bifurcation with slight narrowing of the proximal internal carotid artery (arrow). b) 3D-RA: volume rendered image with similar projection as figure 4a; narrowing and irregularities at the proximal internal carotid artery (arrowhead). c/d) 3D-RA: stenosis and ulcerative characteristics of the internal carotid artery lesion are demonstrated to advantage on this volume rendered image. e) 3D-RA: volume rendered image after stent placement showing complete resolution of the stenosis.

cinefluoroscopic angiographic images allows us to obtain information on flow characteristics.

The time necessary to perform the default 3D-reconstruction and the reconstructive zoom is relatively short (a total of less than five minutes), and should not be considered a loss of time, as the necessity to perform various runs (as with conventional angiography) is lacking with the 3D-RA technique. It has been demonstrated that in the examination of the extracranial part of the carotid artery as well as in imaging of renal transplants, the use of 3D-RA results in a decrease of procedure time [6,7]. As prolonged procedure times increase the risk of complications, 3D-RA has the potential to reduce this [7]. It has to be kept in mind that the initial systems used clinically still need reconstruction times of more than 15 minutes, and that future hardware developments will continue to reduce reconstruction times, finally bringing real-time 3D-imaging [1].

The possibility to perform measurement 'on-line' allows corrections of stent choice during the procedure. This is of paramount importance since over- or undersizing has unwanted sequelae. The unwanted complications of undersizing of a stent

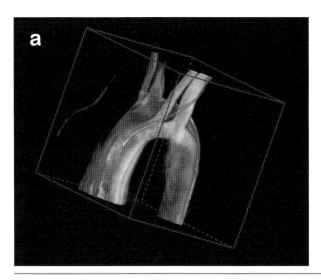 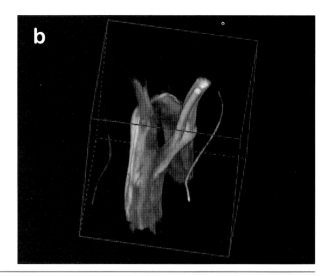

Figure 5. a/b) 3D-RA: volume rendered reconstructive zoom of the aortic arch (5a-LAO projection; 5b-craniocaudad view), demonstrating the presence of a double aortic arch and branching vessels.

placed for stenotic or occlusive peripheral arterial disease speak for themselves: insufficient dilatation or incomplete deployment of the stent has been identified as a possible cause for restenosis [21], or migration of the stent. In the case of treatment of aneurysms with covered stents, undersizing will lead to (type I) endoleaks [2,7,22,23]. Underdeployment of a stent can not always be discerned on conventional angiographic studies alone [5,10,11,21,23-27]. Oversizing of the stent may have deleterious effects on the vessel wall, leading to pseudoaneurysm formation. Very simple techniques (using the movement of the guidewire in a digitally subtracted image), have been proposed as a reliable measurement tool [28], but usually more sophisticated techniques are used, such as intravascular ultrasound (IVUS), calibrated angiography, conventional or spiral CT, CT angiography and MR imaging. With modern CT workstations it is possible to do measurements of diameter, length and volume and make three-dimensional reconstructions and 'central lumen line' length measurements. The disadvantage of this method is that these workstation reconstructions are very time-consuming and all measurements have to be made 'manually', and can not be done in the interventional suite during the procedure.

A disadvantage of the 3D-RA technique is non-visualisation of thrombus. The same is true for conventional angiography. Calcification, however, can

be demonstrated with 3D-RA using either the source images showing some indirect signs of the presence of thrombus (discrepancy between angiographic lumen and location of calcification), or the calcified plaque software.

The disadvantage of any two-phase acquisition (either the technique used to obtain the 3D-images or to acquire the calcification view), is the limitation caused by patient movement (eg. breathing, swallowing, and haemodynamic movement), leading to a lower spatial resolution or blurring of images [1].

Logistical limitations in performing the technique can occur in morbidly obese patients, where the C-arm can not rotate freely around the patient [5].

Like conventional digital subtraction angiography, and unlike CT and MRI, 3D-RA is not hampered by image artifacts caused by metallic stents or coils. In fact, 3D-RA is capable of demonstrating stent anatomy and conformability as well as adaptation of the stent to the vessel wall. Additional advantages of the 3D-RA technique as perceived by us and others [2] is the capability to reveal findings such as stenosis of the inferior mesenteric artery or aberrant arteries (made possible by the availability of true lateral projections) and detection of an inadvertent subintimal course of the guidewire and/or catheter, mal-alignment of intravascular stents, and even holes in the fabric of aortic stent grafts [1,2,20]. The virtual angioscopy tool (also called the 3D fly-through technique), allows visualisation of stenosis and ulcer-like abnormalities [1,2]. Finally, 3D-RA has the ability to obtain orthogonal views in the plane of any vessel (eg. renal artery) [5,16], or true cranio-caudad views of vasculature (eg. aortic arch; Figure 5).

In conclusion, 3D-RA can be used in peripheral endovascular interventions, providing useful additional data on target vessel and lesion morphology, allowing the interventionalist to better understand anatomic relationships and complex pathological states. Because of the short reconstruction times currently available it allows the physician to make adjustments during the procedure, in order to ensure optimal outcome, without additional procedure time.

Summary

◆   3D-RA length and diameter measurements are highly accurate.
◆   The use of 3D-RA in peripheral vascular interventions offers the possibility to reduce radiation dose, contrast volume and procedural time.
◆   3D-RA helps in understanding complex anatomy and due to short acquisition times can be used in the interventional suite during vascular procedures.

References

1. Klucznik RP. Current technology and clinical applications of three-dimensional angiography. *Radiol Clin North Am* 2002; 40(4): 711-28, v.

2. Unno N, Mitsuoka H, Takei Y, *et al.* Virtual angioscopy using 3-dimensional rotational digital subtraction angiography for endovascular assessment. *J Endovasc Ther* 2002; 9(4): 529-534.

3. Bridcut RR, Winder RJ, Workman A, Flynn P. Assessment of distortion in a three-dimensional rotational angiography system. *Br J Radiol* 2002; 75(891): 266-270.

4. Fahrig R, Fox AJ, Lownie S, Holdsworth DW. Use of a C-arm system to generate true three-dimensional computed rotational angiograms: preliminary *in vitro* and *in vivo* results. *Am J Neuroradiol* 1997; 18(8):1507-1514.

5. Prestigiacomo CJ, Niimi Y, Setton A, Berenstein A. Three-dimensional rotational spinal angiography in the evaluation and treatment of vascular malformations *Am J Neuroradiol* 2003; 24(7): 1429-1435.

6. Bosanac Z, Miller RJ, Jain M. Rotational digital subtraction carotid angiography: technique and comparison with static digital subtraction angiography. *Clin Radiol* 1998; 53(9): 682-687.

7. Hagen G, Wadstrom J, Magnusson A. 3D rotational angiography of transplanted kidneys. *Acta Radiol* 2003; 44(2): 193-198.

8. Froelich J, Barth KH, Lutz RJ, Lossef SV, Lindisch D. Injection characteristics and downstream contrast material distribution of flush aortography catheters: *in vitro* study. *J Vasc Intervent Radiol* 1992; 3(4): 713-718.

9. Kemkers R, op de Beek J, Aerts H. 3D-rotational angiography: first clinical applications. In: *Proceedings in computer assited radiology and surgery.* Lemke HU, Vannier MW, Inamura K, Farman A, Eds. Elsevier Science, Amsterdam, 1998: 182-187.

10. Bidaut LM, Laurent C, Piotin M, *et al.* Second-generation three-dimensional reconstruction for rotational three-dimensional angiography. *Acad Radiol* 1998; 5(12): 836-849.

11. Piotin M, Gailloud P, Bidaut L, *et al.* CT angiography, MR angiography and rotational digital subtraction angiography for volumetric assessment of intracranial aneurysms. An experimental study. *Neuroradiology* 2003; 45(6): 404-409.

12. Kumazaki T. Development of rotational digital angiography and new cone-beam 3D image: clinical value in vascular lesions. *Comput Methods Programs Biomed* 1998; 57(1-2): 139-142.

13. Missler U, Hundt C, Wiesmann M, Mayer T, Bruckmann H. Three-dimensional reconstructed rotational digital subtraction angiography in planning treatment of intracranial aneurysms. *Eur Radiol* 2000; 10(4): 564-568.

14. Anxionnat R, Bracard S, Ducrocq X, *et al.* Intracranial aneurysms: clinical value of 3D digital subtraction angiography in the therapeutic decision and endovascular treatment. *Radiology* 2001; 218(3): 799-808.

15. Hochmuth A, Spetzger U, Schumacher M. Comparison of three-dimensional rotational angiography with digital subtraction angiography in the assessment of ruptured cerebral aneurysms. *Am J Neuroradiol* 2002; 23(7): 1199-1205.

16. Endo H, Shimizu T, Kodama Y, Miyasaka K. Usefulness of 3-dimensional reconstructed images of renal arteries using rotational digital subtraction angiography. *J Urol* 2002; 167(5): 2046-2048.

17. Elgersma OE, Buijs PC, Wust AF, van der GY, Eikelboom BC, Mali WP. Maximum internal carotid arterial stenosis: assessment with rotational angiography versus conventional intraarterial digital subtraction angiography. *Radiology* 1999; 213(3): 777-783.

18. Pozzi MF, Pecenco R, Calderan L, Pozzi MR. Rotational angiography of the carotid artery bifurcation: technical aspects and preliminary results. *Radiol Med* (Torino) 2002; 104(3): 157-164.

19. Yamamoto K, Maeda S, Kameoka N, Komatsu S, Ishikawa T. Rotational Digital Angiography for the Evaluation of Iliac Artery Disease. *Int J Angiol* 1999; 8(1): 11-15.

20. van den Berg JC, Moll FL. Three-dimensional rotational angiography in peripheral endovascular interventions. *J Endovasc Ther* 2003; 10(3): 595-600.

21. Arko F, McCollough R, Manning L, Buckley C. Use of intravascular ultrasound in the endovascular management of atherosclerotic aortoiliac occlusive disease. *Am J Surg* 1996; 172(5): 546-549.

22. White GH, May J, Waugh RC, Chaufour X, Yu W. Type III and type IV endoleak: toward a complete definition of blood flow in the sac after endoluminal AAA repair. *J Endovasc Surg* 1998; 5(4): 305-309.

23. van den Berg JC, Overtoom TT, de Valois JC, Moll FL. Using three-dimensional rotational angiography for sizing of covered stents. *Am J Roentgenol* 2002; 178(1): 149-152.

24. Buckley CJ, Arko FR, Lee S, *et al.* Intravascular ultrasound scanning improves long-term patency of iliac lesions treated with balloon angioplasty and primary stenting. *J Vasc Surg* 2002; 35(2): 316-323.

25. White RA, Donayre CE, Kopchok GE, Walot I, Mehringer CM. Utility of intravascular ultrasound in peripheral interventions. *Tex Heart Inst J* 1997; 24(1): 28-34.

26. Scoccianti M, Verbin CS, Kopchok GE, *et al.* Intravascular ultrasound guidance for peripheral vascular interventions. *J Endovasc Surg* 1994; 1: 71-80.

27. Navarro F, Sullivan TM, Bacharach JM. Intravascular ultrasound assessment of iliac stent procedures. *J Endovasc Ther* 2000; 7(4): 315-319.

28. Snow TM, Bennetts M. Technical report: A low cost technique for vessel sizing in angioplasty. *Clin Radiol* 1998; 53(12): 929-931.

Contrast-enhanced magnetic resonance angiography: current indications and new developments

James FM Meaney, FRCR FFR(RCSI), Consultant Radiologist

Gerard E Boyle, PhD, Principal Physicist

St. James's Hospital, Dublin, Ireland

Historical perspective

Over the last 20 years, it has become apparent that flow phenomena, rather than solely presenting an unwanted contribution to artifacts, could be harnessed to generate diagnostic images of blood vessels [1-3]. Initial approaches Time-of-Flight (TOF) and Phase Contrast Effect (PCA) relied on the inherent properties of flow, and were accepted with great enthusiasm. However, limitations related primarily to long scan time and flow-related artifacts limited the acceptance of these techniques into clinical practice. With the introduction of contrast-enhanced techniques, a whole new diagnostic vista was realized [4]. Contrast-enhanced MRA (CE-MRA) offers the significant advantages of high resolution, high signal-to-noise and freedom from artifacts that are required to establish an MRA technique as the clinical routine. It is now the standard of reference for MRA against which all new techniques must be measured and in many instances offers information that is not available from catheter angiography.

Difference between catheter angiography and MRA

There are several important fundamental differences between conventional angiography and MRA, as follows:-

- MRA employs strong magnetic fields to generate angiographic images and there is no exposure to ionizing radiation.
- Contrast agents, if used, have negligible toxicity. In particular, there is no nephrotoxicity at standard doses used in clinical practice.
- The MR angiographic display is almost always in the form of a three-dimensional projectional image - the Maximum Intensity Projection (MIP). This relies on extraction of high-signal vascular data from a series of cross-sectional images, in which the arteries have been rendered bright by virtue of the technique used (TOF/PCA/contrast injection).
- For contrast-enhanced MRA (the most widely accepted and exploited approach to MRA), contrast agent is delivered intravenously. Because the site of injection into a peripheral vein is remote from the region of interest, accurate timing of scan data in relation to peak arterial enhancement is crucial.
- Unique features of k-space can be exploited to improve the quality of CE-MRAs. Specifically, the central lines of k-space (which determine image contrast) must be synchronized with the arterial peak of contrast enhancement which gives optimal signal-to-noise ratios. Also, in cases

where a robust method of scan timing is available (eg. real-time MR fluoroscopy), sampling of central k-space lines, if performed at the start of the scan, allows acquisition of higher resolution images as completion of peripheral k-space data (during the venous phase) does not result in venous contamination.

Non-contrast versus contrast-enhanced techniques

The aim of MRA is to generate images with high intra-signal intensity within the lumen of the vessel. This high signal is then re-projected into a (pseudo) three-dimensional image, using a powerful computer algorithm (the Maximum Intensity Projection - MIP), that selectively extracts high signal data from the images. The goal of generation of high intravascular signal can be achieved by exploiting:-

◆   a Time-of-Flight effect (TOF) [1,2];
◆   a Phase Contrast Effect (PCA) [3];
◆   a T-1 shortening effect (contrast-enhanced MRA) [4].

With the first two methods (TOF and PCA), intravascular signal depends on inherent properties of flow, and scan parameters must be tailored accordingly. For example, in the case of TOF MRA, scan data must be acquired perpendicular (ideally orthogonal) to the direction of flow, and the time between the radiofrequency (RF) pulses (the repetition time [TR]), must be sufficiently long to allow adequate 'inflow' of fully relaxed protons into the imaging slice between successive TRs. For PCA, scan data can be acquired in any plane. However, the velocity-encoding-gradient (Venc), must be tailored to the blood velocity in the artery of interest. This assumes a priori knowledge of the blood flow within the relevant artery, which constitutes one of the significant drawbacks of this technique. Although the velocity can be rapidly measured directly by acquiring a series of 2D PC images with different phase-encoding values, this is time-consuming and different velocities frequently exist within the arteries enclosed within a single field of view which introduces artifacts.

Time-of-flight MRA methodology and limitations

TOF angiography relies on the fact that the blood enters the volume with relatively high velocity and traverses the volume in a short time period so that it receives very few RF pulses. In order to maintain highest possible inflow effect, all protons within the imaging volume must be replenished between successive TRs, although maximal inflow may not be necessary in clinical practice and some trade-offs can be accepted. An oblique course of a blood vessel in relation to the slice orientation and short TRs both affect SNR unfavourably, as protons under these conditions experience more RF pulses whilst in the imaging slice, and as a result, saturation of signal.

Images were prone to artifactual over-estimation of the degree and length of stenosis, because of intra-voxel dephasing secondary to turbulent, slow and pulsatile flow.

TOF MRA has failed to offer a viable non-invasive screening test to conventional arteriography, and has not had a major impact on clinical practice.

Advantages of contrast-enhanced MRA?

CE-MRA is a flow-independent technique that relies on paramagnetic contrast agent induced T1 shortening for generation of intra-vascular signal. The unique nature of k-space data lends itself to some modifications that can be exploited to generate superior quality CE-MRAs. Because central k-space data governs signal-to-noise ratio (SNR) (and peripheral k-space governs resolution), images with unrivalled SNR are rapidly generated provided the contrast-defining central lines of k-space are synchronized with peak arterial enhancement [5]. As images are independent of 'inflow-effects' 3D data-sets can be acquired in the coronal plane (which affords the greatest anatomical coverage for any combination of field of view, number of slices and slice thickness) and the shortest available TR can be used (gives shortest scan time). As selective arterial images are generated by appropriate timing of the 3D data-set in relation to the arterio-venous window, neither saturation bands (that may impair SNR in 2D TOF

MRA) nor ECG triggering (that prolongs scan time), are required. Because of these combined advantages of freedom of acquisition geometry, speed of acquisition, freedom from artifacts, absence of requirement for cardiac triggering and superior SNR, CE-MRA has largely replaced non-contrast methods for evaluation of most vascular territories.

CE-MRA: technique

The technique of CE-MRA is highly operator-dependent. Therefore, in order to generate high-quality CE-MRAs, the operator must pay careful attention to detail. Unlike other MR applications, the operator must interact with the patient and address region-specific issues at several levels. For example, the 3D scan must be carefully tailored to the region of interest to facilitate use of highest possible resolution; also, the scan time must be tailored to the patient's breath-hold capability (for thoracic and abdominal imaging); lastly, initiation of 3D scan data collection must coincide with onset of arterial enhancement to ensure a selective arterial phase study. Meticulous planning of the following steps ensures highest quality CE-MRA.

1. Acquire a localizer.
2. Plan a 3-D scan that is sufficiently short to allow completion of imaging during the arterio-venous window and during breath-holding with sufficiently high resolution to allow accurate evaluation of the vessel of interest (higher resolution implies longer scan time).
3. Inject a sufficient volume of contrast agent to make the arteries the brightest structures on the image.
4. Time the start of the 3D scan to coincide with peak arterial enhancement.
5. Post-process data-set.

Planning the 3D scan: importance of the localizer

Although there is little or no diagnostic information inherent in the localizer, imaging during the arterial phase and during a breath-hold can only be achieved if a relatively small 3D imaging volume can be prescribed. This implies that an 'outline' of the vessels must be provided by the localizer. We advocate a low-

resolution gradient-echo time-of-flight scan in the axial plane which highlights the arteries because of 'inflow'. This localizer takes approximately one minute per location, and lateral and antero-posterior MIPs generated from the axial data-set allow accurate 3D volume placement. This approach is appropriate for all anatomic sites.

Optimizing the 3D scans: spatial resolution and scan time considerations

A fast 3D spoiled gradient echo acquisition is used (see Table 1 for technical parameters). Despite advances in MRA, images are still limited in terms of spatial resolution compared to conventional arteriography. This is not because high resolution images cannot be acquired, but rather due to the fact that a sufficient number of slices of highest available resolution cannot be acquired within the breath-hold capability of the patient, as increase in in-plane resolution (in the phase-encode direction) and increase in the slice direction (higher number of thinner slices) leads to increased scan time.

Therefore, in order to ensure optimized resolution (and therefore scan time), the four parameters that govern scan time must be addressed, as given by the following equation:-

SCAN TIME = TR x Np x Ns x NSA

TR: For CE-MRA applications, short TRs must be available. Short TRs are available on most modern scanners, although it is the gradient performance and not the field strength that governs how short the TR can become.

NSA: This is always one or less (usually 0.6-0.8 as partial Fourier imaging is implemented in almost every case).

Np and Ns: The matrix size in both the phase- and frequency directions governs in-plane resolution. However, the number of frequency-encoding steps does not affect scan time, and therefore, high resolution can be achieved in the frequency-encoding direction without time penalty (eg. 400mm FOV/512 samples gives a head-foot resolution of 0.78mm, compared to a head-foot resolution of 1.56mm for a 256 matrix for the same scan time). Ideally, the resolution in the frequency-encode direction should

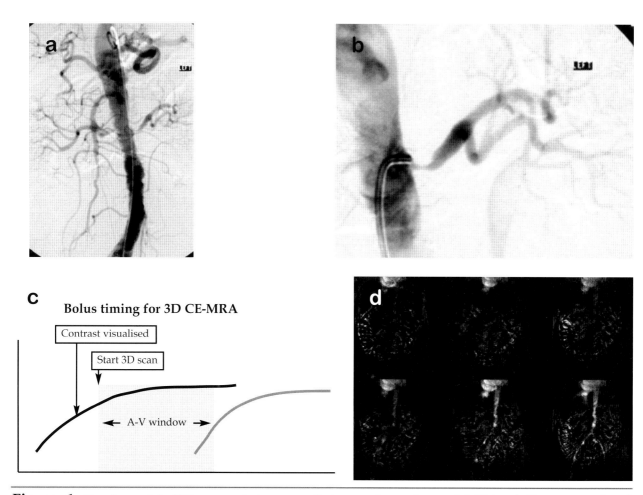

Figure 1. Fundamental differences between catheter angiography and MRA. a) For conventional angiography, contrast is delivered intra-arterially to the region of interest. b) Catheterisation of individual arteries allows selective visualisation of specific regions of interest. However, for CE-MRA, contrast is delivered intravenously. A method that ensures collection of scan data coincident with the arterial peak and prior to onset of venous enhancement initiation of the 3D scan, must be implemented, i.e. during the arterio-venous window, as shown graphically in c). Otherwise, images will suffer from a 'ringing' artifact (if the 3D scan is initiated too early) or overlapping venous enhancement (if initiated too late). d) This emphasises the importance of scan timing, which is optimally performed with direct visualisation of contrast arrival within the arteries of interest with MR fluoroscopy. When MR fluoroscopy is combined with 'centric' phase-encoding, venous contamination is eliminated in virtually all cases.

be matched by identical resolution in both the phase-encode and slice-encode directions, and both should be 1mm or less. However, achieving this (use of 512 phase-encode steps, and use of 1mm thick slices) substantially increases scan time and places scan time out of the breath-hold range. Therefore, in order to prescribe a scan that can be completed within the breath-hold capability of the patient, the resolution in both the phase-encode (Np) and slice-encode directions (Ns) must be sacrificed in favour of shorter scan time. In practical terms, in-plane resolution for most areas within the body (apart from the carotid arteries and pedal arteries), is usually 0.6-1mm x 1.5-2mm with slice thickness of 1-4mm depending on location. However, it is essential to note that within the abdomen (particularly renal artery imaging), a lower resolution scan successfully completed within a breath-hold is infinitely better that a high resolution scan acquired without breath-holding.

Table 1. Parameters for CE-MRA.

TR	<5msec	Shorter TRs give shorter scan time, higher resolution or a combination of both.
TE	<3msec	Typically <2msec. Lower values give less dephasing.
Flip angle	30-45deg	Optimally predicted by Ernst equation. However, higher flip angles give better background suppression.
Matrix size	512 x 128-256	Higher matrix in frequency direction does not increase scan time but gives higher resolution (and lower SNR). The resolution in the phase-encode direction must be carefully tailored to allow a sufficiently short scan time.
Slice thickness	1-4mm slices	Thinner slices give higher resolution but need higher number of slices for same anatomic coverage which gives longer scan time.
Bandwidth	+/- 32-64KHz	Narrower bandwidths give higher SNR but longer scan times. Wider bandwidths give shorter scan times but higher SNR.
NSA	1 or less	Partial Fourier almost always used. Typically 0.6-0.9.

Exploiting the unique aspects of k-space to diminish the risk of venous contamination of MRAs:

By mapping central k-space data as soon as contrast arrives in the artery of interest (a software modification routinely available on almost all current systems), the risk of venous enhancement is reduced or eliminated, even if venous enhancement appears late in the scan [5]. This feature is typically exploited for all CE-MRAs as follows:-

◆ To guarantee arterial phase images with highest possible SNR providing bolus-detection is used to allow the operator to initiate the 3D scan.

◆ By collecting central k-space data at the start of the scan, there will be maximal artery-vein signal difference which minimises venous contamination of the images.

In some instances, typically applications where breath-holding is not required (eg. carotid artery and pedal MRA), image resolution can be increased by continuing to collect peripheral k-space data beyond the duration of the arterio-venous window, without increasing the likelihood of venous-enhancement. This allows the operator to prescribe a long (eg. 40-60 seconds) high resolution scan for the smaller arteries of the legs.

Contrast agent issues: how much and how fast?

Remember that MRA relies on the simple principle of rendering the arteries the brightest structure on the image, so that the MIP algorithm reprojects the arteries, and no other tissue on the final processed image. As fat is the brightest structure on T1 weighted images, the T1 value of the contrast-enriched blood must be substantially lower than that of fat so that fat is 'windowed' out on the MIP images (the aim is to reduce the T1 of arterial blood on first pass to 50msec or less compared to a T1 of fat of approximately 230msec) (ignoring the fact that fat may also be subtracted by subtraction of a pre-contrast mask) [6]. This can be achieved with a flow rate of approximately 1cc per second. However, if fat is eliminated (by subtraction), lower infusion rates can be used (injection rates of 0.3-2cc/sec have been reported in the literature). For abdominal and thoracic CE-MRA we use 30cc (of 0.5M contrast agent), injected at 1-2cc/sec. However, the duration of the bolus should at least approximate the scan duration. The fact that this varies from 10secs (a rapid renal MRA) to 60secs (a three-station moving-table CE-MRA), explains the widely differing infusion rates and infusion duration reported in the literature.

The importance of timing

This issue emphasizes one of the fundamental differences between conventional catheter arteriography (where contrast agent is injected at or close to the region of interest) and CE-MRA (where contrast agent is injected intravenously, remote from the region of interest). In order to ensure that 3D scan data is collected during the arterial peak, three methods have been used widely in clinical practice, as follows:-

Empiric (best-guess)

Assumes that the circulation time falls with a short range predictable on the basis of age and cardiovascular status (no longer widely practised due to superior methods being available).

Timing bolus

A small volume of contrast agent (the 'test-dose', typically 1cc), is injected at the same rate as planned for the total injection, and followed by a long (30cc) saline flush. Scans are dynamically acquired over the region of interest (ROI) with a temporal resolution of 1/sec. The scan delay time is set according to the following calculation:-

Scan delay time = bolus arrival time - injection time/2 - scan time/2

Automated bolus-detection

There are two approaches:-

'Black-box' approach (eg. SMARTPREP, GE Medical Systems) [7]:

'Fluoroscopic' triggering (eg. BOLUSTRAK, Philips Medical Systems, CAREBOLUS, Siemens Medical Systems) [8]. A time resolved single thick 2D slice reconstructed and displayed in real time allows visualisation of contrast arrival within the region of interest.

Post-processing/image display

The MIP forms the basis of image display. Other reconstruction algorithms such as surface-shaded display and video 'angioscopy' (fly-through) have not established a clear role in clinical practice.

The following format is widely accepted:-

◆ Data should be interrogated on a 3D workstation using multi-planar reformatting, whole volume and sub-volume MIP as appropriate.
◆ An overview of the whole anatomy images is usually generated.
◆ For each artery, selective multi-planar or MIP reformats that best demonstrate the arterial anatomy should be generated.
◆ Video (rotated) MIPs are useful for many areas (especially carotid and pedal arteries).

Clinical results, current applications, limitations and future potential

CE-MRA has been applied to and has established a major role in imaging of virtually all vascular territories in the body, with the exception of the coronary arteries. A brief discussion of the relevant areas follows.

Renal arteries

CE-MRA has become the technique of choice for evaluation of the renal arteries [4,9]. Although most papers report that it is highly accurate for detection of and grading of renal artery stenosis, there is little functional information inherent in the images. Methods for 'grading' the severity of renal artery stenosis (RAS), in borderline cases include:-

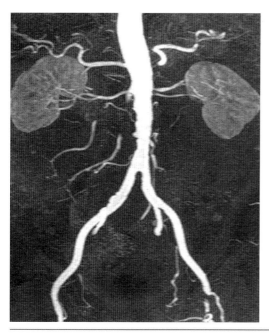

Figure 2. Renal MRA acquired with bolus detection, centric phase-encoding, and resolution optimized to the breath-holding capability of the patient. Note excellent visualisation of the abdominal aorta, its visceral branches and iliac arteries.

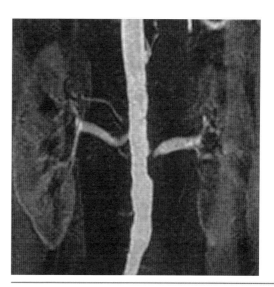

Figure 3. Sub-volume MIP targeted to the upper abdominal aorta and renal arteries demonstrates severe left renal artery stenosis.

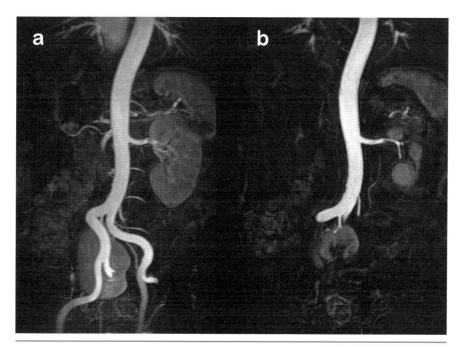

Figure 4. Whole volume MIP demonstrates a normal left kidney and normal left renal artery. The right kidney is absent from the renal fossa, and lies in ectopic position within the right pelvis. A sub-volume MIP confirms that the artery arising from the inferior aspect of the proximal right common iliac artery just beyond the bifurcation represents the right main renal artery.

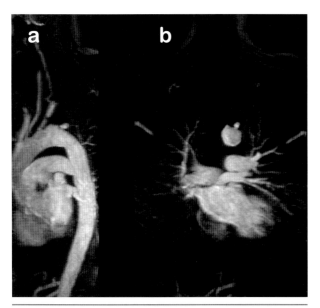

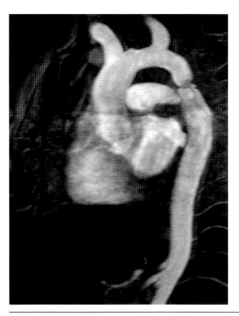

Figure 5. a) Lateral MIP of the thoracic aorta demonstrates a small out-pouching of contrast agent beyond the great vessel origins. b) This is confirmed as a penetrating ulcer of the thoracic aorta on a sub-volume coronal MIP. Further images (not shown) demonstrated mediastinal haematoma.

Figure 6. Lateral MIP of the thoracic aorta demonstrates focal narrowing due to coarctation.

◆ Measurement of renal size.

◆ Inspection of the 'density' of the nephrogram, which is almost always reduced in significant RAS.

◆ Use of a phase-contrast method, either 3D PCA where significant stenosis on CE-MRA is always associated with signal drop-off within the proximal artery on PCA, or 2D cine PCA where flow can be directly measured [10].

CE-MRA is also highly accurate for evaluation of transplant RAS. In this instance, there is the significant advantage of not having to acquire images during breath-holding, as the transplanted kidney does not move with respiration due to its fixed location within the iliac fossa. Higher resolution images can therefore be obtained.

Abdominal aorta

CE-MRA is an excellent modality for visualising the abdominal aorta and side branches [11-14]. However, in most centres, contrast-enhanced CT has become the technique of choice prior to endovascular stenting despite similar accuracy of CTA and MRA. The main

drawbacks of MRA are failure to visualise calcification within the aortic wall, and poorer depiction of the external dimensions compared to CTA unless further imaging (eg. post-contrast T1w imaging), is performed. However, MRA has the advantage of having no nephrotoxicity associated with the contrast agent, an important factor to consider in the large group of patients with impaired renal function.

Mesenteric arteries

Although PCA has been reported for suspected chronic mesenteric ischaemia [15], CE-MRA is now the technique of choice for detection of mesenteric artery stenosis on patients with suspected chronic mesenteric ischaemia [16-18]. Chronic mesenteric ischaemia rarely occurs unless the superior mesenteric artery is severely stenosed or occluded. Pseudostenosis of the coeliac trunk (crus compression) is common and should not be confused with pathological narrowing (occurs when images acquired in full inspiration, therefore repeating the scan in expiration helps to differentiate true from artifactual narrowing). Asymptomatic inferior mesenteric artery stenosis or occlusion is also common in patients with severe vascular disease. Therefore, as asymptomatic mesenteric artery stenosis is extremely common, findings on MRA must be closely correlated with the clinical scenario. Functional evaluation may provide further useful information [19]. CE-MRA is rarely performed in patients with acute mesenteric ischaemia as this usually constitutes an urgent abdominal emergency requiring immediate surgery. CE-MRA has also been exploited to determine resectibility of pancreatic carcinoma [20]. However, in most institutions this is accurately performed with contrast-enhanced CT.

Pulmonary arteries

Three prospective studies validate CE-MRA for detection of pulmonary embolism (PE) [21-23]. Despite this, CE-MRA has not been widely implemented in clinical practice, primarily because of the widespread acceptance of spiral CT [24]. An important limitation of MRA compared to CTA is that MRA images are severely degraded by motion artifact, whereas CT suffers less from motion artifact, an important factor to remember considering the fact that the majority of patients with suspected PE have limited breath-hold capability [24]. The issue of limited breath-holding potential in the majority of patients undergoing imaging for suspected PE has an important bearing on choice of imaging parameters and scan plane. For example, although the importance of sub-segmental PE is uncertain, visualisation of the arteries to sub-segmental level is a goal of imaging [24]. In order to achieve this goal, if images are acquired in the coronal plane, a larger number of slices than can be accommodated within a breath-hold must be used. Therefore, the scan volume must be limited in the AP plane, thus excluding subsegmental vessels both anteriorly and posteriorly [21,22]. A second, and probably superior approach, is to use a higher resolution sagittal acquisition for each lung individually, with a separate injection for each lung [23]. This satisfies the requirement to image at a higher resolution but has the drawbacks of requiring two injections and having a slightly longer examination time.

Carotid arteries

In order to image the carotid arteries at high resolution, a long scan time is required. However, the carotid-jugular AV transit time is short, approximately 8-12 seconds only, because the intact blood brain barrier does not allow parenchymal extraction of gadolinium chelates. Because of the unique nature of k-space, selective arterial phase high resolution

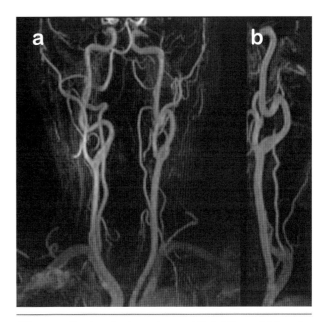

Figure 7. a) Whole volume AP MIP and b) sub-volume MIP of the right carotid artery demonstrates normal appearance.

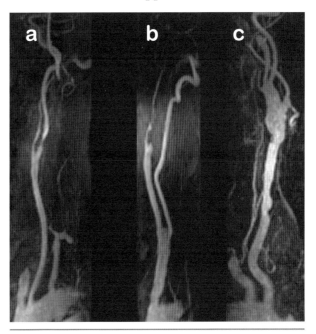

Figure 8. a) Severe left internal carotid artery stenosis, b) occlusion of the right internal carotid artery from its origin and c) post-endarterectomy appearance (three different patients).

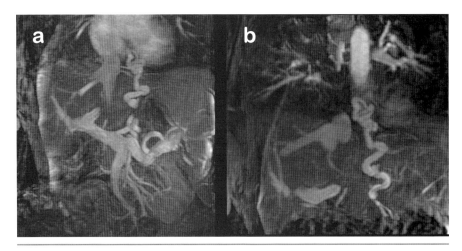

Figure 9. a) Sub-volume MIPs in the venous phase demonstrate enlargement and patency of the portal, superior mesenteric and splenic veins in a patient with portal hypertension. b) Note the enlarged coronary vein.

imaging of the carotids can be performed providing firstly, that the central lines of k-space are acquired at the start of the scan and secondly, that 3D scan data is initiated as soon as contrast arrives within the carotid arteries. Essentially, this mandates use of fluoroscopic triggering because of the critical nature of scan timing.

CE-MRA is useful for differentiating sub-total from total occlusion (string sign) and gives excellent visualisation of the head and neck arteries from arch to circle of Willis [25]. Despite use of a 'high' resolution (1mm isotropic voxels), this resolution remains limited in comparison to catheter angiography, and probably cannot differentiate for example, a 65% stenosis from a 70% stenosis [25].

Peripheral arteries

Most limitations of peripheral artery MRA have been overcome. For example, the issue of limited spatial coverage in the cranio-caudal direction has been addressed by implementation of a moving-table approach [26-30]. The issue of limited spatial resolution has been addressed by tailoring imaging parameters for each 3D volume individually to the artery of interest [30]. Although venous enhancement within the third imaging location remains an issue in some

patients, this issue is being addressed (eg. ever-increasing acquisition speed, by implementation of 2D/3D hybrid techniques, by use of parallel imaging techniques, and by use of tourniquets to slow onset of venous enhancement). Several meta-analyses have established the role of CE-MRA in peripheral vascular disease [31-33].

Magnetic Resonance Venography

Non-contrast techniques suffer from the same drawbacks in the venous system as compared to the arterial system. CE-MRV can be performed as follows:-

◆ Indirect CE-MRV. Images are acquired in the 'venous' phase after collecting arterial phase data or by applying a longer scan delay time. This technique is suitable for evaluation of all venous territories, and is particularly useful for evaluation of the spleno-portal system [34,35].

◆ Direct CE-MRV. This is applicable to territories where the contrast can be injected 'upstream' of the region of interest, therefore limiting its usefulness to the upper and lower extremities only. In order to avoid the severe susceptibility artifact which results from injection of undiluted contrast directly into veins, contrast must be

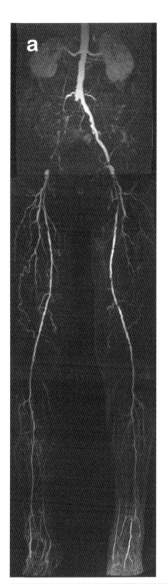
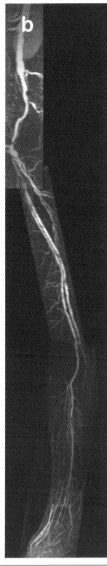

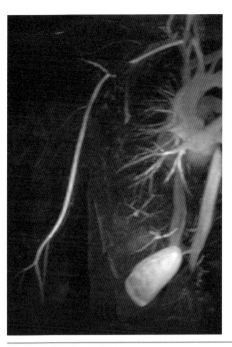

Figure 11. 3D CE-MRA in a patient extremity following a motor vehicle accident. There is abrupt cut-off of the axillary artery, with reconstitution of flow distally. The appearance is typical of acute traumatic dissection.

Figure 10. Moving table three-station contrast-enhanced MRA from the level of the upper abdominal aorta to the pedal arteries in the a) AP and b) lateral projections. There is excellent depiction of the arteries throughout. Note occlusion of the right common and external iliac arteries, diffuse atheroma throughout the right superficial femoral artery and occlusion of the right anterior tibial artery in the mid calf. The right posterior tibial artery is also occluded, the right peroneal artery is of good calibre and gives rise to the dorsalis pedis artery. Note that 3D volumes optimised to the region of interest were employed. This allows the scan parameters to be individually tailored to the arteries, which get smaller from aorta to foot. Note that the largest 3D volume is used for the third station (legs) so as to include the pedal arch within the imaging volume.

diluted to between 2-10% (1-5cc 0.5M contrast agent in 50cc saline). This overcomes the T2* induced signal drop-off whilst still maintaining adequate T1 shortening [36].

◆ In the future, blood pool agents will give persistence of venous signal over a long time period, and thus allow high quality MRV [37].

Future directions

Continual increases in gradient speed facilitate higher resolution, shorter acquisition times or a combination of both. 3T imaging opens new horizons. Parallel imaging, which increases speed/resolution by a factor of 2-4 is making inroads into clinical practice [38]. New contrast agents, improved coil design and efficiency and the future potential for functional imaging offer enormous possibility for future improvements. Isotropic 1mm resolution studies for all regions of interest with a functional component are anticipated within the next few years, and new applications are constantly being added [39].

Summary

- Contrast-enhanced techniques have supplanted non-contrast techniques for almost all applications.
- CE-MRA requires fast scanner capability (fast gradients).
- Attention to detail with CE-MRA is paramount, in particular 3D data must be synchronized with the arterial peak.
- CE-MRA has been validated for aortic, renal, mesenteric and carotid artery evaluation.
- CE-MRA of the peripheral arteries requires use of a moving-table technique to give extended anatomic coverage from renal arteries to pedal arteries. Peripheral MRA has been validated in several studies and several meta-analyses.
- Because of limitations related to the arterio-venous window and to limited breath-holding capability, scan resolution is often sacrificed for shorter scan times.
- This emphasizes the need for higher spatial resolution, in order to match more closely that of catheter angiography. This can be achieved by a combination of increased acquisition speed, use of parallel imaging methods and novel pulse sequences.
- Introduction of 3T imaging into the clinical arena offers enormous potential for higher quality MRA in clinical practice.

References

1. Lenz G, Haacke E, Masaryk T, Laub GA. Inplane vascular imaging: pulse sequence design and strategy. *Radiology* 1988; 166: 875-882.

2. Keller PJ, Drayer BP, Fram EK, Williams KD, Dumoulin CL, Souza SP. MR angiography with two-dimensional acquisition and three-dimensional display. *Radiology* 1989; 173: 527-532.

3. Dumoulin CL, Souza SP, Walker MF, Wagle W. Three-dimensional phase contrast angiography. *Magn Res Med* 1989; 9: 139-149.

4. Prince MR, Narasimham DL, Stanley JC, *et al*. Breath-hold gadolinium-enhanced MR arteriography of the abdominal aorta and its major branches. *Radiology* 1995; 197: 785-792.

5. Mezrich R. A perspective on k-space. *Radiology* 1995; 195: 297-315.

6. Kopka L, Vosshenrich R, Rodenwaldt J, Grabbe E. Differences in injection rates on contrast-enhanced breath-hold three-dimensional MR angiography. *Am J Roentgenol* 1998 Feb;170(2): 345-8.

7. Prince MR, Chenevert TL, Foo TK, Londy FJ, Ward JS, Maki JH. Contrast-enhanced abdominal MR angiography: optimization of imaging delay time by automating the detection of contrast material arrival in the aorta. *Radiology* 1997; 203(1): 109-14.

8. Riederer SJ, Bernstein MA, Breen JF, *et al*. Three-dimensional contrast-enhanced MR angiography with real-time fluoroscopic triggering: design specifications and technical reliability in 330 patient studies. *Radiology* 2000 May; 215(2): 584-93.

9. Vasbinder GB, Nelemans PJ, Kessels AG, Kroon AA, de Leeuw PW, van Engelshoven JM. Diagnostic tests for renal artery stenosis in patients suspected of having renovascular hypertension: a meta-analysis. *Ann Intern Med* 2001; 135(6): 401-11.

10. Zhang HL, Schoenberg SO, Resnick LM, Prince MR. Diagnosis of renal artery stenosis: combining gadolinimum-enhanced three-dimensional magnetic resonance angiography with functional magnetic resonance pulse sequences. *Am J Hypertens* 2003 Dec; 16(12): 1079-82.

11. Douek P, Revel D, Chazel S, Falise B, Villard J, Amiel M. Fast MR angiography of the aorto-iliac arteries and arteries of the lower extremitiy: value of bolus-enhanced, whole volume subtraction technique. *AJR* 1995; 165: 431-437.

12. Haulon S, Lions C, McFadden EP, *et al*. Prospective evaluation of magnetic resonance imaging after endovascular treatment of infrarenal aortic aneurysms. *Eur J Vasc Endovasc Surg* 2001; 22(1): 62-69.

13. Ludman CN, Yusuf SW, Whitaker SC, *et al*. Feasibility of using dynamic contrast-enhanced magnetic resonance angiography as the sole imaging modality prior to endovascular repair of abdominal aortic aneurysms. *Eur J Vasc Endovasc Surg* 2000; 19(5): 524-530.

14. Lee VS, Morgan GR, Teperman LW, *et al*. MR imaging as the sole preoperative imaging modality for right hepatectomy: a prospective study of living adult-to-adult liver donor candidates. *Am J Roentgenol* 2001; 176: 1475-1482.

15. Li KCP, Whitney WS, Mc Donnell C, *et al*. Chronic mesenteric ischemia: evaluation with phase-contrast cine MR imaging. *Radiology* 1994; 190: 175-179.

16. Meaney JF. Non-invasive evaluation of the visceral arteries with magnetic resonance angiography. *Eur Radiol* 1999; 9: 1267-1276.

17. Meaney JFM, Prince MR, Nostrand TT, *et al*. Gadolinium-enhanced magnetic resonance angiography in patients with suspected chronic mesenteric ischemia. *J Magn Reson Imaging* 1997; 7: 171-176.

18. Ernst O, Asnar V, Sergent G, *et al*. Comparing contrast-enhanced breath-hold MR angiography and conventional angiography in the evaluation of mesenteric circulation. *Am J Roentgenol* 2000 Feb;174(2): 433-9.

19. Li KC, Dalman RL, Chen IY, *et al*. Chronic mesenteric ischemia: use of *in vivo* MR imaging measurements of blood oxygen saturation in the superior mesenteric vein for diagnosis. *Radiology* 1997; 204: 71-77.

20. Gaa J, Wendl M, Georgi M. New concepts in MR imaging of pancreas carcinoma: the 'all-in-one' approach. In: *High power gradient MR imaging*. Oudkerk M, Edelman RR, Eds. Blackwell Publishing, Oxford, 1997: 425-430.

21. Meaney JF, Weg JG, Chenevert TL, Stafford-Johnson D, Hamilton BH, Prince MR. Diagnosis of pulmonary embolism with magnetic resonance angiography. *N Engl J Med* 1997 May 15; 36(20): 1422-7.

22. Gupta A, Frazer CK, Ferguson JM, *et al*. Acute Pulmonary Embolism: Diagnosis with MR Angiography. *Radiology* 1999; 210: 353-359

23. Oudkerk M, van Beek EJ, Wielopolski P, *et al*. Comparison of contrast-enhanced magnetic resonance angiography and conventional pulmonary angiography for the diagnosis of pulmonary embolism: a prospective study. *Lancet* 2002 May 11; 359(9318): 1643-7.

24. Stein PD, Woodard PK, Hull RD, *et al*. Gadolinium-enhanced magnetic resonance angiography for detection of acute pulmonary embolism: an in-depth review. *Chest* 2003 Dec; 124(6): 2324-8.

25. L Remonda, O Heid, Schroth G. Carotid artery stenosis, occlusion, and pseudo-occlusion: first-pass, gadolinium-enhanced, three-dimensional MR angiography - preliminary study. *Radiology* 1998; 209: 95-102.

26. Ho KY, Leiner T, de Haan MW, Kessels AG, Kitslaar PJ, van Engelshoven JM. Peripheral vascular tree stenoses: evaluation with moving-bed infusion-tracking MR angiography. *Radiology* 1998; 206: 683-92.

27. Meaney FM, Ridgway JP, Chakraverty S, *et al*. Stepping-Table Gadolinium-enhanced Digital Substraction MR Angiography of the Aorta and lower extremity Arteries: Preliminary Experience. *Radiology* 1999; 211: 59-67.

28. Lee HM, Wang Y, *et al*. Distal Lower Extremity arteries: evaluation with two-dimensional MR digital subtraction angiography. *Radiology* 1998; 207: 505-512.

29. Wang Y, Winchester PA, Khilnani NM, *et al*. Contrast-enhanced peripheral MR Angiography from abdominal Aorta to the pedal arteries. Combined dynamic two-dimensional and bolus-chase three-dimensional acquisition. *Invest Radiol* 2001; 36:170-177.

30. Leiner T, Ho KY, Nelemans PJ, de Haan MW, van Engelshoven JMA. Three-Dimensional Contrast-Enhanced Moving-Bed Infusion-Tracking (MoBI-Track) Peripheral MR Angiography With Flexible Choice of Imaging Parameters for Each Field of View. *JMRI* 2000; 11: 368-377.

31. Nelemans PJ, Leiner T, de Vet HCW, van Engelshoven JMA. Peripheral arterial disease: meta-analysis of the diagnostic performance of MR Angiography. *Radiology* 2000; 217: 105-114.

32. Visser K, Hunick MG. Peripheral arterial disease: gadolinium-enhanced MR angiography versus color-guided duplex US - a meta-analysis. *Radiology* 2000; 216: 67-77.

33. Koelemay MJ, Lijmer JG, Stoker J, Legemate DA, Bossuyt PM. Magnetic resonance angiography for the evaluation of lower extremity arterial disease: a meta-analysis. *JAMA* 2001; 285: 1338-45.

34. Stafford-Johnson DB, Hamilton BH, Dong Q, *et al*. Vascular complications of liver transplantation: evaluation with gadolinium-enhanced MR angiography. *Radiology* 1998; 207: 153-160.

35. Pandharipande PV, Lee VS, Morgan GR, *et al*. Vascular and extravascular complications of liver transplantation: comprehensive evaluation with three-dimensional contrast-enhanced volumetric MR imaging and MR cholangiopancreatography. *Am J Roentgenol* 2001; 177: 1101-1107

36. Ruehm SG, Wiesner W, Jörg F. Debatin Pelvic and Lower Extremity Veins: Contrast-enhanced Three-dimensional MR Venography with a Dedicated Vascular Coil-Initial Experience. *Radiology* 2000; 215: 421-427.

37. Lahti KM, Lauffer RB, Chan T, Weisskoff RM. Magnetic resonance angiography at 0.3 T using MS-325. *MAGMA* 2001 May; 12(2-3): 88-91.

38. van den Brink JS, Watanabe Y, Kuhl CK, *et al*. Implications of SENSE MR in routine clinical practice. *Eur J Radiol* 2003; 46(1): 3-27.

39. Wentz KU, Frohlich JM, von Weymarn C, Patak MA, Jenelten R, Zollikofer CL. High-resolution magnetic resonance angiography of hands with timed arterial compression (tac-MRA). *Lancet* 2003 Jan 4; 361: 49-50.

PART VII. Venous disease

Chapter 29

Radiofrequency ablation in the treatment of varicose veins

Sriram Subramonia, MS FRCS, Clinical and Research Fellow

Tim A Lees, MD FRCS, Consultant Vascular Surgeon

Michael G Wyatt, MSc MD FRCS, Consultant Vascular Surgeon

Crispian Oates, MSc BSc MIPEM AVS, Head of Regional Vascular Ultrasound

Northern Vascular Centre, Freeman Hospital, Newcastle-upon-Tyne, UK

Introduction

Varicose veins of the lower limb are a common problem in the Western World affecting approximately 15% of men and 25% of women [1]. Although they are not life-threatening they can impact considerably on the physical and psychological health status of those affected leading to impairment in quality of life [2]. The commonest underlying pathophysiology is incompetence of the long saphenous system and this is frequently treated by surgery. This conventionally involves disconnection of the vein at the saphenofemoral junction, stripping of the thigh segment of the vein and stab avulsions. However, surgery itself may cause significant early morbidity, such as bruising, pain, haematoma formation, and cutaneous nerve injury, and patients may need several weeks off work following such surgery [3].

Radiofrequency ablation of the long saphenous vein is one of a number of new techniques emerging which has the potential to improve the outcome of treatment for varicose veins. Early attempts at destroying the long saphenous vein without stripping were aimed at producing intraluminal thrombosis by application of direct current externally to the vessel wall [4]. Later on, intraluminal application of high-frequency alternating current achieved luminal thrombosis within a few seconds. However, this was usually followed by recanalisation and therefore was not successful. A new technique has been developed which employs heat generated by radiofrequency energy. Initial experience with this technique has been encouraging.

Heat created with radiofrequency energy has been used in surgery for many years primarily to coagulate small blood vessels during an operation. Harvey Cushing was the first to use radiofrequency ablation for creating small central nervous system lesions in 1920. Since then radiofrequency energy has been used in the treatment of cancer, joint disorders, bone growths, arrhythmias, nerve ablation in chronic pain, sleep apnoea and faecal incontinence. The VNUS Closure procedure (VNUS Medical Technologies Inc., California), developed as a minimally invasive alternative to vein stripping, was first used in Europe in 1998 and became available in the United States in 1999. It involves the application of radiofrequency energy to the vein wall via electrodes placed at the tip of an intraluminal catheter (Figure 1) to obliterate the vein lumen. This has the potential to reduce operative trauma whilst achieving the same result as stripping.

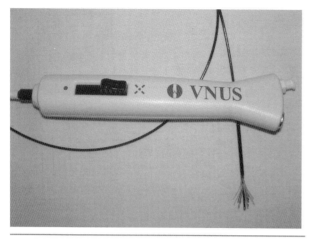

Figure 1. VNUS Closure® Catheter with collapsible bipolar electrodes.

Principles of radiofrequency energy

Electromagnetic radiation consists of waves of electric and magnetic energy moving together through space at the speed of light. All forms of electromagnetic energy are referred to as the electromagnetic 'spectrum' (Figure 2). Radiofrequency energy or 'radiowaves' is one form of electromagnetic energy and forms that part of the spectrum where electromagnetic waves have frequencies in the range of about 3 kilohertz (3 kHz) to 300 gigahertz (300 GHz).

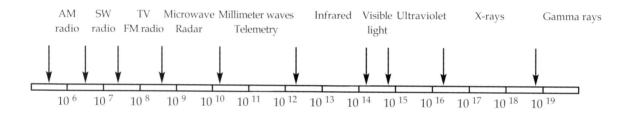

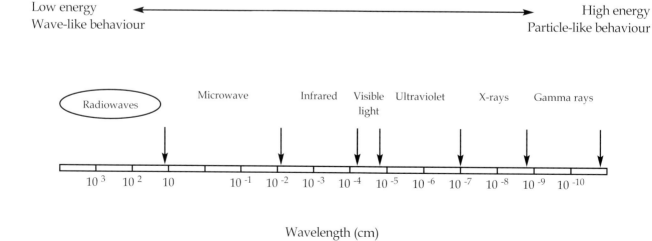

Figure 2. The electromagnetic spectrum.

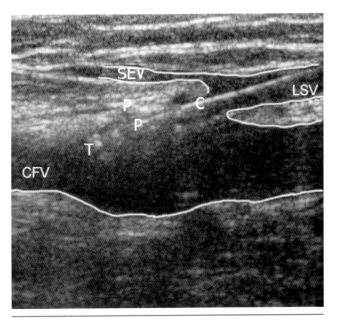

Figure 3. The ablation catheter is passed into the common femoral vein under duplex ultrasound control.

CFV = Common femoral vein
LSV = Long saphenous vein
SEV = Superficial epigastric vein
C = Ablation catheter
P = Prongs at the end of the catheter
T = Tip of the electrode

Radiofrequency ablation

Ablation or luminal obliteration is achieved with radiofrequency-resistive heating of the vein wall that is controlled by a feedback system for venous wall temperature and impedance as well as for power consumption by the system. The VNUS Closure® system (VNUS Medical Technologies Inc., California), comprises a computer-controlled bipolar thermal energy generator and catheters with sheathable electrodes. The generator supplies radiofrequency energy at 460 KHz to intraluminal bipolar catheter electrodes.

The high frequency alternating current flowing from the active electrode causes the ions in the tissue about the electrode tip to vibrate at very high speeds as the ions attempt to follow the changes in direction of the alternating current. This ionic agitation produces frictional heating and drives the water from the cells leading to desiccation and coagulative necrosis. Heat causes venous spasm and denaturation and irreversible shrinkage of vein wall collagen with intimal destruction. The feedback controlled heating ensures precise destruction of venous tissue and maximum lumen contraction with preservation of vein integrity. This leads to vein wall thickening and rapid organisation, forming a fibrotic seal of the lumen with minimal thrombus formation. The contraction of the vein wall minimises the likelihood of recanalisation.

Technique of venous ablation

The authors' practice is to perform ablation under general anaesthesia, combined with stab avulsions, although the procedure may be done under local anaesthesia with or without sedation [5]. Duplex ultrasound is used to guide the entire procedure. The course of the long saphenous vein is first mapped out on the skin from the sapheno-femoral junction to the level of the knee. The long saphenous vein is accessed at the knee level either percutaneously or via a small cut-down (access can sometimes be obtained more easily at ankle level but in the authors' experience, passage of the catheter from this level may be more difficult). A sheath is inserted over a guidewire, which is then removed. The sheath required is either 6 or 9 French depending on the catheter used; catheters are available in two sizes, 6 French and 8 French, to allow for obliteration of veins from 2-12mm in diameter. The ablation catheter is passed through the sheath up the long saphenous vein into the common femoral vein under ultrasound control (Figure 3). The tissue immediately surrounding the long saphenous vein in the thigh is then infiltrated with 0.9% saline, which may be combined with local anaesthetic (20ml of 1% lidocaine with 1:200,000 adrenaline diluted in 500ml of 0.9% saline). This helps to achieve vein compression and to reduce the risk of skin burns, and paraesthesia from saphenous nerve injury. Following infiltration the patient is placed with a 30° Trendelenberg tilt, the leg is elevated and the part to be treated (the thigh) is wrapped in an Esmark bandage in order to compress the vein around the catheter (Figure 4). Manual compression is applied between the upper limit of this bandage and the

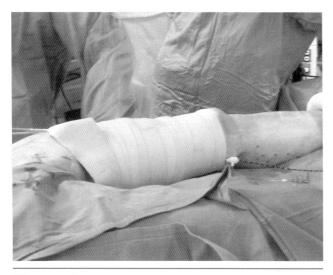

Figure 4. The thigh is wrapped in an Esmark bandage prior to ablation.

saphenofemoral junction. Under ultrasound control the catheter is then withdrawn from the common femoral vein into the long saphenous vein, usually to a position just inferior to the superficial epigastric vein. The electrodes are unsheathed and wall contact tested by measuring the impedance. The power level, maximum temperature and duration of treatment are then selected. The target temperature is set at 85°C. Ablation is performed from just below the saphenofemoral junction (usually leaving in circulation to the superficial epigastric vein) to the level of the knee maintaining the target temperature at 85°C ± 3°C withdrawing the catheter at a rate of approximately 2.5cm/min. To avoid thrombus formation on the electrodes, heparinised saline is infused continuously into the catheter via a central lumen that can also accommodate a small guide wire if required. After completion of treatment, a duplex scan is performed and re-treatment of any patent segment carried out until satisfactory vein shrinkage is achieved. At this stage there will be minimal flow but not yet complete occlusion of the vein. Stab avulsions are carried out using phlebectomy hooks at previously marked sites to complete the operation.

Selection of patients for venous ablation

Patients with duplex ultrasound confirmed incompetence of the long saphenous vein, which may

be primary or recurrent, are potential candidates for radiofrequency ablation. At present the authors consider the following criteria as unsuitable for ablation:-

◆ A vein diameter that is <2mm (too small to cannulate) or >12mm (poor impedance) in the supine position.
◆ A very tortuous vein above the knee (unsuitable for catheterisation).
◆ Thrombus in the long saphenous vein.
◆ Patients with a pacemaker or internal defibrillator.

The authors do not treat short saphenous vein incompetence due to the potential risk of sural nerve injury.

Current results of venous ablation

The results of radiofrequency ablation published from various centres including our own are summarised below [5-13]. The follow-up period in these studies varies from six weeks to two years.

Vein occlusion rate

The acute vein occlusion rate at one week following the procedure is between 88-100% [5,6,8,9,11,12]. At two years, 85-90% of those treated remain occluded [5,8,13].

Symptom improvement and patient satisfaction

Complete absence of symptoms or a significant improvement was observed in 94-100% of patients [6-8,11,13]. Patient satisfaction ranged between 92-100% [5,7,8,10,12].

Recurrent reflux and varicose veins

Doppler-confirmed reflux in the treated vein was observed in approximately 10% at two years [5,7,13]. Recurrent varicose veins were noted in 5-13% at two years [5,7,9,13]. Most of the recurrences have occurred in original anatomic failures and only a fraction of these have required re-treatment. No significant differences in recurrent reflux rates were shown between conventional high ligation and radiofrequency ablation without high ligation [14].

Recurrence and neovascularisation

Studies have previously reported the significance of neovascularisation in the development of recurrence after vein stripping [15,16]. The VNUS Closure procedure maintains normal venous flow from the superficial epigastric vein through the terminal segment of the long saphenous vein and avoids a groin dissection, thereby providing no stimulus for neovascularisation. This may help to prevent the development of collaterals and potentially reduce long-term recurrence rates. No neovascularisation was observed two years after radiofrequency ablation in a recently published series [13].

Randomised controlled trials

The first randomised trial [10] comparing endovenous radiofrequency ablation with conventional stripping and high ligation involving 28 patients revealed lesser postoperative pain, earlier return to normal activities and shorter sick leave in patients undergoing ablation, with similar complication rates in both groups. It also suggested that the closure procedure could be cost-saving for society particularly in the employed group.

A second multicentre trial involving 85 patients [11] showed significantly better outcomes in terms of time to return to activities and work, postoperative pain and quality of life scores in patients undergoing ablation.

Complications

Intraoperative complications include perforation of the vein and thermal injury to the skin or saphenous nerve. Inadequate vein compression, leading to poor impedance, may cause failure to achieve adequate ablation and in this circumstance the vein is unlikely to occlude. Thrombus accumulation at the tip of the catheter may also lead to inadequate ablation.

Bruising, erythema, haematoma, purpura and clinical phlebitis may be clinically significant in a small proportion of patients. More major complications include paraesthesia (0-19%), thermal injury to skin overlying the vein (0-3%), deep vein thrombosis (1%) and pulmonary embolism (<1%) [5,6,8,9,11,12]. Incidence of the latter two is comparable to conventional surgery. The incidence of paraesthesia seems to be much less when treatment is limited to the thigh and upper leg. Infiltration of saline or local anaesthetic around the vein may reduce the risk of paraesthesia and skin burns. Increasing experience with the procedure also tends to decrease the incidence of these complications.

Cost of venous ablation

The actual treatment cost of ablation is higher than conventional surgery due to the use of the generator, the catheter (single patient use at approximately £550 per catheter), the use of intraoperative duplex ultrasound and possibly longer operating time. This may appear to place an additional burden on the financial outlay of hospitals and health services. However, an earlier return to normal activity and work may significantly reduce the number of lost working days and potentially increase productivity. Seen in this context, ablation could arguably be cost-beneficial for society. Indeed, though the numbers involved were small, results of a recent randomised trial suggests that radiofrequency ablation could be cost-saving for society particularly in the employed group if indirect costs from lost working days are considered [10].

NICE guidance on radiofrequency ablation of varicose veins

Based on currently available safety and efficacy data, the National Institute for Clinical Excellence (NICE) has issued a guidance document [17] supporting the use of radiofrequency ablation as an alternative to sapheno-femoral ligation and stripping, provided that normal arrangements for consent, audit and clinical governance are in place.

Summary

◆ Radiofrequency ablation of the long saphenous vein using the VNUS Closure technique appears to be a safe and effective minimally invasive alternative to conventional surgery with a better short-term outcome and a comparable 2-year recurrence rate in selected patients.

◆ It may potentially reduce long-term recurrence by avoiding a stimulus for neovascularisation.

◆ The higher cost of initial treatment may be offset by a more rapid recovery and return to work.

◆ Further randomised controlled trials are required to determine clinical and cost-effectiveness before ablation becomes an established procedure.

References

1. Callam MJ. Epidemiology of varicose veins. *Br J Surg* 1994; 81: 167-173.

2. Smith JJ, Garratt AM, Guest M, *et al*. Evaluating and improving health-related quality of life in patients with varicose veins. *J Vasc Surg* 1999; 30: 710-9.

3. Mackay DC, Summerton DJ, Walker AJ. The early morbidity of varicose vein surgery. *Journal of the Royal Naval Medical Service* 1995; 81: 42-6.

4. Sawyer PN, Page JW. Bioelectric phenomena as an etiological factor in intravascular thrombosis. *Am J Physiol* 1953; 175: 103-107.

5. Merchant RF, DePalma RG, Kabnick LS. Endovascular obliteration of saphenous reflux: a multicenter study. *J Vasc Surg* 2002; 35: 1190-6.

6. Chandler JG, Pichot O, Sessa C, *et al*. Treatment of Primary Venous Insufficiency by Endovenous Saphenous Vein Obliteration. *J Vasc Surg* 2000; 34: 201-14.

7. Goldman MP, Amiry S. Closure of the greater saphenous vein with endoluminal radiofrequency thermal heating of the vein wall in combination with ambulatory phlebectomy: 50 patients with more than 6-month follow-up. *Dermatol Surg* 2002; 28: 29-31.

8. Weiss RA, Weiss MA. Controlled radiofrequency endovenous occlusion using a unique radiofrequency catheter under duplex guidance to eliminate saphenous varicose vein reflux: a 2-year follow-up. *Dermatol Surg* 2002; 28: 38-42.

9. Banerjee B, Lees TA, Wyatt MG, *et al*. Radiofrequency ablation of the long saphenous vein in the treatment of lower limb varicose veins. *Phlebology* 2003; 18: 51.

10. Rautio T, Ohinmaa A, Perala J, *et al*. Endovenous obliteration versus conventional stripping operation in the treatment of primary varicose veins: a randomised controlled trial with comparison of costs. *J Vasc Surg* 2002; 35: 958-65.

11. Lurie F, Creton D, Eklof B, *et al*. Prospective randomised study of endovenous radiofrequency obliteration (Closure procedure) versus ligation and stripping in a selected patient population (EVOLVeS Study). *J Vasc Surg* 2003; 38: 207-14.

12. Wagner WH, Levin PM, Cossman DV, *et al*. Early Experience with Radiofrequency Ablation of the Greater Saphenous Vein. *Ann Vasc Surg* 2004 Jan 20 (Epub ahead of print).

13. Pichot O, Kabnick LS, Creton D, *et al*. Duplex ultrasound scan findings two years after great saphenous vein radiofrequency endovenous obliteration. *J Vasc Surg* 2004; 39: 189-95.

14. Chandler JG, Pichot O, Sessa C, *et al*. Defining the role of extended saphenofemoral junction ligation: a prospective comparative study. *J Vasc Surg* 2000; 32: 941-53.

15. Nyamekye I, Shephard NA, Davies B, *et al*. Clinicopathological evidence that neovascularisation is a cause of recurrent varicose veins. *Eur J Vasc Endovasc Surg* 1998; 15: 412-5.

16. Jones L, Braithwaite BD, Selwyn D, *et al*. Neovascularisation is the principal cause of varicose vein recurrence: results of a randomised trial of stripping the long saphenous vein. *Eur J Vasc Endovasc* 1996; 12: 442-5.

17. National Institute for Clinical Excellence. Radiofrequency ablation of varicose veins. Interventional Procedure Guidance 8; Sep 2003.

Chapter 30

Alternative endovascular methods for the treatment of varicose veins

Bruce Campbell, MS FRCP FRCS, Professor and Consultant Surgeon

Royal Devon and Exeter Hospital and Peninsula Medical School, Exeter, UK

Introduction

There have been huge shifts in the management of varicose veins in recent years. The general level of professional interest in their treatment has increased and in the UK, varicose veins have increasingly become the province of vascular surgeons, rather than general surgeons. Assessment of varicose veins has evolved beyond recognition - from clinical examination with the use of tourniquets, through regular use of hand-held Doppler, to selective or routine duplex ultrasound scanning. In addition, there has been renewed interest in alternative methods of treating varicose veins, particularly using endovascular techniques designed to reduce the side-effects of conventional surgery.

Standard treatment

The commonest pattern of varicose veins presenting for treatment is with long saphenous vein (LSV) reflux, and this chapter will focus largely on LSV varicose veins. The textbook operation involves three basic principles:-

◆ Ligation of the LSV flush with the femoral vein, including ligation of all tributaries in the groin beyond their first confluences. There is a belief that if tributaries are left intact they may gradually enlarge, causing recurrent reflux in the groin and further varicose veins. Despite thorough surgery of this kind, recurrence can occur as a result of neovascularisation in the scar tissue of the operation: this is the commonest cause of groin recurrence. Surgical measures to reduce neovascularisation have not proved particularly successful.

◆ Stripping of the LSV to a level just above or below the knee. There is good evidence that stripping the LSV produces better results than leaving the vein in place. In comparing results of stripping against new treatments it is important to recognise that methods of stripping vary, and this may have significant effects on early outcomes (specifically haematoma, bruising, pain, and mobility). Many surgeons (including those performing most of the comparative studies) use a traditional 'olive' on the stripper which creates a traumatic passage through the thigh as the vein is stripped (the larger the olive, the larger this passage). It is likely that less trauma is caused if the LSV is stripped by invagination, using a stripper without an olive or large head (the PIN stripper is just one way of doing this: a conventional stripper without an olive is at least as effective). If new methods are to be compared with the best type of standard surgery, then this should include stripping by invagination.

◆ Phlebectomies of all marked varicose veins. Throughout this chapter it is important to bear in mind that dealing with the long saphenous trunk is only one part of a varicose vein operation. For thorough treatment all troublesome varicosities also need to be dealt with. This may be a major part of the procedure (and of the potential morbidity) if varicose veins are extensive and/or large. Surgeons vary in the ways in which they do phlebectomies (the frequently used term 'avulsions' gives a hint of the technique used by some) and this has the potential to affect postoperative haematoma and discomfort significantly.

Sclerotherapy used to be used widely for varicose veins in the UK. In its conventional form (multiple injections of small volumes of sclerosant), sclerotherapy was often inappropriate because veins which would have been better treated by operation, frequently recurred. It remains an option for varicose veins with insignificant proximal reflux, residual varicose veins after operation, and minor recurrent varicose veins. Sclerotherapy may also be used as a planned way of dealing with varicose veins after ablation of truncal reflux, and this can form an important part of the treatment strategy when using endovascular methods for the LSV.

Outcomes of standard treatment

A problem in assessing the clinical effectiveness of any new treatment for varicose veins is the rather poor evidence on outcomes of standard treatments, specifically LSV surgery with phlebectomies. This is rather surprising for an operation which is one of the most frequently performed in the UK health service. Recurrence after standard surgery certainly is common (some 20% of patients presenting with varicose veins have had surgery before), but there are many possible reasons for this which do not

necessarily reflect the efficacy of the operative technique. Assessment may have been incorrect leading to an inappropriate choice of operation, or surgery may not have been done thoroughly. There are few studies in which patients have been followed-up for long periods of time, and the definition of 'recurrence' is elusive.

New treatments

New endovascular treatments are largely aimed at ablating the LSV trunk without the need for a groin incision or stripping of the vein. The leading alternatives are radiofrequency ablation (RFA), laser treatment, and foam sclerotherapy (which in addition aims to seal off the varicose tributaries of the vein). Cryotherapy [1] is another possible method for dealing with the LSV by an endovascular approach, but has not gained any popularity. For the sake of completeness it is worth mentioning transilluminated powered phlebectomies - a new method for performing phlebectomies which has received recent publicity. This is not an endovascular treatment and will not be considered further.

Radiofrequency ablation (RFA)

The equipment consists of a control unit and a radiofrequency catheter with a sheath (through which heparinised saline is infused during the procedure), and specially designed terminal electrodes. Refer to other sources for full descriptions of the technique [2-5]. In summary, the LSV is entered (usually about knee level) by making a small incision over it, or by percutaneous puncture with a needle and sheath. The radiofrequency catheter is introduced into the vein and advanced under duplex ultrasound control towards the saphenofemoral junction. Ablation of the LSV is achieved by heating the vein to 85°C in 3cm segments from groin level distally. Avoidance of damage to the femoral vein is particularly important and heating is therefore started just below the terminal valve cusps [4] or below the entrance of the highest tributary [6]. Pressure is applied during RFA using a compression bandage and additional manual compression. Treatment time, including access, has been reported at around 40 minutes [6]. Tumescent anaesthesia is used, with infiltration of local anaesthetic (60-150ml [4]) around the LSV. The procedure may be done under local or regional anaesthesia, or under general anaesthetic (particularly, if extensive phlebectomies need to be done).

Endovenous laser treatment

This method uses laser as the means of closing the LSV by a technique very similar to that described for RFA [7-9]. The laser fibre is advanced to within 1-2cm of the saphenofemoral junction under duplex ultrasound control, and withdrawn in 1-5mm increments, using laser pulses of around 1 second. The types of laser and the precise settings used vary between different operators. Min [9] has perhaps the largest published experience of the technique and has used 810-nm wavelength laser energy via a 600 micrometre fibre. He describes a policy of laser ablation under local anaesthesia, with subsequent sclerotherapy of varicose veins (although laser can be used to treat varicosities of larger tributaries [8]).

Foam sclerotherapy

This is an adaptation of sclerotherapy in which sclerosant is forcibly mixed with a gas (air or CO_2) so that it spreads widely through the lower limb veins under ultrasound control [10-12]. There are a number of variations in the technique which are well reviewed by Frullini et al [12]. It has the potential advantages of very low cost and short treatment times on an outpatient basis.

Safety, efficacy and effectiveness

For any technique to enter regular use, adequate evidence on safety and efficacy is essential. Safety data are best assessed on large numbers of patients, not necessarily in the setting of randomised controlled trials. Large numbers are necessary to expose less common complications. Whether a procedure is sufficiently safe depends on balancing the number and severity of adverse events against the severity and natural history of the condition being treated.

Varicose veins seldom threaten life or limb, and the majority of patients requesting treatment have minor symptoms. A high risk of serious complications would therefore be unacceptable.

Efficacy means that a procedure does what it is claimed to do. This is different to clinical effectiveness, which includes comparison with other treatments, preferably in the context of randomised controlled trials. Finally, comparisons of cost-effectiveness are desirable if a procedure is likely to disseminate widely in a cash limited system such as the National Health Service.

The National Institute for Clinical Excellence (NICE) issues recommendations about the safety and efficacy of new procedures to the Health Service in England and Wales through its Interventional Procedures Programme. It has recently recommended that the evidence on safety and efficacy appears adequate for both RFA and laser to be used with normal arrangements for clinical governance, consent and audit [13] (but with some reservations about longer-term efficacy). Foam sclerotherapy has yet to be considered by NICE for its safety and efficacy. None of the procedures has been appraised by NICE for its clinical and cost-effectiveness.

Evidence on efficacy and effectiveness of endovascular treatments

Evidence on ablation of the long saphenous vein

Radiofrequency ablation

Immediate success in obliteration of the LSV has been reported in about 95% cases but scans during the first week showed some flow in 16% (seven of 86) proximal segments of the vein in the EVOLVeS study, reported by Lurie et al [6]. Two of these showed no reflux and three had occluded at the time of a scan three weeks after the procedure. At one week 93% (267 of 286) LSVs were completely occluded in the multicentre study reported by Merchant [14]. Weiss et al [4] observed 98% occlusion of 140 LSVs at one week, but 4% (five) had some flow at six weeks: two were treated by sclerotherapy but the remaining three went on to recanalise by six months.

With regard to the longer-term, results of two-year follow-up have been reported by Merchant et al [14]. Duplex scanning showed that 85% (121 of 142) LSVs were completely occluded; 4% showed near complete occlusion (<5cm proximal LSV patent); but reflux was not seen in any of the LSVs. Pichot et al [15] have recently published a detailed description of duplex scan findings in 63 limbs two years after RFA, in which the treatment had been started just distal to the saphenofemoral junction. The commonest duplex finding (in 82%) was of a patent saphenofemoral junction receiving antegrade flow from proximal LSV tributaries through a short (<5cm) patent LSV segment above an otherwise obliterated LSV. In just two cases the patent segment was longer (21 and 27cm) and there was reflux at the saphenofemoral junction in five cases. Overall, the LSV trunk was occluded in 90% cases. In a smaller group of 21 patients followed for two years, Weiss et al [4] found a very similar occlusion rate (90%).

Although no longer-term randomised comparison has yet been done for effectiveness of RFA against standard surgical treatment by stripping, the two-year results described above seem similar [4,15]. In the longer-term, recurrence of varicose veins after surgery is most commonly caused by neovascularisation in the groin. This is likely to be due to growth of new blood vessels in the scar tissue which follows surgical trauma. It has been suggested that this might be less common after RFA and this idea is supported by the two-year observations of Pichot et al [15], who found no evidence of neovascularity on scanning of 63 limbs treated by RFA.

In summary, about 90% LSVs remain ablated at two years after RFA; flow through terminal tributaries is common but seems seldom to matter; and recurrence due to neovascularisation may be less of an issue than after standard surgery.

Endovenous laser treatment

Min [7-9] is one of the foremost proponents of laser treatment and has reported an early success rate of 98% (490 of 499 LSVs). A few recurrences were then observed, especially during the first three months after treatment, but at two years 93% (113 of 121) LSVs remained occluded.

Enthusiasts may debate the details of how laser differs from RFA, but in essence it seeks to ablate the LSV in a similar manner, damaging the interior of the vessel by laser energy rather than radiofrequency heating. It might, therefore, be expected that longer-term results will be similar. Unfortunately, there are simply less good quality reports of its efficacy. A cohort of 141 patients (244 limbs) observed for a mean of 19 months by Chang et al [16] were said to have experienced 'remarkable improvement' in 98% cases but good objective data were not described (it is worth noting that these patients were treated using a 2cm groin incision and an incision at the ankle). In a series of 39 treated short saphenous veins (two treatments were unsuccessful) Proebstle et al [17] observed no re-canalisation during a median follow-up interval of six months.

Larger numbers of patients need to be reported from a variety of units before the evidence on laser treatment matches that of RFA, but it seems likely that the longer-term results will be similar.

Foam sclerotherapy

Early success rates, assessed by duplex scanning have been reported as 88% in 167 'medium or large veins' using the Monfreux method and 93% in 196 patients with the Tessari method (some smaller veins included) [12]. Dealing specifically with the LSV, Cabrera et al [10] reported the results of at least three years of follow-up after treatment of 500 limbs. Details of the follow-up protocol were sparse, but they described obliteration of the vein in 81% cases. One injection had been required for 86% LSVs, while 10.5% had required two injections and 3.5%, three injections.

These results are somewhat difficult to compare directly with standard surgery, RFA, or laser. The fact that foam sclerotherapy can be repeated means that failure to obliterate the LSV completely is less of an issue. Treatment can be repeated on an outpatient basis: the results of Cabrera et al [10] show that second or third injections can produce satisfactory results. In addition, foam sclerotherapy has the potential to ablate other veins, which would require individual attention by phlebectomies, selective use of RFA or laser, or subsequent sclerotherapy if the LSV were dealt with by any of the other methods. These considerations mean that foam sclerotherapy has to be judged in a somewhat different light to the other treatment modalities, and objective comparisons will only be possible if well controlled comparative trials are conducted (including cost-effectiveness comparisons).

It is perhaps worth noting that Belcaro et al [18] have reported five and ten-year results after a number of sclerotherapy regimes, including foam sclerotherapy. However, they did not describe treatment of the LSV, but simply results of obliteration of a variety of primary varicose veins. Patients were followed-up by annual duplex scans. New veins were noted after foam sclerotherapy in 44% at five years and apparently in 51% after ten years. However, the numbers of patients reaching these follow-up times were not clear, nor was it clear exactly how many required repeated treatments.

Recovery and return to activity

More rapid recovery and return to full activity are important aims of the new endovascular treatments. In a randomised study of 85 patients, Lurie et al [6] found significantly more rapid return to normal activities after RFA (mean 1.2 days) compared with stripping (mean 3.9 days) and in return to work (4.7 versus 12.4 days). They reported significant differences in favour of RFA for global quality of life and pain scores especially during the first postoperative week.

Another randomised comparison reported by Rautio et al [5] compared 15 patients treated by RFA and 13 patients treated by conventional stripping. They observed significantly less pain after RFA but average pain scores on a linear analogue score (maximum ten) were only 0.7 (RFA) versus 1.7 (stripping) at rest and 1.8 versus 3.0 on walking, with differences most marked between the 5th and 14th postoperative days. Analgesic requirements were also

significantly less in the surgical stripping group, but the average daily dose was only 1.3 tablets of ibuprofen. Return to work and patients' assessment of their required duration of sick leave was significantly shorter for RFA (mean 6.5 versus 15.6 days); however, it was not clear what the patients were advised in this regard, and expectations can be an important influence in determining when patients return to full activity. The greater delay in return to work in the stripping group did not seem commensurate with their reported degrees of pain or analgesic requirements.

Overall, RFA seems to result in less pain and more rapid return to full activity than stripping in the first few days after operation. It might be expected that laser would have similar effects to RFA but more and better reports of outcomes after laser treatment are needed.

Complications

Comprehensive data on complications after standard surgical treatment by stripping the LSV are elusive, but saphenous nerve damage is probably the commonest. This is less of a problem if stripping is done to knee level (rather than to the ankle) and Critchley et al [19] observed a 7% incidence of 'minor neurological disturbance' in a series of 599 patients. By comparison, the incidence of nerve damage after RFA from a multicentre registry was 5% at two years (initially 15% at one week) while in their randomised trial, Lurie et al [6] observed paraesthesiae at three weeks in 16% after RFA and 6% after stripping. (The only significant differences they observed were in the ecchymosis and haematoma: results in favour of RFA). After laser treatment, paraesthesiae have been reported in 37% (92 of 252) at three weeks, 7% at six months and none at two years by Chang et al [16]. Min [9] too observed no instances of paraesthesiae at two years.

Damage to the femoral vein or artery are rare but serious complications of standard surgery. The one concern about major vessel damage using RFA or laser is that of thermal/laser damage to the femoral vein; occasional cases have been reported but have been attributed to faulty technique or inexperience (this highlights the importance of training and audit).

For sclerosant foam treatment there is a potential danger of sclerosant entering the deep veins (causing local deep vein thrombosis or effects in distant parts of the body), but proponents claim that this is not an issue when the technique is done properly with good imaging (another caution about training and audit if this technique starts to disseminate more widely). Deep vein thrombosis is also a risk of any treatment which involves general anaesthesia, more than half an hour on an operating table, or postoperative immobility. Occasional cases of phlebitis have been reported after each of the treatment methods.

Damage to the skin is another concern which applies to all the endovascular treatments. Experience seems important in avoiding skin burns with RFA. Merchant et al [14] described a 4% incidence at one week in the first 143 LSV treatments reported to their registry but none in the second 143. Chang et al [16] reported superficial burns/scarring in 5% at three weeks; 2% at six months; and none at two years (but completeness of follow-up was not clear). Min and his coworkers found no evidence of burns either early on [8] or after at two years [9]. Skin necrosis is a risk of foam sclerotherapy, reported in four of 257 (2%) patients by Frullini et al [12], but adverse outcomes have been rather poorly reported in other series.

Publicity versus evidence

The new endovascular treatments have been popularised largely by publicity and advertising in the media, rather than by measured assessment in the medical literature. This has stemmed from a desire to use them in private practice by convincing patients that they offer significant advantages over conventional treatment. Unfortunately, financial motives often have a negative influence on publication of good scientific data, and there can be scepticism about results reported from the private sector. Acquisition of good randomised controlled data is therefore important, but factors other than scientific data on outcomes are likely to influence implementation of these treatments in a health service setting.

Factors in implementation of new endovascular treatments

Radiofrequency ablation and laser

It is reasonable to consider these two techniques together because they aim to achieve similar ends in a similar way: at present the evidence for RFA is simply better. Both aim to avoid a groin wound, to reduce haematoma, and to minimise early postoperative pain, so achieving earlier return to full activity. Either can be accompanied by phlebectomies or followed by sclerotherapy, just like surgical stripping. In the context of health service treatment, each would require the facilities of a day-case unit and usually the services of an anaesthetist. Concomitant phlebectomies are the usual practice in the health service: only one treatment visit is required and if a team of two or more surgeons is operating these can be done synchronously with LSV dissection and stripping. The duration of such surgery is generally much shorter than that reported in publications of RFA or laser.

RFA and laser both require the following, over and above the requirements for standard surgery:-

◆ Purchase of a generator unit, of radiofrequency or laser catheters, and servicing costs.
◆ Presence of a duplex ultrasound machine in theatre (not generally available in most operating theatres).
◆ Presence of a skilled ultrasound technologist (in short supply in the NHS).
◆ Increased operating time.

All of these would increase the cost and burden on an already overstretched UK health service, in which waiting times for varicose vein treatments are long, and in which many hospitals place restrictions on varicose vein referrals because they cannot manage the demand. Making varicose vein operations more expensive and lengthy seems to makes little sense in these circumstances, when the potential gain is a modest reduction in postoperative discomfort and perhaps an earlier return to work (a theoretical benefit to society, but not one which reflects in any tangible way on health services resources). The considerations are different in private practice, where purchase costs of equipment and disposables, and longer operating times are manageable if they are associated with fee-paying patients. Restrictions on capacity which limit the numbers of patients who can be treated in the NHS do not apply. Good and persuasive cost-effectiveness data will be necessary if these treatments are to diffuse widely into health service practice.

The published evidence on pain and activity notwithstanding, it is important to remember that many patients suffer little discomfort after standard surgical treatment. Those who are slim and have few varicose veins usually do particularly well. Evidence on patient selection might well assist in the appropriate diffusion of endovascular techniques into health service practice, by targeting those patients who have most to gain (perhaps those with LSVs which are large or which have obvious big thigh tributaries, the more obese, or those with residual LSV trunks after previous groin surgery).

Anaesthesia

Use of local or regional anaesthesia is one of the particular advantages claimed for RFA and laser treatment. The feasibility of these depends heavily on the extent of varicose veins which need to be treated, and on treatment strategy. If extensive phlebectomies need to be done at the same procedure then general anaesthesia is the most satisfactory option. Phlebectomies under local anaesthesia are difficult for big, adherent veins. If very few phlebectomies are needed, or if there is a strategy to deal with the LSV surgically and then to perform sclerotherapy, local or regional anaesthesia may be entirely appropriate. The way patients are counselled and their personal preferences are also important considerations.

Whether patients have one or both legs treated at the same procedure may also have an influence on choice of anaesthesia. Patients with bilateral varicose veins would generally prefer to have both legs treated at the same time [20].

Training and expertise

The published results on all the new techniques have been produced by enthusiasts. As described above these endovascular treatments are likely to be used for the foreseeable future in private practice, where practitioners tend to work in isolation without pressure for peer group audit and where the temptation exists to work with minimal paid assistance (eg. without a vascular technologist for scanning). This raises concern about the possibility of poorer results and unreported complications. Good training, regular practice and reporting of outcomes should be encouraged by specialist peer groups.

Summary

◆   RFA produces results similar to stripping for ablation of the LSV. It seems that neovascularisation does not occur after RFA, and this might lessen recurrence in the long-term.

◆   Laser treatment appears to have similar results to RFA but the data are less robust.

◆   Discomfort is somewhat less and recovery is quicker after RFA and laser than after stripping, but the size and extent of varicose veins requiring treatment and the way these are dealt with (by phlebectomies or by subsequent sclerotherapy) may have important effects on discomfort and recovery.

◆   Dissemination of RFA and laser in a health service setting will be influenced by the facts that they take longer, require additional personnel and equipment, and they cost more than standard surgery, for marginal gain. Good cost-effectiveness data are needed.

◆   Foam sclerotherapy offers an outpatient method for dealing with both truncal and other varicosities. Recurrence appears more common but treatment can be repeated. More good quality studies are required.

◆   Proper training is important. Good audit and honest reporting of complications are vital, particularly in the private sector, where these methods are likely to be used most in the foreseeable future.

References

1.   Cheatle TR, Kayombo B, Perrin M. Cryostripping the long and short saphenous veins. *Br J Surg* 1993; 80: 1283.

2.   Chandler JG, Pichot O, Sessa C, *et al*. Treatment of primary venous insufficiency by endovenous saphenous obliteration. *J Vasc Surg* 2000; 34: 201-14.

3.   Manfini S, Gasbarro V, Danielsson G, *et al*. Endovenous management of saphenous vein reflux. Endovenous Reflux Management Study Group. *J Vasc Surg* 2000; 32: 330-42.

4.   Weiss RA, Weiss MA. Controlled radiofrequency endovenous occlusion using a unique radiofrequency catheter under duplex guidance to eliminate saphenous vein reflux: a 2-year follow-up study. *Dermatol Surg* 2002; 28: 38-42.

5.   Rautio T, Ohinmaa A, Perala J, *et al*. Endovenous obliteration versus conventional stripping operation in the treatment of primary varicose veins: a randomised controlled trial with comparison of the costs. *J Vasc Surg* 2002; 53: 958-965.

6.   Lurie F, Creton D, Eklof B, *et al*. Prospective randomised study of endovenous radiofrequency ablation (closure procedure) versus ligation and stripping in a selected patient population (EVOLVeS Study). *J Vasc Surg* 2003; 38: 207-14.

7.   Min RJ, Zimmet SE, Isaacs MN, Forresta MD. Endovenous laser treatment of the incompetent greater saphenous vein. *J Vasc Intervent Radiol* 2001; 12: 1167-1171.

8.   Navarro L, Min RJ, Bone C. Endovenous laser: a new minimally invasive method of treatment for varicose veins - preliminary observations using a 810nm diode laser. *Dermatol Surg* 2001; 27: 117-22.

9.   Min RJ, Khilani N, Zimmet SE. Endovenous laser treatment of saphenous reflux: long-term results. *J Vasc Intervent Radiol* 2003; 14: 991-6.

10.   Cabrera J, Cabrera JJr, Garcia-Olmedo MA. Treatment of varicose long saphenous veins with sclerosant in microfoam form. *Phlebology* 2000; 15: 19-23.

11.   Tessari L, Cavezzi A, Frullini A. Preliminary experience with a new sclerosing foam in the treatment of varicose veins. *Dermatol Surg* 2001; 27: 58-60.

12.   Frullini A, Cavezzi A. Sclerosing foam in the treatment of varicose veins and telangiectases: history and analysis of safety and complications. *Dermatol Surg* 2002; 28: 11-15.

13.   www.nice.org.uk/ip

14.   Merchant RF, DePalma RG, Kabnick LS. Endovascular obliteration of saphenous reflux: a multicenter study. *J Vasc Surg* 2002; 35: 1190-6.

15.   Pichot O, Kabnick, Creton D, *et al*. Duplex ultrasound scan findings two years after great saphenous vein radiofrequency endovenous obliteration. *J Vasc Surg* 2004; 39: 189-95.

16.   Chang CJ, Chua JJ. Endovenous laser photocoagulation (EVLP) for varicose veins. *Lasers Med Surg* 2002; 31: 257-62.

17.   Proebstle TM, Gul D, Kargl A, Knop J. Endovenous laser treatment of the lesser saphenous vein with 940-nm diode laser: early results. *Dermatol Surg* 2003; 29: 357-61.

18.   Belcaro G, Cesarone MR, Di Renzo A, *et al*. Foam-sclerotherapy, surgery, sclerotherapy and combined treatment for varicose veins: a 10-year prospective, randomised, controlled trial (VEDICO trial). *Angiology* 2003; 54: 307-15.

19.   Critchley G, Handa A, Maw A, Harvey A, Harvey MR, Corbett CRR. Complications of varicose vein surgery. *Ann R Coll Surg of Engl* 1997; 79: 105-110.

20.   Campbell WB, Dimson S, Bickerton D. Which treatment would patients prefer for their varicose veins? *Ann R Coll Surgeons Engl* 1998; 80: 212-4.

Chapter 31

IVC filters, venous thrombolysis and thrombectomy

Fergus Robertson, MRCP FRCR, Specialist Registrar, Radiology

Andrew Platts, FRCS FRCR, Consultant Radiologist

The Royal Free Hospital, London, UK

Inferior vena cava (IVC) filters

Pulmonary embolism (PE) remains a major killer ranking only after cardiovascular and malignancy as a cause of death [1]. Deaths from pulmonary embolism in the UK have been estimated at 30,000-40,000/year [2].

Anticoagulation remains the primary treatment for venous thromboembolic disease with good outcome in 90% of cases. In a minority of patients, anticoagulation is contraindicated, will fail or will result in complications. Surgical interruption of the cava has been superseded by percutaneously sited vena cava filters.

The first endoluminal filter was devised in 1967 - the Mobin-Uddin umbrella filter [3]. Major complications with this device are primarily IVC thrombosis (60%) and migration (0.4%). The first percutaneous insertion of a Greenfield conical filter was performed in 1984 [4,5]. First generation filters were delivered through a 24 French delivery system resulting in a high incidence of insertion site complications. These stimulated the development of modern low profile filters delivered by 6 to 10 French introducer systems that reduce the incidence of complications. Most of the newer generation filters are made of titanium, nitinol or stainless steel alloys that are non- or low

ferromagnetic. These are safe in clinical MRI scanners though producing local imaging artifacts.

IVC filter design

An ideal filter should prevent pulmonary emboli and be easy to insert with few complications. Currently, there is a wide range of IVC filters. Most modern filters can be inserted via small sheaths using the jugular, femoral or brachial vein. Permanent IVC filters come in several forms including the LGM VenaTech filter (B. Braun), the Simon Nitinol filter (Bard), the TrapEase filter (Cordis) and the Titanium Greenfield filter (Boston Scientific) [6]. Others can be retrieved by being withdawn into a sheath introduced from above: Günther Tulip (Cook)(Figure 1), ALN (Pyramed) and Recovery (Bard) all offer the facility of high protection rates with the opportunity of permanent implantation or removal after the acute threat of pulmonary embolus has passed [7]. The Bird's Nest filter (Cook) deploys a tangled mesh of wires which act as an effective filter. It can be deployed in IVC diameters up to 40mm, which is an advantage as other filters will deploy between 28-32mm. It creates a large artifact on MRI [8].

There is currently no prospective data comparing the clinical efficacy and complications of these various

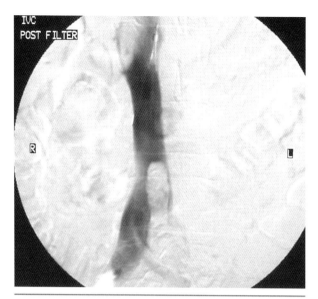

Figure 1. Günther IVC filter above non-adherent caval thrombus. The tip of the filter is slightly tilted and lies at the level of the renal veins.

devices. There are many retrospective case series for each device but meaningful comparison is difficult [1].

Indications and contraindications for IVC filter insertion

Strict criteria should be applied when assessing patients for caval filter insertion, as there are significant associated risks (Table 1). Those with a contraindication to anticoagulation may be managed with a filter alone. In certain cases, combining a filter with anticoagulation may be desirable, as in those with severe cardiopulmonary compromise. The presence of large free-floating iliocaval thrombus is associated with a much higher risk of PE (50%) when compared to occlusive thrombus (15%) [9]. The use of filter protection during deep venous thrombosis (DVT) thrombolysis remains contentious, but is practised in many institutions. The absence of long-term data may make clinicians reluctant to place permanent devices in young patients. Absolute contraindications to IVC filter insertion are complete IVC thrombosis and lack of access to the IVC.

Temporary or retrievable filters

Some patients require temporary protection against thromboembolic events. Indications include protection during thrombolysis, DVT with a short period of contraindication to anticoagulation, prophylaxis after major trauma or 'high-risk' DVT (Table 2). This prompted the development of filters which can be removed once the risk of emboli has passed. Temporary filters remain attached to an anchoring catheter or wire. Models include the Günther Temporary Filter (Cook), the Prolyser (Cordis), and the Tempofilter (B. Braun). The external fixation is a potential pathway for infection and they can distort unless the patient is immobilised.

Table 1. Indications and contraindications for IVC filter insertion [1].

Absolute indications

Contraindication to anticoagulation
Recurrent thromboembolic disease despite anticoagulation therapy
Significant complication of anticoagulant therapy
Inability to achieve adequate anticoagulation (despite patient compliance)

Relative indications

Large, free-floating iliocaval thrombus
Thromboembolic disease with poor cardiopulmonary reserve
Poor compliance with medications
Severe ataxia; at risk of falls on anticoagulation therapy
DVT thrombolysis
Renal cell cancer with renal vein or IVC involvement

Table 2. Indications for a temporary or retrievable IVC filter [1].

Treatment of iliofemoral DVT with catheter thrombolysis
Known DVT with a short period of contraindication to anticoagulant therapy
Prophylaxis after major trauma
High-risk free-floating DVT

Table 3. Indications for suprarenal placement of IVC filters [1].

Infrarenal vena cava thrombosis
Thrombus propagating proximal to infrarenal IVC filter
Renal vein thrombosis
Large patent ovarian vein (pregnancy or childbearing age)

Retrievable filters may be permanently deployed or allow removal when their protective role is no longer required. The Günther Tulip Filter (Cook) requires removal or re-siting within 14 days of implantation [10]. Other retrievable IVC devices include the ALN Filter (Pyramed UK) and the Recovery Filter (Bard UK) [11], both of which can be left *in situ* for up to 60-90 days prior to removal. Problems encountered during filter retrieval include filter adherence and thrombus persisting in the filter. Options for the latter include thrombolysis or leaving the filter deployed as a permanent device.

Prophylactic IVC filters

Indications for prophylactic IVC filters have evolved [12]. These include patients with large 'high-risk' proximal or free floating DVT, particularly if there is poor cardiorespiratory reserve. Currently, there is a trend to place prophylactic IVC filters in patients who are at very high-risk by virtue of associated medical conditions, such as major trauma, stroke or malignancy. Anticoagulants are often contraindicated and the usual conservative measures such as venous compression devices are often impossible. Studies have identified a subgroup of trauma patients who may be at a 50-fold increased risk of thromboembolic events when compared with other trauma patients. These include brain or spinal cord injured patients and those with pelvic or major lower limb fractures [13]. There have been some favourable reports but the results remain inconclusive [14,15,16]. Some argue for prophylactic IVC filter placement in patients with malignancy. Early results indicate a reduction in PE but higher mortality rates [17].

Suprarenal IVC and superior vena cava filters

Filters are classically deployed in the IVC in the immediate infrarenal segment with the filter tip level with the renal veins.

Occasionally, placement of the filter in the normal infrarenal position is impossible or potentially hazardous (Table 3). The filter may safely be deployed in the hepatic caval segment (Figure 2), but the non-circular cross-section of the intrahepatic cava may reduce the clot trapping ability of the device. Small series of superior vena cava (SVC) filter placements have been reported [1]. SVC thrombosis has complicated some of these and further studies are necessary to evaluate this application.

Complications of IVC filter insertion

Clinical recurrent PE occurs relatively infrequently - approximately 2-5% [18, 19, 20, 21, 22]. Many recurrent PEs will be subclinical and the true incidence is likely to be higher. Most IVC filters will trap large, life-threatening clots, but smaller clots may pass through

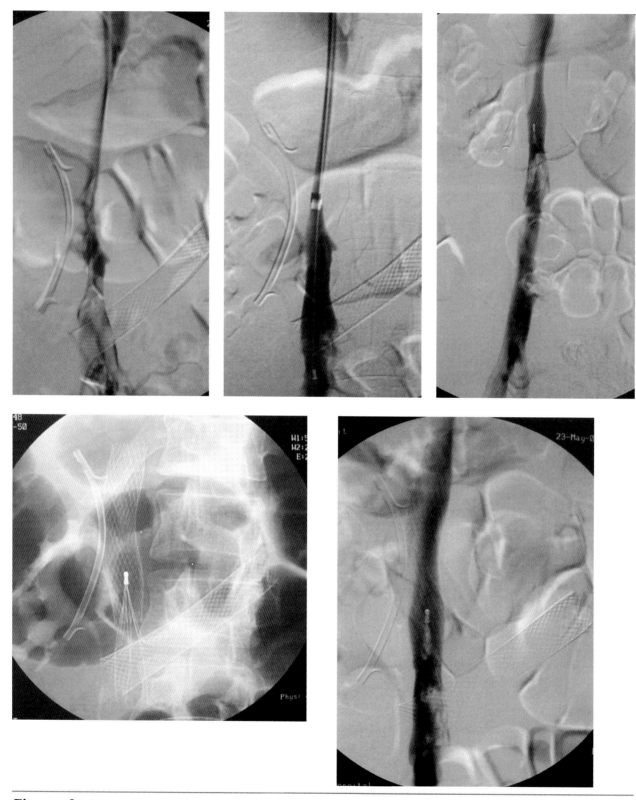

Figure 2. Anasarca secondary to pancreatic cancer metastases compressing the hepatic cava and obstructing the duodenum and biliary tree, both of which are stented. The infrahepatic cava was cleared of thrombus using a Rotarex catheter, a Günther filter was deployed and the hepatic cava stented. (Case courtesy Dr Jon Tibballs).

Table 4. Complications reported with use of IVC filters [1].

Complication	Rate (%)
Pulmonary embolism	2-5
Fatal pulmonary embolism	0.7
Death linked to insertion of IVC filter	0.12
Procedural complications	4-11
Venous access site thrombosis	2-28
Migration of filter	3-69
Penetration of IVC	9-24
Obstruction of IVC	6-30
Venous insufficiency	5-59
Filter fracture	1
Guidewire entrapment	<1

the periphery of the filter where the struts are more widely spaced. Clot formation on the filter itself may also embolise and this should be considered when imaging recurrent PE. Technical failures, such as incomplete expansion, filter tilting or migration may also account for recurrent PE.

The reported incidence of IVC thrombosis varies from 0% to 28% [20]. IVC thrombosis may be asymptomatic in some patients. Insertion site thrombosis has been reported at between 2% and 28% [20]. The incidence may be lower with lower-profile systems.

Procedural complications are reported at between 4% and 11% and include bleeding, infection, pneumothorax, air embolism, delivery system complications (such as guidewire entrapment) and suboptimal filter deployment. Delayed complications include filter detachment and embolisation to the heart, IVC penetration and filter fracture. The reported incidences of these are listed in Table 4 [1].

Recent IVC filter trials

In 1998, Decousus *et al*, performed the first prospective randomised controlled trial using IVC filters [23]. Four hundred patients with venography-proven DVT were randomised to receive anticoagulants alone or anticoagulants with placement of one of four types of IVC filter. The rates of recurrent

venous thromboembolism (DVT or PE), death and major bleeding were analysed at 12 days and two years (Table 5). It was demonstrated that IVC filters are effective in preventing PE but with no improvement in overall mortality. There was a significant two-fold increase in risk of recurrent DVT with an IVC filter at two years. No comparison was made between the four different types of IVC filter used. The data may not apply, however, to the use of IVC filters without anticoagulation.

A number of large, population-based, multicentre studies retrospectively report outcome of IVC filter placement. The Veterans Affairs Medical Centres study (1999) examined 157 filter placements in a group of 4882 patients admitted with PE between 1990 and 1995, finding a non-significant reduction in unadjusted in-hospital mortality from 16.0% to 13.4% [24]. In 2000, a study of Californian Hospitals' discharge data of 3,622 patients treated with filters and 64,333 controls with venous thromboembolism, found no significant difference in readmission rates for PE between filter and non-filter groups [25]. Filter insertion was associated with a significantly higher relative risk of readmission with venous thrombosis in patients initially admitted with PE. A Massachusetts General Hospital study reviewed 1,765 filter insertions, finding a prevalence of 5.6% post-filter PE and 3.7% fatal post-filter PE [26]. IVC thrombosis occurred in 2.7% and major complications occurred in 0.3% of patients after filter insertion. They conclude that IVC filters provide protection from life threatening PE with

Table 5. Results of PREPIC (Prevention du Risque d'Embolic Pulmonaire par Interruption Cave) Study [23].

Result	Anticoagulation alone (n=200)	Anticoagulation and IVC filter (n=200)	Odds ratio (95% CI)	P value *significant
At 12 days				
Recurrent PE	9 (4.8)	2 (1.1)	0.22 (0.05-0.90)	0.03*
Recurrent fatal PE	4 (2.1)	0 (0.0)	-	0.12
Mortality	5 (2.5)	5 (2.5)	0.99 (0.29-3.42)	0.99
Cumulative at 2 yr				
Recurrent PE	12 (6.3)	6 (3.4)	0.5 (0.19-1.33)	0.16
Recurrent fatal PE	5 (2.6)	1 (0.6)	0.22	0.22
Recurrent DVT	21 (11.6)	37 (20.8)	1.87 (1.10-3.20)	0.02*
IVC filter thrombosis	-	16 (9.0)	-	-
Mortality	40 (20.1)	43 (21.6)	1.10 (0.72-1.70)	0.65

minimal morbidity and few complications. In 2001, Greenfield used the Michigan Filter Registry to examine the incidence of recurrent DVT in 465 patients with IVC filters [27]. The overall incidence of DVT was 13.3% with no significant difference between the 241 given anticoagulants (12%) and the 224 who were not (15%). Leg swelling was however, twice as common in the patients who received no anticoagulation (p=.006).

Upper limb venous thrombosis: the Paget-Schroetter syndrome

The Paget-Schroetter syndrome (P-SS) of subclavian and axillary vein thrombosis is also variously described as Primary, Spontaneous, Idiopathic, Effort, Traumatic, Positional and Strain thrombosis. A massive increase in the occurrence of secondary upper limb venous thrombosis, is related to long-term venous access catheters. Axillo-subclavian thrombosis may be secondary to local anatomical venous compression by, for instance, callus from a fractured clavicle or rib, a local tumour or by non-compressive vein wall damage such as radiotherapy.

Changes in flow are the most important factor in the development of P-SS. The subclavian vein passes through the costo-clavicular space where it is liable to extrinsic compression resulting in obstructed flow.

The vein passes between the clavicle and first rib, a space that narrows with arm abduction and external rotation or shoulder depression, causing venous compression. This space is narrowed by the subclavius muscle attached to the undersurface of the clavicle. This increases its bulk when contracted and when the muscle hypertrophies with exercise. Many patients present shortly after vigorous exercise (Figure 3) or after restarting some seasonal sport such as tennis or cricket. The vessel wall may be damaged during repetitive or vigorous arm movement whether occupational or recreational. This leads to thickening of the vein wall and valvular damage, resulting in intraluminal webs and stenoses. Venous valves occur at variable sites in the subclavian vein but when the valve lies at the point of bony venous compression it becomes thickened, and stenosed. This is readily demonstrated after the thrombus has been cleared in some patients who suffer P-SS (Figure 4). Repeated trauma during vigorous exercise damages the vein wall with endothelial denudation and vein wall swelling.

Patients typically present in young adulthood with a short history of arm swelling, discomfort, paraesthesia or pruritis. There will be swelling, mild cyanosis and distended superficial veins. Tender, firm axillary veins may be palpable. The condition is commoner in males and the dominant limb is most frequently affected.

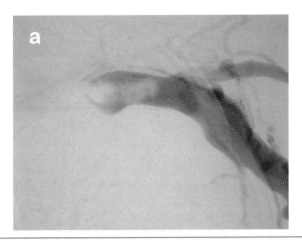

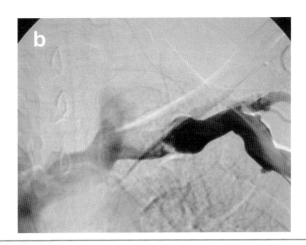

Figure 3. Paget-Schroetter syndrome - acute arm swelling after protracted swimming. a) Venography reveals thrombus within the axillary vein. b) When cleared by thrombolysis a thickened and dysplastic valve lying directly between the clavicle and first rib was revealed. This was dilated and the first rib resected.

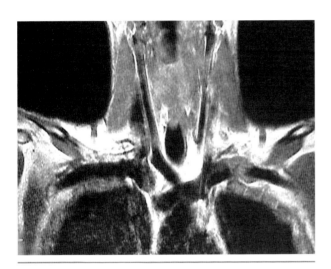

Figure 4. Coronal T1 MRI scan in Paget-Schroetter syndrome. The axillary vein is occluded where it lies between the clavicle and first rib. The underlying valve is engulfed in thrombus.

The diagnosis may be confirmed by Duplex ultrasound, magnetic resonance venography, computed tomography or venography. Historical studies show that conservative treatment by limb elevation results in considerable morbidity with persisting limb swelling and discomfort [28]. Significant numbers of patients are unable to return to work. Anticoagulation prevents propagation of thrombus into collateral veins resulting in benefit compared to conservative management [29, 30]. Up to 10% of patients with upper limb thrombosis develop clinically silent pulmonary embolism [30]. Anticoagulation will not, by itself however, restore normal flow; some veins recanalise, but usually as a late phenomenon. This results in a stenosed vessel with a thickened wall caused by secondary periphlebitis, and abnormal venous flow: the conditions that lead to recurrent thrombosis [31, 32, 33].

Management must address two issues: the acute thrombosis and any underlying local cause. The goal is to restore normal flow and prevent recurrent thrombosis, thereby reducing the morbidity associated with a chronically swollen, uncomfortable, clumsy or easily fatigued arm.

Thrombolysis has been consensually proposed as the preferred treatment [34], though there are no randomised studies. Thrombolysis offers rapid vessel recanalisation and restoration of flow. This reduces secondary periphlebitis resulting in less vein wall damage. Underlying abnormalities are revealed when the vein lumen is clear.

The technique is straightforward. The site of venous occlusion is confirmed using an approach from the arm or the leg. A guidewire is advanced into the occluded segment. If there is no underlying venous stenosis the wire will cross the occlusion. If the wire does not easily traverse the occlusion an underlying web is likely. This should not be traumatised by vigorous manipulation by guidewire or catheter. A catheter is advanced into the thrombus and thrombolysis commenced. The thrombus may well be quite bulky; it is useful to increase the contact surface between the thrombus and lytic agent by forced pulsatile injection or by fragmentation with a shaped catheter. Any effective thrombolytic agents may be used. rtPA given as a 5mg lacing bolus followed by an infusion at 1mg per hour is usually effective within 12-24 hours. Distal injection without impaction of the delivery catheter into the thrombus is ineffective; the drug simply enters the collateral veins. Complications are less frequently reported than with arterial thrombolysis, and the cohort of patients is younger with fewer co-morbidity factors.

When the vein has cleared, venography will show any underlying intrinsic venous pathology. If a venous stenosis, web, or dysplastic valve are shown, then clearly the vein has been chronically traumatised. The venous stenosis can be balloon-dilated, but this alone is ineffective; it should be followed by resection of the first rib with release of scalenus anterior [33]. Division of thickened perivenous tissue and surgical venoplasty can be performed at the same time [35]. There are conflicting recommendations regarding the timing of surgery. Some advocate surgery immediately after thrombolysis, others delay surgery for three months with the patient remaining on anticoagulation in the interim; both report excellent outcome. Patients treated by immediate surgery need not be anticoagulated, but venography should be repeated at three months to demonstrate any venous stenosis and allow treatment by angioplasty.

Metallic stents can temporarily restore venous patency but should not be deployed between an intact clavicle and first rib [30]. Balloon-expanded stents crush irreversibly [36] and self-expanding stents will eventually succumb to fatigue failure. There are numerous anecdotes of stent failure with stent fragmentation, pressure erosion of adjacent bone and local pain.

If there is no venous lesion when the thrombus has cleared, anticoagulation and avoidance of any precipitating activity are effective without surgical decompression. Those with an obvious precipitating activity that they can avoid may be anticoagulated for three months after thrombolysis without surgery.

When the patient is unable to avoid the provoking activity for occupational reasons, or is unwilling to for social reasons, then surgical decompression should be offered. Thrombosis is otherwise highly likely to recur.

Most patients with symptoms of less than eight days will achieve a successful outcome. The substantial majority are able to return to normal work and activity [37]. Those with symptoms of longer duration are less likely to achieve primary success and are more likely to rethrombose and to suffer post-thombotic symptoms [38]. When post-thrombotic symptoms persist, surgical decompression may be beneficial in reducing positional occlusion of collateral veins. Transaxillary, supraclavicular and infraclavicular decompression all have advocates and similar published outcome. Venous bypass by swinging down the jugular vein produces some benefit in cases that do not respond to, or recur after thrombolysis. The temporary creation of an arterio-venous fistula can drive the development of collateral vessels that adequately drain the arm when the fistula is later closed.

Despite the absence of controlled comparative studies, thrombolysis is now extensively used in the treatment of primary subclavian venous thrombosis, P-SS. Primary surgical thrombectomy has largely been abandoned with surgical decompression reserved until thrombus has been cleared and the underlying anatomy demonstrated.

Acute lower limb DVT

Thrombus can form in any part of the venous system, but the vast majority arise in the vein valve pockets in the soleal veins of the calf [39,40]. Proximal extension of isolated calf vein thrombosis occurs in 10-29% of cases. DVT has a clinical spectrum of severity ranging from asymptomatic isolated thrombosis to the life- and limb-threatening phlegmasia caerulea dolens and venous gangrene. The severity of the syndrome depends on the extent of thrombosis in combination with the speed of progression. Anticoagulation with heparin and warfarin remain the mainstay of modern treatment. These halt thrombus propagation, reduce the risk of pulmonary embolism and allow clot resolution by intrinsic fibrinolysis. The natural history of a DVT treated with anticoagulant is for clot lysis and vessel recanalisation over weeks or months. Venous valves may be damaged resulting in chronic venous incompetence and progression to the post-thrombotic syndrome (PTS). There appears to be a relationship between early recanalisation and preservation of valvular competence but this is by no means straightforward. Eklov and co-workers have shown by meticulous duplex ultrasound studies that valvular incompetence is as common in venous segments adjacent to thrombosed calf veins as in thrombosed, recanalised venous segments [41].

Conventional treatment of acute lower limb DVT

Unfractionated heparin and warfarin form the historical mainstay of treatment of DVT and prevention of PE. Low molecular weight heparins provide more convenient, reliable and safe alternatives [42]. A course of anticoagulation can significantly reduce the risk of recurrent venous thrombosis. The incidence of fatal PE following DVT on anticoagulation is very low at 0.4-1.5%. Conventional anticoagulation results in valvular insufficiency and PTS occurring up to 30% at five years. Systemic thrombolysis leads to more rapid and effective recanalisation than anticoagulation alone. An association has been demonstrated between early recanalisation and preservation of venous valvular competence reducing the severity of PTS. The therapeutic paradox is that in order to preserve vein wall and valve function, recanalisation must be accomplished before inflammatory change occurs in the vessel wall. However, the limb is asymptomatic before phlebitis and periphlebitis become established. Thus, by the time the patient develops symptoms it may be too late to restore normal vein function. Thrombolysis for calf vein thrombosis has not been shown to reduce the development of PTS and should not be performed outside the context of a trial.

Iliofemoral DVT

Much confusion surrounds the treatment of iliofemoral DVT. Iliofemoral DVT is one of two diseases. The first occurs when calf vein thrombus propagates centrally to involve the popliteal, femoral and iliac segments. This may propagate to the IVC. The thrombus is poorly adherent to the vein wall and may have a free-floating proximal segment. The potential for massive pulmonary embolisation is high.

The second form of iliofemoral DVT occurs when the thrombus originates in the iliac vein with distal propagation into the femoral vein with or without proximal caval extension. This disease is normally the result of extrinsic compression or by vein wall disease with a venous web or spur. Extrinsic compression is usually caused by the gravid uterus, or enlarged nodes [43].

When this latter disease is restricted to the iliac veins with or without femoral involvement, the potential for PE is small. However, when there is caval propagation the potential for embolisation is high.

Both forms of the disease contain a large volume of thrombus and spontaneous recanalisation with restoration of normal vein function is unlikely. The iliac venous segment is, however, functionally a simple conduit and restoration of a patent channel without obstruction to flow may be sufficient to re-establish normal venous return from the limb.

Systemic thrombolytic therapy

Thrombolytic treatment of calf vein thrombosis does not reduce the incidence of symptomatic pulmonary embolus and in fact, increases the incidence of asymptomatic emboli on V/Q scanning. Systemic thrombolytic therapy in acute DVT has been studied extensively but most studies demonstrate only minor reduction in the incidence of post-thrombotic syndrome when compared with anticoagulation alone. Particularly poor results are seen when systemic thrombolysis starts more than two weeks after the first onset of symptoms. It has had disappointing results in the treatment of extensive iliofemoral thrombosis and phlegmasia caerulea dolens (PCD) where the large volumes of thrombus can rarely be completely lysed [44]. The high risks of bleeding has limited this technique.

Local-regional thrombolytic therapy

This refers to the delivery of thrombolytic agents directly into the thrombus, which maximises the local dose whilst minimising systemic thrombolytic effects. Two approaches have been adopted. The first technique is catheter-directed regional therapy. The thrombolytic drug is infused directly into the clot via percutaneous catheters and infusion wires. One advantage of this method is that the entire venous system may be evaluated before starting therapy. The delivery catheter is placed either from the contralateral femoral vein, internal jugular vein or popliteal vein. Because of the risk of pulmonary embolism during treatment, a temporary IVC filter is used. The infusion catheter can safely be passed through the filter and imbedded into the thrombus. Currently, the most widely used lytic agent is rtPA.

The second technique is flow-directed regional therapy; high-dose thrombolysis is infused into an ipsilateral dorsal foot vein. The flow is directed into the deep venous system using tourniquets. This method is time-consuming, requires high doses of thrombolytics, but allows effective treatment of the smaller crural veins.

The National Venous Thrombolysis Registry of catheter-directed thrombolysis provides the largest published series to date: 287 patients (303 limbs) from multiple centres were followed-up a year after catheter-directed thrombolysis [45]. Complete thrombolysis was achieved in 31% and partial (>50%) thrombolysis in 52% of patients. The procedure was more successful in acute DVT and with no previous history of DVT. There was an 11% incidence of major bleeding (requiring transfusion) and a 16% incidence of minor bleeding with a procedure-related mortality of 0.4%. Twelve-month primary patency was 80%, better in iliofemoral than femoropopliteal segments. The overall rate of valvular reflux was 58%, falling to 28% in those who achieved complete lysis. Complications included sepsis and traumatic valvular incompetence.

Percutaneous mechanical thrombectomy

Percutaneous Mechanical Thrombectomy (PMT) refers to the use of mechanical energy to disperse thrombus using a percutaneous device and includes any combination of mechanical dissolution, fragmentation and aspiration. The combination of catheter-directed pharmacological thrombolytic therapy and PMT has become an effective means of rapid ablation of venous thrombus, particularly in situations where there are contraindications to aggressive or prolonged thrombolytic therapy. In extensive DVT, where rapid venous decompression and restoration of flow is crucial, PMT can restore a venous channel, debulk thrombus and increase the surface area of the thrombus exposed to the pharmacological agent.

PMT carries a risk of fragment embolisation, but aspiration and recirculation techniques, pharmacological thrombolytics and protective IVC filters, reduce the size of the particles reaching the lungs. PMT devices can themselves, however, cause damage to venous valves resulting in chronic venous insufficiency and the post-thrombotic syndrome. A number of commercially available devices have been used extensively in both the arterial and venous systems. Most debulk occlusive thrombus restoring a channel of flow but none completely clear the clot and need to be followed by thrombolysis, anticoagulation or both. There are currently no published randomised trials comparing the efficacy or complication rates of these various devices.

Surgical venous thrombectomy

Venous thrombectomy will successfully clear thrombus from the major veins, relieving the major venous occlusion, but will not clear thrombus in the venular or capillary circulations. Surgical results in severe phlegmasia caerulea dolens (PCD) with venous gangrene are poor [46]. Initial enthusiasm in the 1960s focused on the reduction in risks of pulmonary embolism and of acute venous wall damage, thereby reducing the incidence of post-thrombotic syndromes. Early results of venous thrombectomy performed within ten days of onset in iliofemoral thrombosis reported 85% patency rates and minimal early post-thrombotic symptoms [47]. Later studies found high rethrombosis rates and significant morbidity from late post-thrombotic syndrome on long-term follow-up [48,49].

Poor long-term results and high operative morbidity and mortality led to reduced enthusiasm for surgical treatment. The main remaining indication is failure of thrombolytic therapy [50]. Improved outcomes of venous thrombectomy have been reported utilising adjunctive arteriovenous fistulae and stenting proximal venous obstruction in the common iliac veins [51].

The post-thrombotic syndrome

The post-thrombotic syndrome (PTS) refers to chronic venous symptoms caused by venous hypertension and stasis following a DVT. The syndrome probably only develops when the popliteal or more proximal segments are affected [11]. The clinical picture ranges from oedema, venous varicosities, trophic skin changes and ulceration, to leg pain, heaviness and venous claudication. The pathophysiology is multifactorial involving valvular destruction, venous hypertension and oedema leading to impaired oxygen diffusion and chronic tissue anoxia. PTS is the leading cause of chronic venous insufficiency (CVI), accounting for 33%-75% of cases of venous ulceration. Prevalence of CVI in Western populations is approximately 0.5-1.0% rising to 5% in patients over 80. PTS is therefore a major source of morbidity, with massive socio-economic implications.

Management of post-thrombotic syndrome

Ideally, PTS should be prevented by rapid thromboablation in the acute stage. The mainstays of managing established PTS remain conservative: compression, limb elevation and lifestyle modification. While valvular reflux is the predominant pathology in PTS, in a minority of patients obstruction to venous outflow seems to contribute to symptoms. In refractory patients, endovascular interventions may be considered.

Endovascular management of chronic venous obstructive disease

When thrombosed venous segments fail to recanalise completely, there is fibrotic organisation of thrombus leading to fixed stenoses and occlusions. Balloon dilatation and stenting have a role in the management of these residual stenoses, usually found in the iliocaval segments. Imaging with MR venography, contrast venography or ultrasound is imperative before planning such an intervention. Contrast venography can be combined with invasive pressure measurement prior to treatment of significant stenotic lesions.

May-Thurner syndrome refers to an intraluminal venous spur, web or membrane, the result of chronic pulsatile compression of the proximal left common iliac vein by the overlying right common iliac artery. This common lesion (20% of the adult population) is an increasingly recognised cause of left iliac vein thrombo-occlusive disease. The clinical picture is of left leg venous hypertension or DVT; it is likely to explain the preponderance for left-sided DVT in general. Endovascular treatment with balloon venoplasty and stenting are replacing traditional surgical bypass strategies with good results [52]. Venous stents have been used effectively in the treatment of post-thrombotic iliocaval stenoses. Self-expanding stents seem best suited to this application. They can be oversized to passively expand. They will recoil and re-expand if temporarily deformed or compressed. It is often possible to traverse the diseased or occluded segment of vein with a hydrophilic wire and stiff vessel dilator. Preliminary balloon dilatation and complete stenting of the occluded segment should be performed until any pressure gradient is obliterated. Iliocaval stenting should be followed by at least three months anticoagulation to prevent rethrombosis. Technical success in long standing iliac venous occlusions can be achieved in up to 90% of cases with primary patency at 19 months of 80% [53]. Placing venous stents below the inguinal ligament is not currently recommended, unless the limb is threatened.

Phlegmasia caerulea dolens and venous gangrene

Severe and extensive iliofemoral DVT causes a swollen and painful leg, typically pale but occasionally erythematous - phlegmasia alba dolens (PAD). Phlegmasia caerulea dolens (PCD), is characterised by an acutely swollen, cyanotic limb, classically presenting with extreme constant bursting pain. PCD arises when thrombosis propagates into the venules and capillaries with secondary development of acute arterial ischaemia. Occlusion of the major leg veins alone will not result in PCD [54]. PCD always starts distally, advancing proximally. In up to half of cases, PCD will progress to venous gangrene, also starting distally in the toes and foot and extending proximally [55]. PCD occurs when there is almost total microvascular occlusion of outflow from the limb, resulting in increased capillary hydrostatic pressure and outpouring of fluid with massive interstitial oedema [56]. Pressures in the tissues may increase up to fivefold with plasma sequestration into an affected limb of 6-10 litres, accounting for the shock commonly seen in this condition [57]. Where there is only moderate compromise of the arterial circulation, a reversible syndrome of PCD without venous gangrene develops. Typically however, after 1-2 days and in up to 50% of patients, venous gangrene will supervene secondary to arterial impairment. The mechanism of this arterial compromise seems to be mainly hydrostatic. Capillary flow is further compromised by high interstitial (intramuscular or compartment) pressures overcoming the critical closing pressures of the arterioles and small peripheral arteries resulting in their collapse [56].

PCD develops in hypercoagulable states with an underlying cause being found in 90% of cases [58]. Underlying malignant disease is the major cause of hypercoagulability, particularly where there is venous gangrene and this may be the presenting symptom of a previously unsuspected malignancy [59]. In the absence of a malignant cause, thrombophilia should be suspected. PCD can complicate secondary hypercoagulable states after major surgery or trauma, the puerperal period, radiotherapy, prolonged immobilisation and in chronic inflammatory conditions, particularly relapse of ulcerative colitis [60,61]. PCD is most common in the fifth and sixth decades of life. There is an equal sex distribution and the left leg is involved almost three times more often than the right, probably as a result of the left iliac vein compression syndrome [62]. Untreated, amputation rates of 50% with a mortality of 20% are reported. Pulmonary embolism is common, particularly in venous gangrene, with an incidence of 12-40% [58].

Diagnosis is largely clinical although duplex venography is extremely useful in documenting the extent of venous thrombosis and is now the investigation of choice. Venography is technically extremely difficult and meaningful information in the presence of extensive iliofemoral thrombosis can only

be obtained by descending venography via a contralateral femoral or brachial approach. Angiography is of little diagnostic value usually showing only peripheral arterial constriction in severe cases but is often performed where the diagnosis of PCD and venous gangrene has not been considered or where there is doubt.

Management of phlegmasia caerulea dolens and venous gangrene

PCD is a medical emergency. Initial management is directed at improving tissue perfusion by aggressive resuscitation with intravenous fluids to treat hypovolaemic shock. Bed rest with high limb elevation reduce limb oedema and thus the high interstitial pressures. Anticoagulation with heparin is initiated to achieve and maintain an APTT of 1.5-2.0 to prevent further thrombus propagation. Adequate limb elevation in the early management is vital. The limb must be elevated on a high foam wedge or gallows traction to optimise venous and lymphatic drainage. The use of pillows is not adequate. Conservative treatment together with investigation of an underlying cause will suffice in early cases and prevent progression to venous gangrene. Most cases will improve clinically within 12-24 hours.

Conservative treatment alone is not effective with venous gangrene and more aggressive treatments must be employed [50]. In addition to anticoagulation, thrombolysis and thrombectomy may be necessary. The delivery of thrombolytic agent via intra-arterial catheters to the affected limb have been reported with excellent results in severe PCD [61,63]. This approach delivers thrombolysis to the capillary and venular thrombus. In the small number of patients so treated, relief from pain, swelling and hypotension was rapid (within 6-12hr) and dramatic. Thus, thrombolytic delivery tailored to both components of PCD, namely the large venous occlusions via intravenous catheters and the microvenular occlusions via intra-arterial catheters, is a logical advance and appears to have promising results. Further experience of this combined approach is required to confirm these initial results.

Summary

IVC filters

- ◆ IVC filters are safe and easy to insert.
- ◆ They reduce the risk of fatal PE.
- ◆ They increase the risk of IVC thrombosis and recurrence of leg DVT.
- ◆ Consider the use of removable filter designs in young people.

Venous thrombolysis

- ◆ Thrombolysis restores flow and allows the underlying vein to be imaged.
- ◆ Adjuvant treatment of the vein is needed in most cases.
- ◆ Do not stent the subclavian vein with an intact first rib.
- ◆ Ilio-femoral DVT is a medical emergency. Progression to phlegmasia caerulea dolens carries a high morbidity and mortality.

References

1   Kinney TB. Update on Inferior Vena Cava Filters. *J Vasc Intervent Radiol* 2003; 14: 425-440.

2.   Ansari A. Acute and chronic pulmonary thromboembolism: current perspectives. Part I: glossary of terms, historic evolution and prevalence. *Clin Cardiol* 1986; 9: 398-402.

3.   Mobin-Uddin K, Smith PE, Martines LO, *et al.* A vena caval filter for the prevention of pulmonary embolus. *Surg Forum* 1967; 18: 209-211.

4.   Greenfield LJ, McCrudy JR, Brown PP, *et al.* A new intracaval filter permitting continued flow and resolution of emboli. *Surgery* 1973; 73: 599-606.

5.   Tadarthy SM, Castaneda-Zuniga W, Salomonowitz E, *et al.* Kimray-Greenfield vena cava filter: percutaneous introduction. *Radiology* 1984; 151: 525-526.

6.   Greenfield LJ, Cho KJ, Pais SO, *et al.* Preliminary clinical experience with the titanium Greenfield vena cava filter. *Arch Surg* 1989; 124: 657-659.

7.   Millward SF, Bhargava A, Aquino J, *et al.* Günther tulip filter: preliminary experience with retrieval. *J Vasc Intervent Radiol* 2000; 11: 75-82.

8.   Watanabe AT, Teitelbaum GP, Gomes AS, *et al.* MR imaging of the bird's nest filter. *Radiology* 1990; 177: 578-579.

9.   Ranomski JS, Jarrel BE, Carabasi TA, *et al.* Risk of pulmonary embolus with inferior vena caval thrombosis. *Am J Surg* 1987; 53-101.

10. Millward SF, Oliva VL, Bell SD, *et al.* Günther tulip retrievable vena cava filter: results from the registry of the Canadian interventional radiology association. *J Vasc Intervent Radiol* 2001; 12: 1053-1058.

11. Asch MR. Initial experience in humans with a new retrievable inferior vena cava filter. *Radiology* 2002; 225: 835-844.

12. Proctor MC. Indications for filter placement. *Sem Vasc Surg* 2000; 13: 194-198.

13. Shackford SR, Davis JW, Hollingsworth-Fridlung P, *et al.* Venous thromboembolism in patients with major trauma. *Am J Surg* 1990; 159: 365-369.

14. Khansarinia S, Dennis JW, Veldenz HC, *et al.* Prophylactic Greenfield filter placement in selected high-risk trauma patients. *J Vasc Surg* 1995; 22: 231-236.

15. Rogers FB, Strindberg G, Shackford SR, *et al.* Five-year follow-up of prophylactic vena cava filters in high risk trauma patients. *Arch Surg* 1998; 133: 406-412.

16. McMurty AL, Owings JT, Anderson JT, *et al.* Increased use of prophylactic caval filters in trauma patients failed to decrease overall incidence of pulmonary embolism. *J Am Coll Surg* 1999; 189: 314-320.

17. Rosen P, Porter DH, Kim D. Reassment of vena caval filter use in patients with cancer. *J Vasc Intervent Radiol* 1994; 5: 501-506.

18. Grassi CJ. Inferior vena caval filters: analysis of five currently available devices. *Am J Roentg* 1991; 156: 813-821.

19. Rousseau H, Perreault P, Otal P, *et al.* The 6-F Nitinol TrapEase inferior vena cava filter: results of a prospective multicentre trial. *J Vasc Intervent Radiol* 2001; 12: 299-304.

20. Streiff MB. Vena caval filters: a comprehensive review. *Blood* 2000; 95: 3669-3677.

21. Greenfield LJ, Proctor MC. The percutaneous Greenfield filter: outcomes and practice patterns. *J Vasc Surg* 2000; 32: 888-893.

22. Neuerberg JM, Günther RW, Vorwerk D, *et al.* Results of a multicentre trail of the retrievable Tulip vena cava filter: early clinical experience. *Cardiovasc Intervent Radiol* 1997; 20: 10-16.

23. Decousus H, Leizorovicz A, Parent F, *et al.* A clinical trial of vena caval filters in the prevention of pulmonary embolism in patients with proximal deep-vein thrombosis. *N Engl J Med* 1998 Feb 12; 338(7): 409-15.

24. Kazmers A, Jacobs LA, Perkins AJ. Pulmonary embolism in veterans affairs medical centers: is vena cava interruption underutilized? *Am Surg* 1999; 65: 1171-1175.

25. White RH, Zhou H, Kim J, *et al*. A population-based study of the effectiveness of inferior vena cava filter use among patients with venous thromboembolism. *Arch Int Med* 2000; 160: 2033-2041.

26. Athanasoulis CA, Kaufman JA, Halpern EF, *et al*. Inferior vena caval filters: review of a 26-year single-center clinical experience. *Radiology* 2000; 216: 54-66.

27. Greenfield LJ, Proctor MC. Recurrent thromboembolism in patients with vena cava filters. *J Vasc Surg* 2001; 33: 510-514.

28. Tilney NL, Griffiths HJG, Edwards EA. Natural history of major venous thrombosis of the upper extremity. *Arch Surg* 1970; 101: 792-6.

29. Swinton NW, Edgett JW, Hall RJ. Primary subclavian-axillary vein thrombosis. *Circulation* 1968; 38: 737-45.

30. Adams JT, McEvoy RK, DeWeese JA. Primary deep venous thrombosis of the upper extremity. *Arch Surg* 1965; 91: 29-42.

31. Coon WW, Willis PW. Thrombosis of axillary and subclavian veins. *Arch Surg* 1967; 94: 657-63.

32. Prescott SM, Tikoff G. Deep venous thrombosis of the upper extremity: a reappraisal. *Circulation* 1979; 59: 350-5.

33. Machleder HI. Evaluation of a new treatment strategy for Paget-Schroetter syndrome: spontaneous thrombosis of the axillary-subclavian vein. *J Vasc Surg* 1996; 17: 305-17.

34. Rutherford RB, Hurlbert SN. Primary subclavian-axillary vein thrombosis: consensus and commentary. *Cardiovasc Surg* 1996; 4: 420-3.

35. Thompson RW, Schneider PA, Nelken NA, *et al*. Circumferential venolysis and paraclavicular thoracic outlet decompression for 'effort thrombosis' of the subclavian vein. *J Vasc Surg* 1992 16: 723-33.

36. Bjarnason H, Hunter DW, Crain MR, *et al*. Collapse of a Palmaz stent in the subclavian vein. *Am J Roent* 1993; 160: 1123-4.

37. Urschel HC, Razzuk MA. Neurovascular compression in the thoracic outlet. *Ann Surg* 1998; 228: 609-17

38   Adelman MA, Stone DH, Riles TS, *et al*. A multidisciplined approach to the treatment of Paget-Schroetter syndrome. *Ann Vasc Surg* 1997; 11: 149-54.

39. Nicolaides AM, Kakkar VV, Remmey JTG. The soleal sinuses: origin of deep vein thrombosis. *Br J Surg* 1971; 58: 307.

40. Rollins DL, Semrow CM, Friedell ML, *et al*. Origin of deep vein thrombi in an ambulatory population. *Am J Surg* 1988; 156: 122-5.

41. Masuda EM, Kessler DM, Kistner RL, *et al*. The natural history of calf vein thrombosis; lysis of thrombi and development of reflux. *J Vasc Surg* 1998 Jul; 28(1): 67-73.

42. Breddin HK, Hach-Wunderle V, Nakov R, *et al*. Effects of low-molecular-weight heparin on thrombus regression and thromboembolism in patients with deep venous thrombosis. *N Engl J Med* 2001 Mar 1; 344(9): 626-31.

43. Hurst DR, Forauer AR, Bloom JR, *et al*. Diagnosis and endovacular treatment of iliocaval compression syndrome. *J Vasc Surg* 2001; 34: 106-13.

44. Hill SL, Martin D, Evans P. Massive vein thrombosis of the extremities. *Am J Surg* 1989; 158: 131-6.

45. Mewissen MW, Seabrook GR, Meissner MH. Catheter-directed thrombolysis for lower extremity deep venous thrombosis: report of a national multicenter registry. *Radiology* 1999; 211: 39-49

46. Haimovici H. The ischaemic forms of venous thrombosis. *J Cardiovasc Surg* (TORINO) 1986; 1 (Suppl): 164-73.

47. Haller JA Jr, Abrams BL. Use of thrombectomy in the treatment of acute iliofemoral venous thrombosis in 45 patients. *Ann Surg* 1963; 158: 561-9.

48. Karp RB, Wykie EJ. Recurrent thrombosis after iliofemoral venous thrombectomy. *Surg Forum* 1966; 17: 147.

49. Lansing AM, Davis WM. Five-year follow-up study of iliofemoral venous thrombectomy. *Ann Surg* 1968; 168: 620-8.

50. Weaver FA, Meacham PW, Adkins RB, Dean RH. Phlegmasia caerulea dolens: therapeutic considerations. *South Med J* 1988; 81: 306-12.

51. Eklof B, Kistner RL. Is there a role for thrombectomy in iliofemoral venous thrombosis? *Semin Vasc Surg* 1996; 9: 34-45.

52. Bjarnason H, Kruse JR, Asinger DA, *et al*. Iliofemoral deep venous thrombosis: safety and efficacy outcome during 5 years of catheter-directed thrombolytic therapy. *J Vasc Intervent Radiol* 1997 May-June; 8(3): 405-18.

53. Razavi MK, Hansch EC, Kee ST, *et al*. Chronically occluded inferior venae cavae: endovascular treatment. *Radiology* 2000 Jan; 214(1): 133-8.

54. Haller JA Jr, May ST. Experimental studies on iliofemoral venous thrombosis. *Am Surg* 1963; 29: 567-71.

55. Haimovici H. Gangrene of the extremities of venous origin. Review of the literature with case reports. *Circulation* 1950; 1: 225-40.

56. Qvarfordt P, Eklof B, Ohlin P. Intramuscular pressure in the lower leg in deep vein thrombosis and phlegmasia caerulea dolens. *Ann Surg* 1983; 197: 450-3.

57. Haller JS Jr. Effects of deep femoral thrombophlebitis on the circulation of the lower extremities. *Circulation* 1963; 27: 693-8.

58. Perkins JMT, Magee TR, Galland RB. Phlegmasia caerulea dolens and venous gangrene. *Br J Surg* 1996; 83: 19-23.

59. Adamson AS, Littlewood TJ, Poston GJ, *et al*. Malignancy presenting as peripheral venous gangrene. *J R Soc Med* 1988; 81: 609-10.

60. Woolling KR, Lawrence K, Rosenak BD. Phlegmasia caerulea dolens and ulcerative colitis. Report of a case. *Angiology* 1967; 18: 556-64.

61. Wlodarczyk ZK, Gibson M, Dick R, Hamilton G. Low-dose intra-arterial thrombolysis in the treatment of phlegmasia caerulea dolens. *Br J Surg* 1994; 81: 370-2.

62. Elliot MS, Immelman EJ, Jeffry P, *et al*. The role of thrombolytic therapy in the treatment of phlegmasia caerulea dolens. *Br J Surg* 1979; 66: 422-4.

63. Comerota AJ, Aldridge SC, Cohen G, *et al*. A strategy of aggressive regional therapy for acute iliofemoral venous thrombosis with contemporary venous thrombectomy or catheter directed thrombolysis. *J Vasc Surg* 1994; 20: 244-54.

Chapter 32

Vascular malformations

Peter C Rowlands, BMedSci MRCP(UK) FRCR, Consultant Interventional Radiologist

Royal Liverpool University Hospital, Liverpool, UK

Introduction

Vascular malformations are uncommon but important lesions, with a wide spectrum of appearance and symptoms. They occur in all parts of the body and may present at almost any age. Mis-diagnosis and mis-management of these conditions is common and few vascular centres encounter sufficient cases to allow confident treatment protocols to develop. There seems little doubt that a multidisciplinary approach to management will lead to optimal outcomes. Many vascular specialists, plastic and orthopaedic surgeons will however encounter the occasional case and it is important that appropriate initial assessment is performed. It is even more important that ill-advised treatment is not undertaken, as this is often ineffective and may significantly hamper subsequent therapeutic efforts. Vascular malformations commonly arise within the central nervous system; these are outside the scope of this discussion and will not be considered further.

Classification

Nomenclature of vascular malformations has been confusing and inconsistent. Obsolete terms are still often used, both in clinical practice and in publications. Haemangioma is widely used as a generic description of all varieties of birthmark.

Mulliken initially developed the classification adopted by the International Society for the Study of Vascular Malformations [1]. It was based on presence or absence of endothelial proliferation. Haemangiomas are a variety of benign neoplasm with endothelial proliferation. Cells from haemangioma will grow in tissue culture. Malignant lesions with endothelial proliferation include Kaposi's sarcoma and angiosarcoma.

Lesions without proliferation are classified as vascular malformations. They are further subdivided into:-

◆ Arterial (high flow).
◆ Venous.
◆ Capillary.
◆ Lymphatic.

There is often a mixed tissue of origin such as veno-lymphatic.

There are a number of syndromes whereby a vascular malformation forms part of the clinical

Table 1. Syndromes whereby a vascular malformation forms part of the clinical features.

Syndrome	Vascular malformation	Other features
Klippel-Trénaunay	Port-wine stain Embryonal vein Deep vein hypoplasia	Lymphoedema Hemihypertrophy
Sturge-Weber	Port wine stain	Epilepsy Abnormal cerebral vessels
Kasabach-Merritt	Haemangioma	Consumptive platelet coagulopathy
Osler-Weber-Rendu	Pulmonary AVM Cerebral AVM Facial/intestinal telangiectasia	

features. Some of the more common examples are listed above (Table 1).

Aetiology

Vascular malformations are considered to represent a focal area of persistence of primitive vascular elements. The type of malformation depends on the level of abnormal communication and varies from capillary to arterial connections. The level of the communication is thought to be related to the timing of the developmental failure. There is often an associated neuronal developmental abnormality, which may be seen as localised hyperhidrosis (autonomic dysfunction) or café-au-lait spots, whose origin is neuroectodermal cells [2].

There is now strong evidence of a specific aetiology for haemangiomas. North et al [3,4] demonstrated that a series of 66 haemangiomas showed intense immunoreactivity for factors GLUT1 (normally only expressed at the blood-brain barrier), merosin, LeY and Fcγll. These factors were not found in vascular malformations. The factors are all strongly expressed in placental tissue. Two possible aetiologies were proposed.

1. Invasion of receptive mesenchyme by angioblasts 'switched' to the placental endothelial phenotype by alterations in genome or surrounding conditions.
2. Embolisation of placental endothelial cells via the right to left shunts characteristic of the normal fetal circulation.

Research is ongoing into other causative associations of vascular malformations. Eerola et al [5] have described an association between KRIT1 (KREV1 interaction trapped 1) protein and hyperkeratotic cutaneous capillary-venous malformation, due to a gene mutation.

Boon et al [5,6] have described a familial venous malformation associated with a mutation on the 9p chromosome. It is likely, however, that most vascular malformations are sporadic.

Significance of aetiology

Patients can generally be reassured that vascular malformations and haemangiomas are:-

◆ not neoplastic;
◆ genetically isolated;
◆ rarely genetically transmitted;
◆ often stable lesions requiring no specific treatment [4].

Clinical features

Venous malformation

This usually presents with swelling and pain. The degree of swelling is often variable and is influenced by factors such as ambient temperature, dependency or elevation. The pain may be worsened by pressure from clothes or furniture. Exercise involving the affected muscle may lead to an increase in pain.

Episodes of acute pain may be associated with areas of spontaneous thrombosis. Pregnancy frequently exacerbates symptoms, particularly in lower limb venous malformations. Lesions round the knee frequently give rise to intra-articular haemorrhage. This can be very disabling with significant loss of limb function, especially in children. Limb length inequality may be seen, although less commonly than in arteriovenous malformation (AVM).

Facial venous malformations are common. Sites that are often involved include the tongue, lip and buccal mucosa. They may involve deeper structures such as the parotid gland and masseter. They present with a cosmetic deformity or with a mass. Lesions related to the oro-pharynx may present with recurrent haemorrhage, which may be significant.

The clinical findings may be very minor. There may be visible swelling and sometimes discoloration overlying the lesion, due to subcutaneous haemorrhage or venous hypertension. Large venous elements may be visible in the skin. The lesion may increase in size with compression of the proximal veins or by a valsalva manoeuvre in central lesions. It is usual that the extent of the lesion on imaging studies is much larger than the visible component.

Arteriovenous malformation

Most lesions that are not visceral are noted at birth or in the first year. They present as a firm mass which may pulsate or have a palpable or audible bruit. There is often prominence of the supplying artery and fullness of draining veins. Distal ischaemic changes, atrophy, skin ulceration and oedema may all be seen. The atrophy and ischaemic change seen in the periphery is usually the result of a steal phenomenon, where the periphery is deprived of blood that is instead shunted through the AVM.

Often there is an associated growth abnormality, most usually hypertrophy of an affected limb. The hypertrophy is often both in length and bulk.

AVMs may suddenly increase in size, changing from stable and asymptomatic to significant. Hormonal changes of puberty and pregnancy may accelerate growth and occasionally trauma may lead to a change in activity.

Cardiac failure is often thought to be a common feature of AVM. In a series of 100 AVMs seen at New York University, only three had significant high output state [4-6]. The two settings in which this is generally seen are in lesions of infancy and in large pelvic or abdominal lesions in adults.

Lymphatic malformation

The distribution of lymphatic malformation is similar to that of venous malformation with craniofacial or limb involvement. The lymphatic malformation of the cervical region is often termed cystic hygroma, and may be simple or mutilocular. The lymphatic malformations of the periphery are very similar to venous malformation. Indeed, the two lesions often co-exist in one limb, and are similar on imaging criteria.

Capillary malformation

This condition may involve the head and neck and limbs also. It manifests as a flat dark patch, often termed a port wine stain. The malformation is usually of cosmetic importance only, as pain or other complications are uncommon. It may be associated with venous malformation and is seen almost invariably in Klippel-Trenéaunay syndrome. Facial capillary malformation is associated with epilepsy and cerebral haemorrhage in Sturge-Weber syndrome.

Klippel-Trénaunay syndrome (KTS)

This is mentioned as a separate condition as it is relatively common and has a typical constellation of signs and symptoms [4-7]. These are:-

◆ Cutaneous port-wine naevi. Histologically, they are capillary malformations.
◆ Soft tissue and bony hypertrophy.
◆ Venous anomalies.

Previous workers had described AVM in association with the above; this is felt to be extremely rare. There is a combined lymphatic, venous and capillary malformation. Ninety percent of Klippel-Trénaunay syndrome (KTS) patients have abnormalities present at birth. Ten per cent of KTS is limited to the upper limb, whilst 70% is in the lower limb only. Other congenital anomalies are present in a third of the patients.

The venous anomalies are complex. There is frequent aplasia or hypoplasia of the deep veins of calf and knee. Rarely, the femoral or iliac vein is absent. There are often persisting embryological veins, which include the lateral vein of the thigh and the sciatic vein. These veins are often very large and produce swelling and heaviness of the limb. Severe reflux may be seen in the anomalous vein. Suprapubic veins are seen in a fifth of patients. As well as poor function, the anomalous veins are prone to venous thrombosis. Thrombophlebitis is also common, and cellulitis is also frequently seen.

Limb hypertrophy is the least common of the three main features. It is caused by overgrowth of bone and soft tissue and may be exacerbated by venous or lymphatic dysfunction.

Investigation

A clinical history and examination by an experienced clinician is accurate at making a diagnosis in the majority of cases. Imaging investigations are more often used to determine the extent of a lesion rather than make a specific diagnosis. An assessment of high vs low flow can be made clinically or with hand-held Doppler probe.

Haematological and biochemical investigations are usually normal. In rare cases there may be evidence of haemolysis or platelet destruction and sequestration in large vascular lesions.

Plain films

Plain films are rarely required in the assessment of vascular malformations. Bony involvement may be seen in venous and arteriovenous malformation. Pressure erosion may be seen and there is often periosteal new bone associated with proximity to these lesions. Phleboliths are commonly seen within venous malformations. Leg-length discrepancy may

be associated with hemihypertrophy in AVM and Klippel-Trénaunay syndrome.

Ultrasound

Sonography, combined with colour duplex is useful in the initial assessment of vascular malformation. It is easy to differentiate high and low flow lesions. It also gives the best information available about the size of vascular spaces within the malformation. This allows a decision about the potential use of percutaneous sclerotherapy. This is generally only successful with vascular spaces visible on ultrasound. It is useful in guiding the site of puncture during sclerotherapy.

The major advantage of sonography is that it may be combined with the clinical examination in the outpatient department to allow decisions on treatment and further investigation to be made instantly.

Limitations of sonography are related to the deep extent of a lesion. It may not be possible to assess involvement of deep structures such as muscles and bones, to accurately determine the maximum extent. It would be unwise to plan major surgery without other cross-sectional imaging. Ultrasound is very useful in follow-up, enabling a good assessment of the amount of a lesion that has been successfully occluded.

Computed Tomography (CT)

There is little role for CT in the assessment of vascular malformations. Generally, the ability of magnetic resonance to demonstrate vascular structures and involvement of soft tissues is much superior and is preferred. The higher resolution of multi-detector vascular CT is promising in the assessment of the anatomy of complex arteriovenous malformations. The ability to perform multiplanar reconstructions might well prove useful in planning of complex embolisation.

Magnetic Resonance (MR)

This is the single most useful diagnostic modality in the assessment of vascular malformations. It provides in a non-invasive fashion, exquisitely detailed

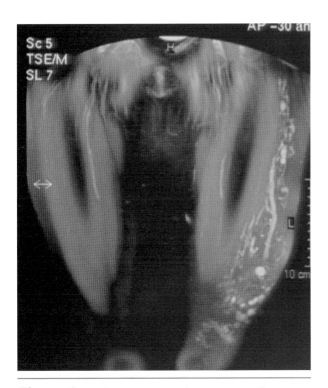

Figure 1. T2 fat suppressed sequence of venous malformation of thigh. This allows the assessment of muscular involvement by the high signal venous malformation.

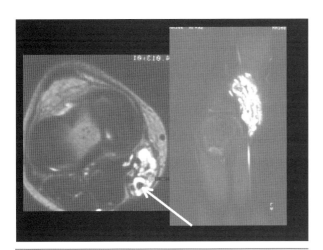

Figure 2. T2 fat suppressed sequence from a nine-year-old boy with recurrent haemathrosis. High signal venous malformation and phlebolith (arrow).

information about the extent of lesions. It allows detailed examination of vascular supply and drainage in arteriovenous malformations. The most useful sequences are T1, for detailed anatomy and fat-suppressed T2, which allows maximum contrast between malformation, demonstrating high intensity signal, and other tissues which are dark (Figures 1, 2 and 3).

An entire limb can be examined within a reasonable length of time; this is especially important in venous malformations where several areas in a single limb may be involved. The multiplanar nature of MR allows an anatomical demonstration of the malformation which may be easily understood by the referring clinician and indeed by the patient.

Intravenous contrast is rarely necessary as the inherent tissue contrast of MR is sufficient to provide all necessary information.

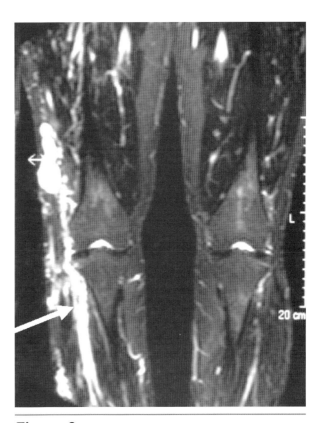

Figure 3. T2 fat suppressed sequence showing the abnormal embryonic vein of Klippel-Trénaunay syndrome.

Venography

Ascending venography is not generally helpful as vascular malformations are rarely filled by this technique. It may be useful if there is a history of venous thrombosis as it is important to avoid sclerotherapy of superficial lesions if there is occlusion of deep veins. Venography may be of value in demonstrating the abnormal venous anatomy in Klippel-Trénaunay syndrome. Generally, MR will provide enough information about deep venous structures.

Direct puncture phlebography is important in demonstration of extent and connections of vascular structures within venous malformation. The direct puncture study is usually combined with the sclerotherapy episode.

Arteriography

Arteriography is rarely required to establish a diagnosis of vascular malformation. This is done by clinical assessment and non-invasive imaging. A road map is required in assessment of arteriovenous malformation. This may be done as part of pre-procedure evaluation or may be the initial stage of an embolisation episode. The technique used in the arteriogram needs to be meticulous, with high frame rates and multiple projections. Selective and superselective catheterisation is necessary. It is essential that the location and supply of the nidus is clearly demonstrated, as this is key to the successful embolisation of the AVM.

It is almost invariable that patients are referred from other centres with angiography. It is recommended that only non-invasive imaging be done prior to referral as invasive imaging does not aid the diagnosis and is often repeated at the specialist centre.

Management of vascular malformations

It is rare that a vascular malformation presents urgently. It is therefore usually possible to assess and image the patients in a relaxed setting. Most publications emphasise a multidisciplinary approach to the management of vascular malformations.

Clinicians that may be included are plastic, vascular and orthopaedic specialists, interventional radiologists and laser practitioners. This allows a discussion of each case in depth and should lead to a rational decision about a management protocol.

It is very important to recognise that a significant proportion of patients attending such a clinic do not require any invasive treatment at all. Frequently, patients will attend a specialist centre having had invasive and non-invasive imaging and surgery or endovascular procedures, but neither knowing the diagnosis nor any idea of prognosis. If the symptoms caused by the malformation are not particularly severe, active intervention may not be indicated. Following an explanation of the nature and cause of the vascular malformation, and an opportunity to see the MR images, with time to ask questions, many patients are reassured and happy to live with minor or moderate symptoms.

Many of the techniques that are subsequently discussed have the potential for moderate or severe complications. It is very unsatisfactory if a patient with a benign condition with symptoms that do not interfere with day-to-day life, finishes with worsening of their condition. Conversely, patients with highly symptomatic lesions are prepared to accept significant risk of complications if a truly informed consent is obtained.

Conservative management

Peripheral vascular malformations are seldom life-threatening and limb loss is rare. Often lesions grow along with the child and stabilise in early adulthood. If the lesion is not particularly symptomatic, and the patient understands cause and outlook, it might be left alone. Advice about early treatment of cellulitis is important. If there is recurrent pain and tenderness in a malformation which is otherwise quiescent, areas of thrombosis are likely. An antiplatelet drug might be considered in this setting.

Surgery

Surgical treatment may be appropriate in certain settings. If a lesion is small and superficial (on imaging rather than clinical grounds) and can be completely resected, operative management is ideal. However, the vast majority of symptomatic lesions are too large to resect and involvement of deep structures risks an outcome that is worse than the lesion left untreated. The recurrence rate of attempted curative surgery in venous and arteriovenous malformation is close to 100%. Better cure rates can be obtained in cervical lymphatic malformation, although the surgery is not without risk. Intralesional suturing, the Popescu technique [8], has some advocates in the management of venous malformation. Other authors question its effectiveness.

Ligation of supplying vessels in AVM is occasionally performed as part of a surgical approach. This is to be avoided at all costs as it may lead to difficulty in access for endovascular techniques.

Radiotherapy

This was occasionally used in the past and is referred to in a few current papers. It is of limited effectiveness and the cosmetic changes induced by radiotherapy are usually unacceptable.

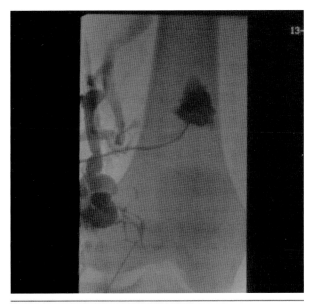

Figure 4. Direct venogram of venous malformation showing chaotic nature of anomalous veins.

Laser

Laser therapy can be very effective in reducing the intensity of colour in the 'port wine' stains that are frequently associated with vascular malformations [9]. Pulsed light systems or flashlamp-pumped pulsed dye laser can treat these in several treatment episodes with minimal complications. Pink coloured lesions respond better than purple ones. Superficial lesions tend to respond better than deeper ones, although newer systems with higher penetration show some promise. Most vascular malformations are situated in subcutaneous fat or muscle and as such are well beyond conventional laser. Bare laser fibres have been inserted into haemangioma; this is not likely to prove more effective than sclerotherapy[10].

Sclerotherapy and embolisation

Most lesions are not amenable to surgery or laser and will present to the interventional radiologist. The application in each lesion type is discussed below.

Venous malformation

Sclerosant agents are effective in the management of venous malformation. They are likely to produce a significant improvement in pain, and sometimes in lesion bulk. The two most widely used agents are sodium tetradecyl sulphate (STD) and absolute alcohol. The technique used involves a preliminary direct venogram (Figure 4). The lesion is filled with contrast and then the contrast is replaced with sclerosant. If there is significant overspill into deep veins, the drainage can be occluded manually or using a tourniquet if the lesion is within a limb. Experts differ as to the relative effectiveness of the two agents. Jackson [11] states that they are of equal effectiveness whilst Yakes [12] believes alcohol to be more effective. There is a significant difference in ease of use. Alcohol is very painful and requires general anaesthesia, while STD can be tolerated using local anaesthesia/sedation.

Risks and complications are relatively low. Deep venous thrombosis is very rare and there is a small risk of skin necrosis. Temporary neurological dysfunction has been described using alcohol.

The treatment is effective, but often several treatment episodes are required. Large series of patients having sclerotherapy have not entered the literature yet, but many operators report high rates of patient satisfaction with the technique. Pappas [13] reported significant clinical improvement in over 90% of venous malformations in the head and neck. More importantly, 95% of patients were satisfied with the outcome of treatment.

Lymphatic malformation

Surgery is often the first choice in cervical lymphatic malformation. If there is recurrence, sclerotherapy using alcohol or OK432 is very effective at treatment. Experts now suggest that sclerotherapy is the primary treatment for the condition. Formerly, lesions with one or several locules were thought most appropriate; more recently, lesions with multiple cysts have been treated with multiple injections with success [8,12,14,15].

Arteriovenous malformations

The management of arteriovenous malformations is the biggest challenge in this group of conditions.

Potential for significant complications is highest and the outcome for ill-advised or poorly planned intervention is highest. In many cases, if symptoms are minor or absent, an explanation of the condition to the patient and occasional review is the best management.

Intervention may be considered if there is significant pain or cutaneous involvement, or if there is peripheral ischaemia due to shunting. Cardiac failure is rarely seen but is another indication for active management.

The key to successful management of these lesions is a clear understanding of the nature of the anatomy that is present and of the location of the nidus, or arteriovenous connection(s).

The work of Houdart allows [16] the anatomy to be divided into three types. The first type is arteriovenous, in which no more than three arteries shunt to the initial venous component. The second type is arteriolovenous, in which there are multiple arteries shunting to a single vein (Figure 5). The third is arteriolovenulous, in which multiple arterioles shunt to multiple draining venules.

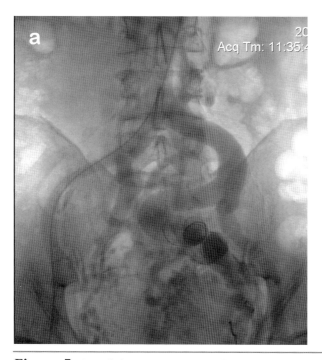 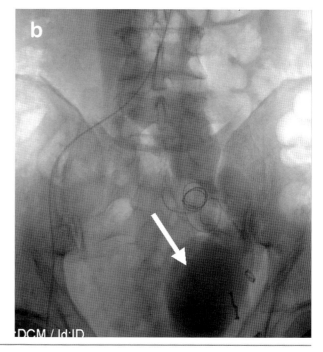

Figure 5. Arteriolovenous AVM of pelvic vessels associated with high output cardiac state. Early (a) and late (b) phases. Note the large venous sac (arrow).

Permanent embolic agents that can be used include coils, cyanoacrylate and alcohol copolymer/ tantalum (onyx - Micro Therapeutics Inc., Irvine, CA, USA). Liquid agents include alcohol and sodium tetradecyl sulphate. Both of these produce a combination of thrombosis and endovascular injury. Particle agents include polyvinyl alcohol.

Arteriovenous lesions can be treated either via an arterial or venous route or by direct puncture. The former is convenient, as arterial access is required to image the AVM. Embolic agent is introduced at the level of the shunt to close the arteriovenous connections. It is very important that the embolisation is limited to the smallest possible area to avoid collateral damage.

Arteriolovenous lesions have a single venous component and it is convenient to treat them via a venous approach, or by direct puncture if not feasible. Embolic agents can be introduced at the level of the fistulae. It is frequently necessary to mechanically occlude the venous outflow to reduce flow and allow the embolic agent prolonged contact with the nidus. An alternative approach is to pack the venous outflow with coils, to occlude the flow through the lesion.

Arteriolovenulous lesions are very resistant to treatment due to the multiplicity of supplying and draining vessels. The results of embolisation are poor and palliation is often all that can be achieved. Particle embolisation may be effective at reducing flow and bulk of these lesions. Particle embolisation may also be used in devascularisation prior to surgical debulking or resection.

Complications of embolisation

The number of potential complications of embolisation in AVM is much higher than venous or lymphatic malformation. Agents and devices such as coils and balloons can pass through the fistulae if incorrectly sized. This should be rare. With liquid agents, there is a risk of overspill into other vessels that are not part of the AVM. This is a particular fear with alcohol as cases of tissue necrosis and nerve damage have been reported [12]. The advances in imaging and the development of superior catheter technologies should allow accurate deployment of embolic materials.

Klippel-Trénaunay Syndrome

KTS is a complex condition, involving soft tissue, skin and venous and lymphatic systems. Much of the management of KTS patients is supportive. It is most important for the patient or carer to have a realistic understanding of the nature of the condition.

Limb swelling is usually a combination of limb overgrowth and lymphoedema. External graduation compression garments may help the symptoms of limb heaviness, but are relatively ineffective. The use of pneumatic compression pumps has been disappointing in most cases. Debulking surgery has also met with indifferent results.

Limb length inequality up to 2cm is usually of no significance. It is uncommon that the inequality is larger than this. Referral for epiphyseal surgery is recommended above this level.

Cutaneous lesions are common in KTS and are usually capillary port wine type lesions. If they are of cosmetic concern, they often respond to laser therapy.

Cellulitis is common in KTS. The patient must be aware of the signs of infection and should use antibiotics at an early stage, as the infection may be very slow to resolve.

Intervention in the venous system is the most difficult decision in KTS. Deep veins are usually hypoplastic and there may be varicose veins or commonly, a persistent embryonic lateral vein. These veins are often very large and functionally poor. There may be marked reflux into the abnormal veins.

Management should be minimalist. A good duplex exam and MR will indicate the extent of the venous abnormality and localise reflux. Targeted surgery to prevent reflux may be very successful. Ligation or excision of anomalous veins may be helpful but care should be taken as the native deep veins are limited functionally. Exclusion and sclerotherapy of anomalous veins has been reported [17].

Summary

◆ Vascular malformations are uncommon.

◆ They may present to many different specialties.

◆ Most require no active investigation or treatment.

◆ They are best assessed in a multidisciplinary setting.

◆ Treatment is best carried out in specialist settings.

References

1. Mulliken JB, Glowacki J. Classification of pediatric vascular lesions. *Plast Reconstr Surg* 1982; 70(1): 120-121.

2. Rosen R, Riles T. Arteriovenous Malformations. In: V*ascular diseases: surgical and interventional therapy.* Strandness E, Van Breda A, Eds. Churchill Livingstone, 1993.

3. North PE, Waner M, Mizeracki A, *et al*. A unique microvascular phenotype shared by juvenile hemangiomas and human placenta. *Archives of Dermatology* 2001; 137(5): 559.

4. Rosen R, Riles T. Arteriovenous Malformations. In: *Vascular diseases: surgical and interventional therapy.* Strandness E, Van Breda A, Eds. Churchill Livingstone, 2004.

5. Eerola I, Plate KH, Spiegel R, Boon LM, Mulliken JB, Vikkula M. KRIT1 is mutated in hyperkeratotic cutaneous capillary-venous malformation associated with cerebral capillary malformation. *Human Molecular Genetics* 2000; 9(9):1351-1355.

6. Boon L, Mulliken JB, Vikkula M. Assignment of a locus for dominantly inherited venous malformations to chromosome 9p. *Human Molecular Genetics* 1994; 3: 1583-1587.

7. Jacob A, Driscoll DJ, Shaughnessy WJ, Stanson AW, Clay RP, Gloviczki P. Klippel-Trénaunay Syndrome: Spectrum and Management. *Mayo Clinic Proceedings* 1998; 73: 28-36.

8. Popescu V. Intratumoral ligation in the management of orofacial cavernous haemangioomas. *Journal of Maxillofacial Surgery* 1985; 13: 99-107.

9. Raulin C, Schroeter CA, Weiss RA, Keiner M, Werner S. Treatment of port-wine stains with a noncoherent pulsed light source: a retrospective study. *Archives of Dermatology* 1999; 135(6): 679.

10. Glaessl A, Schreyer AG, Wimmershoff MB, Landthaler M, Feuerbach S, Hohenleutner U. Laser surgical planning with magnetic resonance imaging-based 3-dimensional reconstructions for intralesional Nd:YAG laser therapy of a venous malformation of the neck. *Archives of Dermatology* 2001; 137(10): 1331.

11. Jackson J. Vascular Malformations. In: *Vascular and Endovascular Surgery,* 2nd edition. Beard J, Ed. Saunders, 2001: 515-528.

12. Yakes WF, Haas DK, Parker S. Symptomatic vascular malformations: ethanol embolotherapy. *Radiology* 1989; 170: 1059-1066.

13. Pappas DC, Jr., Persky MS, Berenstein A. Evaluation and treatment of head and neck venous vascular malformations. *Ear, Nose & Throat Journal* 1998; 77(11): 914.

14. Burrows P. 2003. Ref Type: Personal Communication.

15. Jackson J. Vascular Malformations. In: *Vascular and Endovascular Surgery,* 2nd edition. Gaines PA, Beard J, Eds. Elsevier, 2000: 515-528.

16. Houdart E, Gobin YP, Casasco A, Aymard A, Herbreteau D, Merland JJ. A proposed classification of intracranial arteriovenous fistulae and malformations. *Interventional Neuroradiology* 1993; 35: 381-385.

17. Burrows P. Effectiveness of sclerotherapy in multilocular lymphatic malformation. 2003. Ref Type: Personal Communication.

Chapter 33

Percutaneous endovascular venous valve replacement

Shakeel Ahmed Qureshi, FRCP, Consultant Paediatric Cardiologist

Guy's Hospital, London, UK

Philipp Bonhoeffer, MD, Consultant Paediatric Cardiologist

Great Ormond Street Hospital for Sick Children, London, UK

Introduction

Work has been ongoing in trying to find ways of replacing the valves by non-invasive means for more than three decades, since Hufnagel's attempts at surgically implanting a prosthetic valve in the descending aorta in a patient with severe aortic regurgitation [1]. This valve was implanted in a small series of patients with aortic regurgitation [2]. In 1965, these workers implanted the first catheter mounted valve, a simple cone-shaped inverted parachute [3]. What is the rationale for these attempts which have now reached the stage of being successful with more sustained results? The percutaneous approach may reduce the surgical risk in high-risk patients, may be associated with lower complication rates, and shortens rehabilitation times. The procedure may be cost-effective because of shorter stay in the intensive care unit and a shorter hospital stay. It could be used in patients in whom valve surgery may be contraindicated because of their poor clinical condition.

Transcatheter valve replacement

The interest in transcatheter valve replacement was resurrected by the publication from Andersen et al [4]. They used a porcine aortic valve mounted inside a stainless steel balloon-expandable stent. This was implanted via the abdominal aorta, because the valve had a large profile and required a 41 French sheath for introduction. Nine implantations were successfully made in seven pigs. The valve was implanted in sub-coronary and supra-coronary positions. Haemodynamic evaluation showed no stenosis in any of the valves and mild aortic regurgitation in two. However, not surprisingly, there was restriction of coronary blood flow in three of the pigs. Despite these problems, this study showed that it would be possible to replace the aortic valve by catheter techniques. Almost simultaneously in 1992, Pavcnik et al reported on a transcatheter technique to implant a cage-ball prosthesis, but with important complications [5]. In 1996, Moazami et al reported on the implantation of a collapsible bovine pericardium leaflets mounted inside a stainless steel stent in the ascending aorta via a thoracotomy and cardiopulmonary bypass [6]. This valve was implanted using a 24 French catheter in three pigs in the subcoronary position. In one of the pigs, the valve dislodged because of structural failure. In 2000, Sochman et al, reported on a catheter-based aortic valve consisting of a stent-based valve cage with a locking mechanism and a prosthetic flexible tilting valve disc [7]. Such a valve was implanted in four dogs and functioned well for the duration (three hours) of the experiment.

Pulmonary valve replacement

An extremely important development was published by Bonhoeffer et al in 2000 [8]. A bovine jugular venous valve was harvested and mounted inside a balloon-expandable stent and implanted inside the native pulmonary valve in lambs. This valve functioned well at two months follow-up. The bovine jugular venous valve may be trileaflet or bileaflet and is usually of 18-20mm diameter. This valve has been used surgically (Contegra valve) with acceptable medium-term results [9, 10]. The study by Bonhoeffer et al thus had important clinical implications [8]. Many patients, who have undergone a surgical repair of tetralogy of Fallot or pulmonary atresia, develop progressive pulmonary regurgitation. In some cases, the pulmonary regurgitation results in impairment of right ventricular function, producing limitation of exercise tolerance. In the past, this necessitated surgical replacement of the pulmonary valve usually with a homograft, but occasionally with a prosthetic tissue valve. However, after the report by Bonhoeffer et al, the natural progression was to perform transcatheter replacement of the pulmonary valve in humans. Indeed, this was reported by Bonhoeffer et al also in 2000 [11]. In a 12-year-old boy, with stenosis and regurgitation of a prosthetic conduit between the right ventricle and the pulmonary artery, a valved stent was implanted percutaneously inside the conduit. This resulted in partial relief of the conduit stenosis and complete abolition of the regurgitation. Since then, this valved stent has been implanted as part of a clinical study and the early reports have been very encouraging [12, 13]. Various technical modifications have been required to produce the optimum delivery system for the valved stent. The procedure is usually performed under general anaesthesia and via percutaneous femoral venous entry. The valved stent is mounted on a balloon-in-balloon catheter and passed through a percutaneously introduced 18 French sheath, thus avoiding the need for surgical cutdown for access. After appropriate haemodynamic evaluation and angiography for definition of the morphology and the landmarks, the inner balloon is inflated followed by the outer balloon for the deployment of the valved stent.

The main limitations of this procedure are the size of the patient at which the 18 French sheath can be introduced (usually the patients are >25kg) and the size of the pulmonary trunk (of necessity this needs to be <20-22 mm). The original valved or non-valved conduit or the original pulmonary valve remains in place and the valved stent is inserted within these. The durability of the bovine jugular venous valve is uncertain. In a study from the same institution, seven children and one adult with pulmonary regurgitation and/or right ventricular outflow obstruction had successful implantation of valved stents in the pulmonary valve position. At a follow-up of five to 16 months [12], the results were generally good, but fracture of a weld between the wires of the stent was noted in two stents.

From this initial experience, it seems reasonable to conclude that percutaneous pulmonary valve replacement is feasible, keeping in mind the limitations of the technique and the lack of long-term results of the bovine jugular venous valve. Even if it degenerates as it would eventually, its role may well be to reduce the number of operations a patient requires to treat pulmonary regurgitation.

Aortic valve replacement

Perhaps a greater challenge than transcatheter pulmonary valve replacement is transcatheter replacement of the aortic valve. The reasons for this include the potential for damage to the mitral valve and obstruction of blood flow in the coronary arteries by the valved stent. Several experimental studies have attempted to address the issue of aortic valve replacement.

In an experimental report by Lutter et al in 2002, a porcine aortic valve was mounted by suturing it inside a self-expanding nitinol stent [14]. The outer diameter of the stent ranged between 15mm and 23mm. Six were implanted in the descending aorta and eight in the ascending aorta in pigs. The delivery catheter was 22 French and so was inserted by surgical cutdown onto the iliac artery or the infrarenal aorta. Technical problems with the stent twisting in the aorta occurred in two pigs and one died before the stent could be implanted. Eleven had successful implants with satisfactory haemodynamics in the acute study. They proposed that transcatheter aortic valve implantation in humans would depend on developing techniques for transluminal ablation of the native aortic valve with a low debris rate, a good filtration method which would avoid emboli and an adequate circulatory support system.

A similar experimental study was reported by Boudjemline and Bonhoeffer in 2002 [15]. They attempted implantation of valved stents percutaneously in 12 lambs. After creation of aortic regurgitation, in one group (group I) of lambs, the valved stent was implanted in the descending aorta, in another group (group II), the valve was implanted in the native aortic valve position and in the third group (group III), it was implanted also in the native position but using an orientation mechanism. It was interesting to note that although the valve was implanted successfully, complications were encountered in group II, with the valved stent obstructing the coronary artery flow, causing mitral regurgitation and premature migration of the stent. The obstruction of flow to the coronary arteries was not surprising and will be a challenge for any attempted implants. In their group III, the orientation mechanism allowed perfect alignment of the device without any obstruction of flow to the coronary arteries or damage to the mitral valve. The other limitation to be considered was the 18mm maximum diameter of the valve being implanted in an annulus of more than 22mm.

Almost at the same time as these reports were published, Cribier *et al* reported the transcatheter implantation of the aortic valve in the human [16]. These authors constructed a 3-leaflet valve from bovine pericardium mounted inside a balloon-expandable stent. This was implanted in the aortic valve position in a 57-year-old man with calcific aortic stenosis associated with cardiogenic shock, leg ischaemia and other medical problems, who had undergone balloon dilation previously and who was considered unsuitable for surgical aortic valve replacement. The valved stent was implanted successfully within the native aortic valve using the antegrade trans-septal approach. There was no impairment of the function of the mitral valve or flow into the coronary arteries, but moderate paravalvar aortic regurgitation was present. There was early haemodynamic improvement, which persisted for four months, before progressive ischaemia of the leg resulted in amputation of the leg, followed by infection and death 17 weeks after the valve implantation. This was an important landmark publication showing the feasibility of percutaneous aortic valve replacement, albeit with a bovine pericardial valve. Such a valved stent could be expanded to a diameter of 21mm to 23mm. Although there were concerns about the possibility of the stent

migrating after deployment, as had been encountered in experimental studies by the authors, they thought that the calcified aortic valve in humans would allow the valved stent to remain adherent to the diseased valve.

Since this initial attempt, the same authors have extended their expertise and have recently published their early experience with percutaneously attempted implantation of aortic valve stent prostheses in six patients with inoperable calcific aortic stenosis [17]. The valve was constructed of equine pericardium. An antegrade trans-septal approach was used in all the patients and the valves were deployed through 24 French sheaths. The valve prosthesis was successfully implanted in five patients. One patient died after immediate migration of the valved stent. There was no residual stenosis in any of the patients, but three patients had mild and two had severe aortic regurgitation. All had patent coronary arteries. Although clinical and haemodynamic improvement was noted, three patients died at two, four and 18 weeks after the procedure, whilst the remaining two patients were alive eight weeks after the procedure. This study again confirmed the feasibility of transcatheter aortic valve replacement, but is limited still by technical problems and by performing the procedure only on the sickest patients. Nevertheless, this is also an exciting advance. There will inevitably remain a question mark over the durability of such a valve.

Conclusions

Percutaneous pulmonary valve replacement will have a definite longer-term therapeutic role in a significant population of patients with pulmonary regurgitation, who are not necessarily extremely sick. Percutaneous aortic valve replacement, however, may have a shorter-term palliative role in the sickest inoperable patients, whereas surgical valve replacement will remain the standard treatment in most of the patients with aortic valve disease. This will be a small population of patients with calcific aortic stenosis. However, once the technical concerns and worries about durability are resolved, then aortic valve replacement will be indicated in a large population of patients with severe aortic regurgitation.

Summary

◆ Percutaneous valve replacement may reduce the surgical risk in high-risk patients, may be associated with lower complication rates, and shortens rehabilitation times.

◆ It could be used in patients in whom valve surgery may be contraindicated because of their poor clinical condition.

◆ Experimental studies have confirmed feasibility of valved stent implantation in pulmonary and aortic valve positions.

◆ Excellent results have been obtained with percutaneous pulmonary valve replacement in patients with pulmonary regurgitation.

◆ Short-term studies in humans have confirmed the feasibility of percutaneous aortic valve replacement in sick inoperable patients with severe calcific aortic stenosis.

◆ Further technical developments and studies are needed for these techniques to become widespread.

References

1. Hufnagel CA, Harvey WP. The surgical correction of aortic regurgitaton. Preliminary report. *Bull Georgetown Univ Med Center* 1953; 6: 3-6.

2. Hufnagel CA, Harvey WP, Rabil PJ, *et al.* Surgical correction of aortic insufficiency. *Surgery* 1954; 35: 673-683.

3. Hufnagel CA, Harvey WP, Rabil PJ, *et al.* In the beginning. Surgical correction of aortic insufficiency. *Ann Thorac Surg* 1989; 47: 475-76.

4. Andersen HR, Knudsen LL, Hasenkam JM. Transluminal implantation of artificial heart valves. Description of a new expandable aortic valve and initial results with implantation by catheter technique in closed chest pigs. *European Heart Journal* 1992; 13: 704-8.

5. Pavcnik D, Wright KC, Wallace S. Development and initial experimental evaluation of a prosthetic aortic valve for transcatheter placement: work in progress. *Radiology* 1992; 183: 151-4.

6. Moazami N, Bessler M, Argenziano M, *et al.* Transluminal aortic valve replacement. A feasibility study with newly designed collapsible aortic valve. *ASAIO J* 1996; 42: M381-5.

7. Sochman J, Peregrin JH, Pavcnik D, *et al.* Percutaneous transcatheter aortic disc valve prosthesis implantation: a feasibility study. *Cardiovasc Intervent Radiol* 2000; 23: 384-8.

8. Bonhoeffer P, Boudjemline Y, Saliba Z, *et al.* Transcatheter implantation of a bovine valve in pulmonary position: a lamb study. *Circulation* 2000; 102: 813-6.

9. Breymann T, Thies WR, Boethig D, *et al.* Bovine valved venous xenografts for RVOT reconstruction: results after 71 implantations. *Eur J Cardiothorac Surg* 2002; 21: 259-60.

10. Corno AF, Hurni M, Griffin H, *et al.* Bovine jugular vein as right ventricle-to-pulmonary artery valved conduit. *J Heart Valve Dis* 2002; 11: 242-7.

11. Bonhoeffer P, Boudjemline Y, Saliba Z, *et al.* Percutaneous replacement of pulmonary valve in a right ventricle to pulmonary artery prosthetic conduit with valve dysfunction. *Lancet* 2000; 356: 1403-5.

12. Bonhoeffer P, Boudjemline Y, Qureshi S, *et al.* Percutaneous insertion of the pulmonary valve. *J Am Coll Cardiol* 2002; 39: 1664-9.

13. Boudjemline Y, Agnoletti G, Piechaud JF, *et al.* Percutaneous pulmonary valve replacement: towards a modification of the prosthesis. *Arch Mal Coeur Vaiss* 2003; 96: 461-6.

14. Lutter G, Kuklinski D, Berg G, *et al.* Percutaneous aortic valve replacement: An experimental study. 1. Studies on implantation. *J Thorac Cardiovasc Surg* 2002; 123: 768-76.

15. Boudjemline Y, Bonhoeffer P. Steps toward percutaneous aortic valve replacement. *Circulation* 2002; 105: 775-8.

16. Cribier A, Eltchaninoff H, Bash A, *et al.* Percutaneous transcatheter implantation of an aortic valve prosthesis for calcific aortic stenosis. First human case description. *Circulation* 2002; 106: 3006-8.

17. Cribier A, Eltchaninoff H, Tron C, *et al.* Early experience with percutaneous transcatheter implantation of heart valve prosthesis for the treatment of end-stage inoperable patients with calcific aortic stenosis. *J Am Coll Cardiol* 2004; 43: 698-703.